ABUNDANT HEALTH

ABUNDANT HEALTH

Expounding the

LEARN-HOW-TO-BE-WELL

System of Daily Living

By
JULIUS GILBERT WHITE

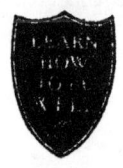

TEACH Services, Inc.
P U B L I S H I N G
www.TEACHServices.com

Facsimile Reproduction

This book played a formative role in the development of Christian thought and the publisher feels that this book, with its candor and depth, still holds significance for the church today. Therefore the publisher has chosen to reproduce this historical classic from an original copy. Frequent variations in the quality of the print are unavoidable due to the condition of the original. Thus the print may look darker or lighter or appear to be missing detail, more in some places than in others.

Copyright © 2005 TEACH Services, Inc.
ISBN-13: 978-1-57258-314-6
Library of Congress Control Number: 2005931597

Published by

TEACH Services, Inc.
P U B L I S H I N G
www.TEACHServices.com

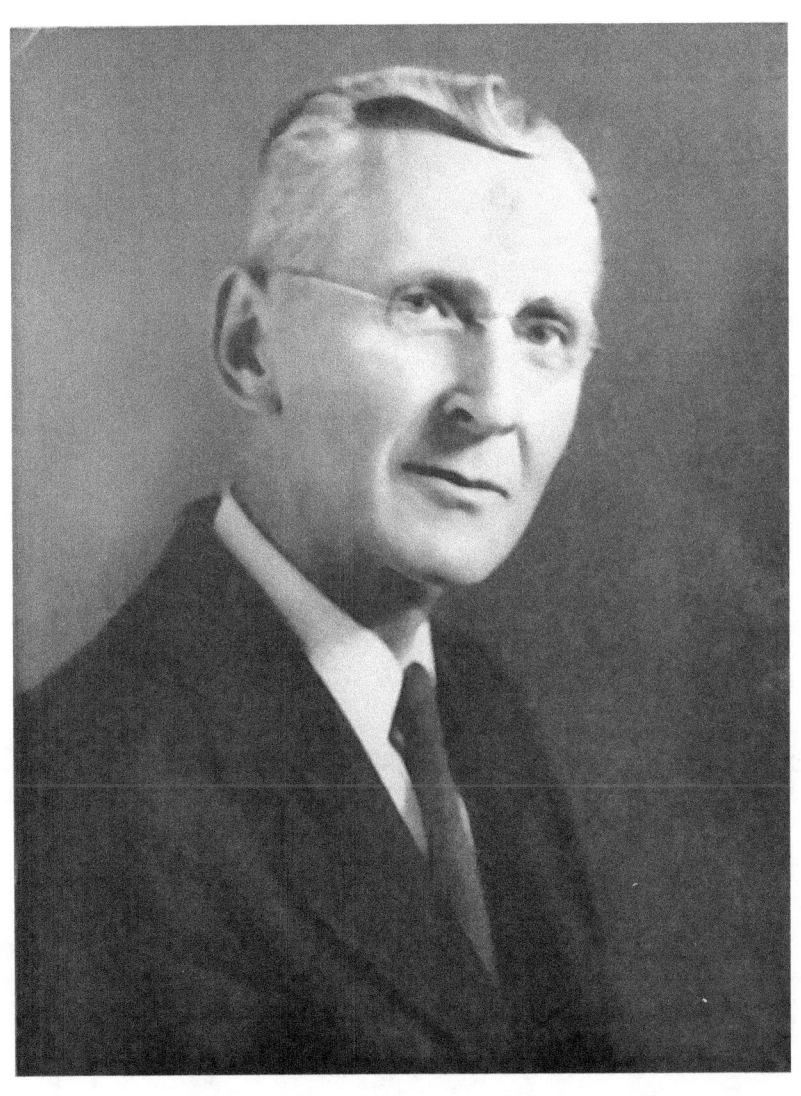

JULIUS GILBERT WHITE

Introduction

Julius Gilbert White was for eleven years at the head of the Lecture Bureau at Madison College, Tennessee. The purpose of the Bureau was to disseminate knowledge of the principles of health and wholesome living.

During those years I was closely associated with him, and he each season conducted a Health Institute in connection with Madison College. He helped to train young men and women in the principles of healthful living and for the lecture platform in this field of endeavor.

He prepared himself for this type of work by serious study and research in the science of health, diet, and nutrition, and has gathered a wealth of material for this work. He has also enjoyed a life-long affiliation with a movement which for more than sixty years has been prominent in advancing a knowledge of rational health principles, and has thus had the privilege of drawing his guiding principles from the original sources of that movement.

His work has been well received by educators, business men, church workers, and officials. He has lectured before large audiences in both schools and churches in many states. His presentations are clear and direct, and pleasing alike to youth and adults.

E. A. SUTHERLAND, M.D.

"THE HEALTH SHOULD BE
AS SACREDLY GUARDED AS
THE CHARACTER"—*"Medical
Ministry,"* page 77.

Acknowledgement

The author is deeply indebted to a large number of writers who have made priceless information available to the reading public; and he is hereby seeking to widen the influence of the truths they have presented. The list of authors who should be mentioned is too long to present here, but they duly appear in the bibliographies throughout the book. So far as he is able to judge, the author is giving the consensus of opinion of the best authorities on the subjects discussed.

Foreword

Why have I written this book?
A series of purposes prompted the preparation and sending forth of this book.

FIRST.—*More Health Needed*

Notwithstanding all that is being done and said and written, the world is still in dire need of better health; very few people are really well. Hundreds of thousands of people are sick who might be well if they could learn how to live. We need to provide more abundant health for more people.

SECOND.—*Lengthen the Prime of Life*

Although more babies are being piloted through the hazards of childhood and youth to the age of maturity, fewer people are reaching maximum ages than fifty years ago. The degenerative diseases are increasing in severity at younger ages so that the useful period of life is shortening while it should be prolonged.

THIRD.—*Use Only the Good*

The needs of the body, including its living processes, are provided for largely by elements deliberately put in from the outside; and the average person does not give his body as efficient supplies as he might, and he puts in many things which he ought not.

FOURTH.—*Natural Nutrition in Modern Science*

Everyone knows that sound bodies cannot be built without food; yet, notwithstanding this, and all the efforts put forth, the true science of nutrition is but little understood, and is still in its infancy. Standards of correct nutrition were established at the origin of the race, but they have been popularly abandoned for so long that they are now but dimly perceived. Many of the recent "discoveries" of "science" are but modern recognitions of principles and food values which have existed since the day man was made. This book is an effort to place natural foods in the true setting of modern science.

FIFTH.—*Increase Natural Immunity*

The philosophy of this book is to make use of those foods which aid in restoring a measure of the natural immunity to disease which man possessed in the long ago—to use foods, as far as possible, that build up the health and keep down disease—so as to greatly lessen the need for unnatural, artificial immunity procedures, which are expensive and not very satisfactory in the end.

SIXTH.—*Food as Medicine*

The science of fighting disease with the "medicinal values" of foods has been but little investigated, although it is the strongest weapon we have. On the other hand many people eat in a way that encourages disease. We need to learn how to eliminate every harmful thing and to make wise use of the very best and purest foods to be found in nature, and so get all of the benefit and leave out all of the handicaps and thus reach the optimum of health.

SEVENTH.—*A Balanced Ration*

Not only do we need to select the best foods, but even they must be in proper proportions, or in balance, as we say. A carburetor may be fed with perfect gasoline and perfect oxygen but in wrong proportions, and the car will be "dead."

Furthermore, a balanced ration needs to be expounded in terms which will be understood by all, and the reasons for its components made so plain that none can doubt the correctness.

This also needs to be done in a manner to clear away the fog of confusion which arises from the variety of conflicting teachings which are on every hand today. That may seem to be an impossible task, but the doubter is only asked to read "Abundant Health" with an open mind.

EIGHTH.—*A Complete Way of Living*

There is an unalterable relation between the physical, mental, and spiritual phases of human experience. For any one of the three to be normal, all three must advance in coordinate unison. Only in this way can we reach our own highest ideals and the eminence intended by the Creator; only in this way can we find a complete, harmonious way of life. This is the higher order of living.

NINTH.—*Complete Obedience*

All body functions reveal inexorable laws which were designed and established by a Mind and Power infinitely greater than man. They reveal the thought, planning, and purpose of the Ruler of the Universe. Every function of each cell within the body responds with loyal obedience to that Sovereign Will, with the single exception of the human will, which the Sovereign Will gave man the power to exercise for weal or woe. Many people stubbornly exercise the will in ways which undermine the physical and mental powers, and in doing so convert themselves into rebels against Divine Authority. The knowledge of the fact that every process and cell, except the will, obeys the Sovereign Will should challenge the owner of each human will to yield it to God and so make the obedience in the body and life complete.

TENTH.—*The Gateway to Life*

The open-minded reader of "Abundant Health" will discern from its presentation of physiology that he is "fearfully and wonderfully made." He will find mysteries which no scientist claims to fathom. The author hopes that as the reader discerns the laws of the Creator in his own physical body and becomes obedient to them, this experience shall become the gateway to the still higher experience of completely accepting the plans of the Creator for every detail of life, and so contribute to the solution of the problems pertaining to life here and hereafter.

JULIUS GILBERT WHITE

Table of Contents

PART ONE

PART TWO

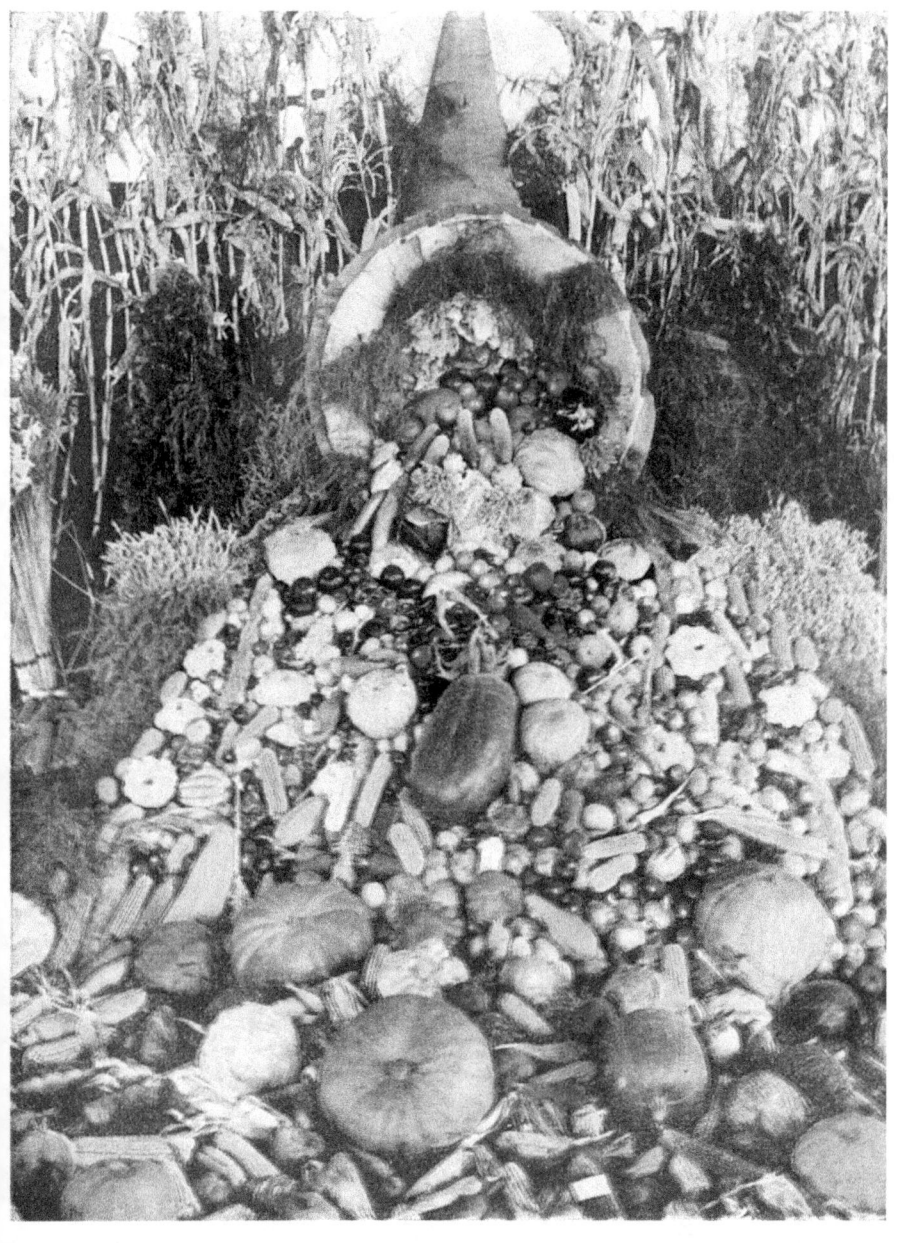

THE FOUNTAIN OF LIFE

We "Need to understand the deep truth underlying the Bible statement that with God 'is the fountain of life.' (Ps. 36:9) Not only is He the originator of all, but He is the life of every thing that lives. It is His life that we receive in the sunshine, in the pure sweet air, in the food which builds up our bodies and sustains our strength. It is by His life that we exist, hour by hour, moment by moment. Except as perverted by sin, all His gifts tend to life, to health, and joy." —Education pp. 197, 198.

LIKE HEAVEN

"By His own working agencies God has created material which will restore the sick to health. If men would use aright the wisdom God has given them, this world would be a place resembling heaven."—"Medical Ministry," page 121.

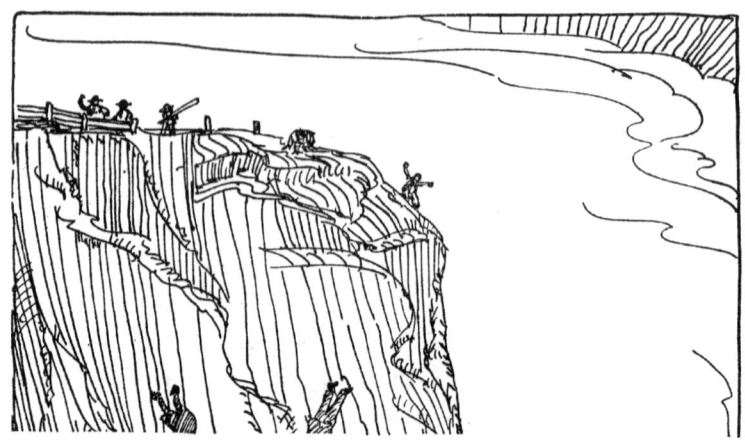

The Fence or the Ambulance

'Twas a dangerous cliff, as they freely confessed,
  Though to walk near its crest was so pleasant:
But over its terrible edge there had slipped
  A duke and many a peasant;
So the people said something would have to be done,
  But their projects did not at all tally:
Some said, "Put a fence round the edge of the cliff";
  Some, "An ambulance down in the valley."

But the cry for the ambulance carried the day,
  For it spread to the neighboring city;
A fence may be useful or not, it is true,
  But each heart became brimful of pity
For those who had slipped o'er that dangerous cliff,
  And the dwellers in highway and alley
Gave pounds or gave pence, not to put up a fence,
  But an ambulance down in the valley.

"For the cliff is all right if you're careful," they said;
  "And if folks even slip or are dropping,
It isn't the slipping that hurts them so much
  As the shock down below—when they're stopping."
So day after day when these mishaps occurred,
  Quick forth would the rescuers sally
To pick up the victims who fell off the cliff
  With their ambulance down in the valley.

Then an old man remarked: "It's a marvel to me
  That people give far more attention.

To repairing results than to stopping the cause,
  When they'd much better aim at prevention.
Let us stop at its source all this mischief," cried he,
  "Come, neighbors and friends, let us rally;
If the cliff we will fence, we might almost dispense
  With the ambulance down in the valley."

"Oh, he's a fanatic," the others rejoined;
  "Dispense with the ambulance? Never!
He'd dispense with all charities, too, if he could:
  No, no! We'll support them forever.
Aren't we picking up folks just as fast as they fall?
  And shall this man dictate to us? Shall he?
Why should people of sense stop to put a fence,
  While their ambulance works in the valley?"

Thus this story so old has beautifully told
  How our people, with best of intentions,
Have wasted their years and lavished their tears
  On treatment, with naught for prevention.

But a sensible few, who are practical, too,
  Will not bear with such nonsense much longer;
They believe that prevention is better than cure,
  And their party will soon be the stronger.
Encourage them, then, with your purse, voice, and pen,
  And (while other philanthropists dally)
They will scorn all pretense, and put up a stout fence
  On the cliff that hangs over the valley.

—Joseph Malines

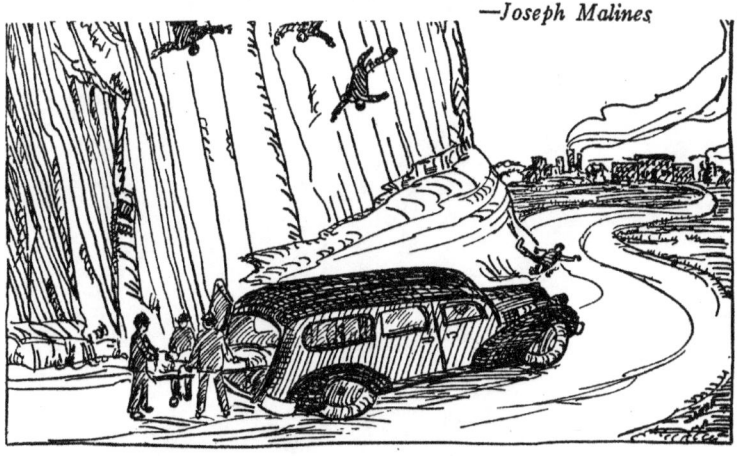

PART I

First Principles

HEALTH AND DISEASE

The reader is asked to approach the study of health and disease with a mind prepared to understand the true meaning of both. Health is a natural, normal state. A "diseased" condition develops when we fail to maintain health; it is the absence of health. Disease is not always some entity which drives out and overcomes health. The true science of conquering disease is to do so by restoring the health rather than to expect to restore the health by conquering disease. Health is maintained by forces which are always persistently at work, which need to have all hindrances to their work removed and all possible assistance given.

Possibly too much attention has been given to the study of disease, and not enough to the study of health—that the study of health has been approached from the standpoint of disease. It is certain that the study of sick, diseased bodies is much more common than the study of sound, healthy ones. To propose reversing this may seem to be like asking one to "stand on his head to get a right point of view," and yet, that change in outlook is the very thing that is needed. A very noted writer on health subjects has defined disease as follows:

"Disease is an effort of nature to free the system from conditions that result from a violation of the laws of health. In case of sickness, the cause should be ascertained. Unhealthful conditions should be changed, wrong habits corrected. Then nature is to be assisted in her efforts to expel impurities and to re-establish right conditions in the system." (1)*

PREVENT SICKNESS

At least 90 per cent of human illness could be prevented if people knew the laws of life and observed them. And yet, of the

---

* See bibliography at the end of the chapter.

millions of dollars spent each year in the United States for medical care it is estimated that not over 3 per cent is spent for the prevention of disease. (2) In other words, the money is spent after the people become sick when it should have been spent before the illness and avoided pain, loss of time and expense. "An ounce of prevention is worth a pound of cure." A little money spent on prevention will pay large dividends in lessening sickness expense. For it to be most effectual we must begin before sickness comes,— while we are still well, and perhaps do not feel the need of safeguarding the future.

Some of the diseases which are known to have been produced in part, at least, by departing from right ways of living are given below for serious reflection. A little information which costs little would prevent much sickness which costs much.

If you are suffering it may be your own fault.

Acid stomach	Diarrhea	Hyperacidity	Piles
Acidosis	Dermatitis	Impure blood	Pleurisy
Acne	Dropsy	Indigestion	Pneumonia
Adenoids	Ear infections	Influenza	Psoriasis
Anemia	Eczema	Insanity	Pyorrhea
Apoplexy	Epilepsy	Insomnia	Reproductive or-
Appendicitis	Gall bladder	Irritability	gan diseases
Arthritis	troubles	Liver cirrhosis	Rickets
Asthma	Gangrene	Loss of hair	Scurvy
Auto-intoxication	Gastritis	Low blood	Shingles
Beriberi	Gland troubles	pressure	Sinusitis
Blood disorders	Goiter	Malnutrition	Sour stomach
Boils	Halitosis	Mental sluggish-	Stomach ulcer
Bright's disease	Hardening of the	ness	Stone in bladder
Bronchitis	arteries	Nervousness	Tapeworm
Cancer	Hay fever	Neuralgia	Tired feeling
Catarrh	Headache	Neuritis	Tonsillitis
Colds	Heart disease	Nose infections	Tooth decay
Colitis	Hemorrhoids	Overweight	Tuberculosis
Constipation	High blood	Pellagra	
Diabetes	pressure	Pep lacking	

The need of the hour is not for more hospitals, surgery, and drugs, but for more information about how to live to be normally well—how to prevent the 90 per cent of prevalent disease. Therefore health education is of first importance as the chief preventive measure.

The forces and methods which constitute that which we call "immunity" will be presented from many viewpoints in this book. There are two kinds of immunity; one natural and the other artificial. Not enough attention has been given to the former in proportion to that given to the latter.

dEATH is mostly EAT

Many eminent authorities confirm the truth of this serious pleasantry. A few notable examples are given here.

Dr. Mikkel Hindhede, Denmark

"The two chief causes of disease are food and drink." (3)

The Mayo Clinic

The Mayo clinic records reveal that from 80 to 90 per cent of all the surgical work done in their hospital is done upon the stomach, intestines, and related organs. (4)

Dr. Harvey W. Wiley

"I believe I would not be far out of the way to say that diet may be said to be a factor in every disease to which man is heir." (5)

Dr. Osler

The late Sir William Osler, eminent English physician, said: "Ninety per cent of all conditions outside of acute infections, contagious diseases, and traumatisms, are directly traceable to diet." (6)

Sir Arbuthnot Lane

Sir Arbuthnot Lane, noted London physician, says: "The food question is infinitely the most important problem of the present day, . . . and if properly dealt with must result in the disappearance of the vast bulk of the disease, misery, and death." (7)

Dr. J. H. Kellogg

"At least nine-tenths of all chronic maladies with which doctors are called upon to deal might be successfully treated without the use of drugs by a physician well acquainted with the varied resources afforded by the science of nutrition." (8)

G. K. Abbott, A.B., M.D., F.A.C.S.

"Man's diet conduces to the occurrence of diseases representative of nearly all the most common and prominent of human ailments." (9)

Haven Emerson, M.D.

"We could actually add more years to the average expectancy of man's life by suitable variety and amount of food than by eliminating any of the prevalent communicable diseases such as tuberculosis and syphilis." (10)

T. F. Arbercrombie, M.D.

"I maintain that if all human beings were well nourished, every cell in the body as God intended it should be, we would have most of our public health and medical problems solved." (16)

George R. Minot
"With faulty food, there is faulty nutrition, faulty function, faulty structure, disease." (17)

Sir Robert McCarrison
Sir Robert McCarrison, M.D., LL.D., D.Sc., F.R.C.P., London, by feeding pigeons, guinea pigs, and monkeys upon "deficiency foods," such as are commonly consumed in civilized countries, induced in them every known disease of the digestive tract, and disease in all their organs.

When serving as Director of Nutritional Research, Pasteur Institute, Coonoor, India, Major General Sir Robert McCarrison, Kt., C.I.E., LLD., F.R.C.P., I.M.S., said: "I found . . . that no organ or tissue of the body escapes the effects of faulty food deficient in vitamins or in other elements and complexes necessary for normal nutrition; and that animals fed on such faulty food are prone to be invaded by microbes of all kinds. . . . Properly fed animals remain remarkably free from disease, while improperly fed animals are remarkably subject to it. Do these discoveries apply equally to human beings? The answer is undoubtedly in the affirmative." (11)

Diseases Produced Under Control

Among the morbid conditions produced by Sir Robert McCarrison, M. D., in animals by improper feeding he names these: pneumonia, pleurisy, bronchitis, infections of the nose, adenoids; infections of the ear; infections of the eye; diseases of the stomach; —growths, ulcer and cancer; inflammation of the small and large intestine including ulcers and colitis, dysentery, diarrhea and constipation; inflammation and stone in the bladder, Bright's Disease; diseases of the skin such as loss of hair, dermatitis and abscesses; gangrene of feet and tail; disease of male and female reproductive organs; premature birth of young or death before birth; anemia; dropsy; enlarged, cystic and suppurating glands; goiter; neuritis; nervousness; irritability; beriberi; scurvy; decaying teeth; rickets; diseases of the heart; inflammation and degeneration of nervous tissue; feeble growth; poor appetite; lassitude; weakness; ill-temper; and ferocity. "All these states of ill-health had a common causation; faulty nutrition with or without infection." (12)

In the address from which the above statement is taken, Dr.

McCarrison made the following profound announcement:

Food Is the Chief Medicine

"Of all the medicines created out of the earth, food is the chief."

In some of the ancient dynasties of China there was an Imperial Dietitian as well as an Imperial Physician. Hu Se-Hui, who occupied this position from 1314 to 1330 A.D., wrote a book called "The Principles of Correct Diet." He gave sixty-two different diets which would supply the vitamins of the B group. The motto of his book was, "Food alone cures many diseases."—J. and L. G. Needham in Journal A.M.A. 117:1418, 1941.

Eat for Health

When meals are planned at home or selected at a public eating place, do you ever raise the question, Does this food contain the elements needed by the heart, brain, nerves, and all the organs and their processes? No! Nine-tenths of the people never give a thought to this. They ask but one question, Do I like this food? That and that alone determines what we will or will not eat. Yet it is more important to us that we know how to nourish our bodies and those of our children than to understand the inner workings of an automobile, the mysteries of the radio, the latest fashion or movie, or to learn all the languages of the earth, the doings of the ancients, the depths of the fourth dimension, or the marvels of the atom. To be sure, these matters are important, but they are of absolutely no value without health.

Inasmuch as "the disease and suffering which everywhere prevail are largely due to popular errors in regard to diet" (13), the chief purpose of this book is to make plain the manner of properly nourishing the body as the major factor in possessing normal health and natural immunity.

CONFUSION ABOUNDS

There is an ever-increasing variety of teachings about foods and how the body should be nourished. They come from many sources —health educators, promoters of the sale of foods and special products, popular writers, and others. Many of the theories propounded contain helpful instruction but are incomplete and often are conflicting. People hear one, another, and another, and perhaps try to follow all of them and so become confused. Or they select one theory and exclude the others and so obtain a partial benefit.

The situation is much as it is in the field of religion which ought to be the simplest thing to understand and which should exert the most uplifting and hallowed influence of all teachings on the earth; and yet, there is such a variety of conflicting religious teachings offered the people that sometimes they become so confused they wonder if any of them are true.

So it is with health teachings; the people try one thing and another and are continually seeking for something they have not found.

The writer wishes to make the right way of living so plain that no one can misunderstand or doubt it, and so easy to follow that all may practice it and enjoy the boon of health. Read and be convinced.

FADS AND FANCIES VERSUS A BALANCED RATION

There are certain fads and fancies which come and go like the waves of the sea. Often they contain much that is good, but too often they are lacking in something and so are not balanced.

Fasting

For instance, fasting will give a tired stomach a rest, and will give the body time to dispose of an overload of starch, sugar, fat and protein. For this reason a short fast is often very helpful, but it is not a permanent correction of any condition because fasting does not correct an unbalanced ration which most likely was the cause of the trouble; it can only prepare the body for the balanced ration which is to supply every need of the body and so produce health. Some people fast one day each week. That is a good plan if one lives so "fast" the other six days that the digestive organs need the seventh in which to catch up their work. If one will eat correctly and conservatively every day he will never need to spend a period of time in fasting. There are those who fast a little every day by taking a very light evening meal. That gives the digestive organs an opportunity to complete their work every day and rest before the next day arrives. Many people would be greatly benefited by doing this.

Raw Foods

Raw foods cannot be a "cure-all" unless a balanced ration can be secured from them, which is difficult for most people; however, there is an important place for certain raw foods daily in every balanced ration. The Automatic Menu Planner (a few pages forward) explains this.

Juice Therapy

There are several herbs which can be used to make delightful and healthful drinks. However, there is an element of danger in stressing the use of some certain herb drink, in that people are liable to place too much dependence upon it to correct their ills and so neglect to secure a balanced ration. In that case an herb drink becomes only a deception, and disappointment.

The same may easily be true of the use of fruit and vegetable juices, both of which are very useful as supplementary foods, but which may crowd out or hinder the digestion of a complete ration. This result is often seen today. Their proper use will be indicated in following pages. See Index for "Juice Therapy."

Vitamin and Mineral Concentrates

Among the most common dietary deficiencies are those of vitamins and minerals. The discovery of this fact has opened a vast field for exploitation by manufacturers of concentrates. Two million pounds of vitamin concentrates are sold in one year in the United States. Some of them are helpful for certain conditions but there is a very definite danger that the people will learn to depend upon these manufactured concentrates, believing that their use actually makes up for the deficiencies in their diet, when such is not the case, because no synthetic ration can be concocted by man which will be equal to the marvelous balance of all the food elements to be secured in natural foods eaten in right proportions. Concentrates are second choice foods. They are infinitely superior to drugs, but as a rule their use should be temporary while helping to make up a deficiency in the ration, but one should not permanently depend upon them and so excuse himself for continuing to use devitalized foods. Nothing can equal nature's own arrangement of minerals and vitamins in natural foods used in a balanced manner. In selecting concentrates of minerals or vitamins preference may well be given to those made direct from foods rather than those made by synthetic processes.

Cleansing Programs

If one has allowed his elimination to be poor and his system to become toxic, or clogged his system with food elements which have not been properly handled in the body, or with poisons deliberately put in, a cleansing program is necessary. Water is the basis of such a process but it is greatly aided by minerals and vitamins. For this purpose the juice therapy in connection with certain cleansing foods is appropriate. However, the ideal plan is to live normally every day so that such a cleansing is never needed. That is the goal of this book.

Physical Culture

To follow a program of healthful living one does not have to try to be an athlete or do stunts in physical exercise; he does not of necessity have to specialize in muscle development. There ought to be a health program which is within the reach of the ordinary work-a-day men and women in the common walks of life. A good amount of exercise is a necessary part of such a daily program. The most helpful exercise is walking or useful labor in the open air.

A BALANCED PROGRAM

There ought to be a way of daily living which will keep its adherents in good health so that they may perform the ordinary duties of life with ease and without undue fatigue, that the daily rounds of life may be one continuous pleasure rather than a struggle to "keep going" from the sheer force of necessity.

Such a happy way of living consists of a balanced program, which must include among other items:

(1) Perfect nutrition—natural foods, raw and cooked, proportioned to provide the right amount of protein to repair the body cells, starch, sugar and fat to supply heat and energy for the body and its activities, with water, minerals, and vitamins to sustain all of the life processes—a program of feeding which will nourish every organ, gland and cell in the body.

(2) A proper amount of exercise to maintain good circulation of the blood that it may promptly bring fresh supplies of oxygen and food to the body cells and quickly transport their wastes to the skin, lungs, and kidneys for elimination so that toxins will not be allowed to accumulate in the body.

The burden of this book is to provide an organized program of daily living so that every nutritional need of the body will be met every day and so make possible the enjoyment of optimum health every day, and to make the right way of living so plain, so consistent, and so manifestly true that no sincere reader will doubt its correctness, and so desirable that all who read will want to follow it.

The plan of living herein described is a digest of the findings of some of the most eminent and successful investigators in the world —highly respected authors from various countries.

THE BODY'S LIFE

The body is built of cells. All body functions are associated with the function of cells. If the cells are normal, the organs and body are normal, and that is health.

The life is in the cell. The continuance of the life and functions of cells is made possible by forces which reside in air, sunshine, water, and food.

Plants can attain perfect development only when all of the elements they need for life and growth are in the soil.

"A plant, in order to obtain perfect growth, must find in soil a certain minimum of each of many elements. Consider, for example, the element potassium. Suppose only half of the necessary amount of potassium be present, then no matter how abundant may be all the other soil and air constituents, their normal utilization is limited to one-half. The rate of growth and the ultimate development of the plant are consequently depressed. Applying this principle to food absorption, showing that the lack of any one mineral requirement in the body will, to the extent it is lacking, thereby deprive the system of the ability to utilize all of the minerals present." (15)

This is similar to the maxim the sages gave us long ago,—"a chain is no stronger than its weakest link." This seems to be so clear that it is useless to dispute it, and yet, when applied to a balanced ration it is almost revolutionary.

Animals—cows, horses, pigs, chickens, etc.—are the most profitable when fed scientifically.

The average farmer knows more about fertilizing the soil that it may bring forth proper crops; the feeding of a balanced ration to the hens that they will lay a goodly number of eggs, and to the cows that they may give a profitable supply of milk, than he does about feeding those for whom all these things exist—himself and family.

The average mother knows less about the foods needed to nourish the inside of the bodies of her children than about the style of the clothes for the outside. She does not discern that the body is more than the raiment.

Animals in the laboratory can be kept in good health or fall ill with common ailments and diseases similar to ours, according to the food given them.

The engine of the automobile is "fed" scientifically to secure the greatest efficiency and the longest service.

Man alone—he who is lord of all living creatures and of every mechanical device, and who holds their destiny in his hands, too often eats according to the caprice of appetite and does not use as good judgment concerning his own health as he does in the protection of the animate and inanimate things under his care.

The Life-Span Is Decreasing

Man is the only creature given to the practice of self-destroying habits. Because of such habits degenerative diseases of the vital organs are rapidly increasing with a consequent shortening of the span of life. The much-lauded reports that human life is lengthening are deceptive in that they give a false impression. Through better care of babies and their mothers, and by better control of contagious and infectious diseases, more children grow to adult life than formerly; but when they reach adult life—age forty—they have already indulged in so many life-destroying habits that, on the average, they will not live as long as their grandparents did. "The young live longer but the old die sooner." People do not live longer, but more babies grow up to adult life and this increases the average length of all lives. The age limit is lowering at the same time the average length of life is increasing. We cannot continue indefinitely to add to the average length of life by conquering infectious diseases, because when they are wiped out there will be no more to conquer, but degenerative diseases are increasing with accelerating rapidity. One authority has said that if cancer continues to increase at its present rate it alone will depopulate the earth.

"The span of human life has not been lengthened, and there is no prospect that it soon will be. The average duration of life is all that has been altered, and that has been accomplished chiefly by giving more babies a fairer start in life's journey than they used to have. Because more of them get by the early and very difficult hurdles, absolutely more of them survive to later ages. But the terms of the bet that any individual man aged seventy today can safely say that he will be alive at ninety appear to be not quite as good as they were fifty years ago." (14)

This book is designed to lead the reader away from the degenerative diseases and to indicate how to attain the highest possible degree of immunity to infectious and contagious diseases and so add to the length, usefulness and joy of life. Inasmuch as the indulgence of the sense of taste is foremost among the causes of degeneracy, this book will faithfully indicate these practices and point the way to a higher order of living. It is hoped that the reader may discern the path to abundant health and happiness and walk therein.

BIBLIOGRAPHY

(1) "Ministry of Healing," page 127.

(2) "The Commentator," November, 1938, page 100.

(3) Hindhede, quoted by G. K. Abbott, M.D., in "High Blood Pressure," page 10.

(4) "Life and Health," April, 1924.

(5) Wiley, in personal letter to J. G. White.

(6) Osler, quoted by Risley and Walton in "Foods, Nutrition, and Clinical Dietetics," page 13.

(7) Lane, in "The Motive," June, 1925.

(8) Kellogg, in "Good Health," June, 1940, page 69.

(9) Abbott, "High Blood Pressure," Second edition, page 164.

(10) Emerson, in "Clean Life Educator," Nov.-Dec., 1938.

(11) McCarrison, quoted in "Madras Mail," March 16, 1935.

(12) Published in "Madras Mail," March 16, 1935, and in the "Wheel of Health," by G. T. French, M.D., pages 36-38. The two lists combined. Similar list published in "The Lancet," London, May 23, 1931.

(13) "Ministry of Healing," page 295.

(14) Prof. Raymond Pearl, in "The Search for Longevity," in "Scientific Monthly," May, 1938.

(15) Dr. F. G. Hoskins, Cambridge University.

(16) T. F. Arbercrombie, M.D., Director Georgia Dept. Public Health. The Land Vol. 3, No. 4, Organ of Friends of the Land.

(17) Research Publications Association 22:29, 1943.

The Body and Its Needs

The chart on this page gives the chemical composition of the body and the approximate amount of each kind of element found in it. It necessarily follows that the body must be nourished by the same elements as those of which it consists—replacement of losses must be of like kind. Therefore, beside the man is a column showing the amount of each element needed daily to maintain health. This is a balanced ration in broad outline: moisture, 8 lbs.; protein, 2½ ozs.; fat, 2 8-10 ozs.; carbohydrate, 16 ozs.; mineral salts, .4 oz. Vitamins will be discussed later.

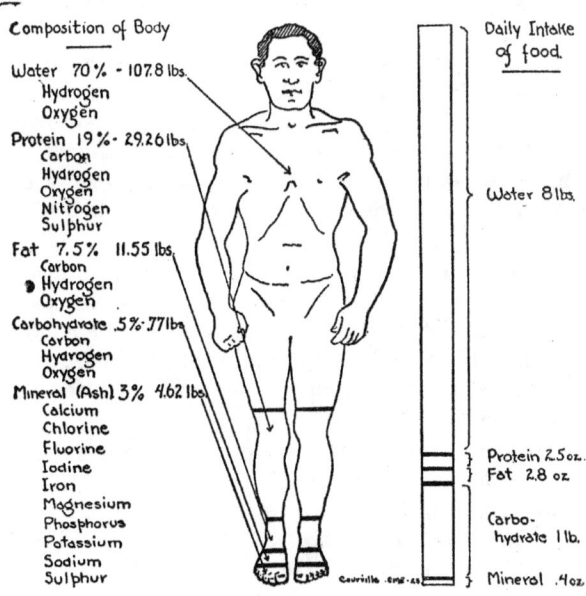

Composition and Food Requirements
of a 154 Pound Man.

Composition of Body

Water 70 % - 107.8 lbs.
  Hydrogen
  Oxygen

Protein 19 % - 29.26 lbs.
  Carbon
  Hydrogen
  Oxygen
  Nitrogen
  Sulphur

Fat 7.5 % 11.55 lbs.
  Carbon
  Hydrogen
  Oxygen

Carbohydrate .5 % .77 lbs.
  Carbon
  Hydrogen
  Oxygen

Mineral (Ash) 3 % 4.62 lbs.
  Calcium
  Chlorine
  Fluorine
  Iodine
  Iron
  Magnesium
  Phosphorus
  Potassium
  Sodium
  Sulphur

Daily Intake
of food

Water 8 lbs.

Protein 2.5 oz.
Fat 2.8 oz.

Carbo-
hydrate 1 lb.

Mineral .4 oz.

Good Health from Good Food

A noted author has set forth this principle in the following profound statement:

"Our bodies are built up from the food we eat. There is a constant breaking down of the tissues of the body; every movement of every organ involves waste, and this waste is repaired from our food. Each organ of the body requires its share of nutrition. The brain must be supplied with its portion; the bones, muscles and nerves demand theirs. It is a wonderful process that transforms the food into blood, and uses this blood to build up the varied parts of the body; but this process is going on continually, supplying with life and strength each nerve, muscle, and tissue." (1)

There are 92 elements known to chemists which are constituents of the physical world, (living and non-living). "Investigators are not yet entirely agreed as to how many of these elements are essential to our nutrition." (6)

The latest the writer has seen as this book goes to press is the following:

"There have been some fifty to sixty essential nutrients isolated from food—and the end is not yet." (7)

For the purpose of this book it seems most practical to use only the basic 16 elements shown in the foregoing diagram. Should we endeavor to trace 40 more of them back into their food sources both the writer and the reader would get lost on the way. Consider wheat as an example. Chemists have found in the wheat kernel dozens of elements which are never mentioned when wheat is discussed as a food.

It will be noted from the chart on the previous page that the body consists of certain definite substances often spoken of as the "sixteen elements of life" (not to mention the vitamins). If these all are secured in the daily intake in proper amounts, and no other substances are put in to hinder their work, manifestly the body will be well nourished.

Next in order the reader should note that these sixteen elements all find their places in five groups of substances: first, water; second, protein; third, fat; fourth, carbohydrate; fifth, a group of minerals. Now that these sixteen have been resolved into five groups, it will be easier to locate them in foods.

Let us now turn our attention to foods and see from which ones these five groups of substances can be obtained.

Grains

The U. S. Department of Agriculture has issued charts showing the analyses of grains as follows:

	Water	Protein	Fat	Carbo-hydrates	Ash (Minerals)
Wheat	10.6	12.2	1.7	73.7	1.8
Oats	11.0	11.8	5.0	69.2	3.0
Corn	10.8	10.0	4.3	73.4	1.5
Rye	10.5	12.2	1.5	73.9	1.9
Buckwheat	12.6	10.0	2.2	73.2	2.0
Rice	12.0	8.0	2.0	77.0	1.0

How wonderful is that! Behold, all of the five groups of elements needed by the man for food are found in every grain that grows! Evidently the same Mind planned the man and the food to nourish him.

It does not follow that grains are a perfect food, but it is plain that they are an ideal food and adapted to be a staple article of man's diet.

The proportions of these elements in the grains are not the same as in the man, and they also vary in the different grains. Therefore, the first step in securing a proper balance of food elements is to use a variety of the grains rather than confine oneself to a single grain.

Vegetables

The same charts show the content of the

	Water	Protein	Fat	Carbo-hydrate	Ash
Potato	78.3	2.2	0.1	18.4	1.0

Then the charts go on to show the composition of other vegetables and that they usually contain the same five groups of elements.

Manifestly they, too, are planned to be food for the man.

The second step in getting a proper balance is to add vegetables to the grains; and the third step is to use a variety of vegetables and not be limited to a certain few.

The Creator has provided a great variety of foods to afford man much pleasure in partaking of them, and in doing so protects man from malnutrition because in a wide variety of food he obtains a wide variety of elements, which is an important feature of a balanced ration.

Legumes

The charters also reveal that the legumes are composed of similar groups of elements. Consider a sample:

	Water	Protein	Fat	Carbo-hydrate	Ash
Shelled Beans	58.9	9.4	0.6	29.1	2.0

And so it is, with varying proportions, with all of the other legumes. Thus the fourth step in securing a balanced ration is to add a variety of legumes to the variety of grains and vegetables already obtained.

Fruits

A further study of the charts shows that the fruits also contain the same five groups in still different proportions. Here are two examples:

	Water	Protein	Fat	Carbo-hydrate	Ash
Apple	84.6	0.4	0.5	14.2	0.3
Banana	75.3	1.3	0.6	22.0	0.8

The fifth step in getting a balanced ration is to add the fruits to the other foods, and then, because of the variation in the content of the fruits, use a variety and so tend always toward a balance of all elements when we have finally encompassed all of the foods.

Nuts

Next we study the charts of the nuts and find the same five groups once more, but with quite a variation in the different nuts. Two examples will suffice.

	Water	Protein	Fat	Carbo-hydrate	Ash
Walnut	2.5	16.6	63.4	16.1	1.4
Chestnut	5.9	10.7	7.0	74.2	2.2

Logically the sixth step toward a proper balance is to add a variety of nuts to the fruits, legumes, vegetables and grains.

A Complete Ration

Inasmuch as each of these classes of foods contains the same substances as does the body of the man, if the man will but learn to know the right quantity of grains, of vegetables, of legumes, of fruits, and of nuts to use in each day's rations, and will change his selection from the various groups now and then to get the variety, every nutritional need of his body will be met; every muscle, nerve, gland, cell, and secretion will have the wherewithal to carry on normal processes of life, and that means health.

The foregoing foods are the true and primary sources of nutrition. There are secondary foods such as milk, cream, butter, and eggs, all of which, with the exception of eggs, contain the same five groups of elements in varying proportions; but there is no element in these secondary foods which was not first found in the primary foods—grains, vegetables, legumes, fruits, and nuts.

By the process of a very little thinking it will be recognized by every reader of these lines that in the ultimate, all animal life, man included, is sustained by the vegetation of the earth. Even those animals which eat other animals are but getting vegetation second hand because the animals so eaten had lived on vegetation. Were there no vegetation on the earth all animal life would cease.

Therefore, if a child or adult is allergic to milk, butter, or eggs, such a person may have a balanced ration without those foods. Or, if one wishes to be a strict vegetarian, it is evident that he can do so and be perfectly nourished by giving attention to the foregoing instructions concerning a balanced ration, and to the following portions of this book in which more explicit directions will be given.

Without Animal Products

That it is possible to secure a balanced ration without any animal product, and that no health hazard is involved if one is well informed, has been definitely stated by no less an authority than E. V. McCollum, Ph.D., Professor of Biochemistry of the School of Hygiene and Public Health, Johns Hopkins University, Baltimore, Maryland.

"From the foregoing (a preceding discussion) it will be evident that both human and animal experience with the fleshless diet, and the result of modern scientific studies on foods and nutrition, afford abundant evidence that meats are not necessary in the diet. It is even possible, if the food is selected with a thorough knowledge of the defects of individual foods, and of their supplementary values—their power to make good each other's deficiencies—to secure a human dietary which would be fairly satisfactory without either milk or eggs, but there is a certain hazard to health in attempting to do so without expert knowledge." (2)

"Animal foods, including dairy produce, are not necessary in the diet. Not only are vegetable foods sufficient, but they are more conducive to health." (5)

During recent years there has been a widespread hunt for proteins, and the food scientists are surprising themselves by discovering that many common foods contain proteins of high biologic quality which they previously thought were to be found only in meats, eggs, and milk. Among the foods now listed as containing excellent proteins are potatoes, the soybean, wheat, corn, rice, as well as certain nuts and leafy vegetables. An example of statements now appearing in public print is the following, found in *Time*, September 27, 1943:

"Soybeans. Rivaling meat in protein and other food elements, the edible varieties of soybeans can be served in a great variety of dishes, from milk shakes to steak (Properly minced soybeans may sometimes be mistaken for meat loaf). Soybeans are only one-fourth as expensive as beefsteak."

This point will be much more fully discussed in later chapters in this book.

Over forty years ago the dangers and problems of the present day were forecast and counsel was given concerning them.

In 1902 the following instruction was published for the guidance of those who are working in the front ranks of reform in living in the interest of better health:

"Let the diet reform be progressive. Let the people be taught how to prepare food without the use of milk or butter. Tell them that the time will soon come when there will be no safety in using eggs, milk, cream, or butter, because disease in animals is increasing in proportion to the increase of wickedness among men. The time is near when, because of the iniquity of the fallen race, the whole animal creation will groan under the diseases that curse our earth." (3)

Two Levels of Living

Many people are allergic to milk or to eggs; many babies cannot tolerate cow's milk; there are many adults with whom milk does not agree for various reasons, some of which will be discussed in this book.

There are still other people who, because of the increase of diseases among animals, and possibly other reasons, prefer not to use any animal product—milk, cream, butter, or eggs—and are earnestly looking for detailed information showing them how to obtain a scientifically complete ration without such animal products. This treatise undertakes to provide such a program of living without danger of deficiency. The author believes that this way of living is a protection against disease. The Automatic Menu Planner on a later page covers both ways of living. Those who do not wish to use any animal product will find substitute foods listed in the same groups, so that every user of the Menu Planner may live according to the method of his choice.

Doubtless the food presenting the most serious obstacles to those who consider deleting it from their menus is cow's milk. In the Menu Planner, soybean milk is offered in its place. A more detailed discussion of the problems involved in the milk question will be found in a later section of this book. Soybean cream is now available in place of dairy cream; soy cheese may be substituted for cottage cheese. Commercial butter substitutes are increasing in variety.

Adventures in Food Flavors

When making changes from foods to which we have long been accustomed, to a new way of living, we should not expect to duplicate the flavors of the foods we leave behind, but should look for new flavors and delights. If we look for exact duplicates of the old tastes, we may be disappointed; but if we are looking for something new, we will find flavors in the new foods every bit as delightsome as the old ones, and some of them far better. It is like entering upon a new adventure.

Students of this higher order of living will want to secure a new cookbook to guide them in the preparation of all kinds of food to make the meals tasty, healthful, and attractive. We are just now beginning to learn about foods, their values and ways of combining and using them to secure their highest biologic values and most charming flavors. A vast new field awaits our investigation and experimentation.

It is now in order that we view the entire field of natural foods and see what an abundance of delectable delights await us.

NATURAL FOODS

Suitable for the Average Person

Fruits

Blackberries	Mulberries	Raisins	Prunes
Loganberries	Persimmons	Bananas	Melons
Gooseberries	Nectarines	Peaches	Pears
Strawberries	Grapefruit	Oranges	Plums
Pomegranates	Pineapple	Guavas	Dates
Huckleberries	Avocados	Mangoes	Limes
Raspberries	Apricots	Apples	Figs
Blueberries	Cherries	Lemons	
Cranberries	Quinces	Grapes	

Vegetables

Watermelon	Greens of every	Parsnips	Garlic
Muskmelon	kind	Tomatoes	Celery
Cantaloupe	Brussels sprouts	Broccoli	Okra
Artichokes	Water chestnut	Beet tops	Beets
Watercress	Peppers, green	Parsley	Citron
Rutabagas	Swiss chard	Pumpkin	Kale
Asparagus	Cauliflower	Spinach	Leek
Lily bulbs	Cucumbers	Endive	Squash
Dandelions	Eggplant	Carrots	Onions
Sweet potatoes	Radishes	Turnips	Chives
Irish potatoes	Lettuce	Salsify	
Sprouts of beans	Kohl-rabi	Cabbage	

Wild plants suitable to use as greens, particularly in the Spring of the year when the shoots are new and tender:

Dandelion	Red root	Marsh marigold	Summer mustard
Watercress	Lamb's quarters	Winter cress	Purslane or
Pig weed or	Narrow dock	Chicory	Pursley
Mountain Spinach	Wild lettuce	Pokeweed (root	(8)
Denver spinach	Cow-slip or	is poisonous)	

Legumes

Peas	Garbanzas	Lima beans	Green beans
Lentils	Soy beans	Kentucky beans	Dry beans
Cowpeas	Navy beans	String beans	
Split peas	Wax beans	Soy bean meal	

Grains

Whole corn meal	Oatmeal	Brown rice	Bread 100%
Whole grain	Popcorn	Green corn	whole wheat
wheat	Rye crisp	Rolled oats	Bran (emergency
Unleavened bread	Barley	Whole wheat	food only)
Shredded Wheat	Corn bread	zwieback	
Wheat flakes	Rye meal		

Nuts

Almonds	Butternuts	Malted nuts	Beechnuts
Chestnuts	Cocoanuts	Pistachios	Litchi (Chinese
Peanuts	Brazil nuts	Pine nuts	hazelnut)
Filberts	English walnuts	Pecans	
Black walnuts	Hickory nuts	Cashews	

When making foods with nut contents the proportion of nuts to other food substances should not exceed one-tenth to one-sixth part of the whole. (6)

Liquids

Water	Soy bean milk	Grain soups	Cultured butter-
Milk	Malted milk	Cream soups	milks
Cream	Lemonade	Vegetable soups	Acidophilus,
Buttermilk	Grape juice	Fruit-juice drinks	homemade

Miscellaneous

Cottage cheese	Tapioca	Eggs	Butter or vege-
Ripe olives	Molasses	Sago	table substitute
Soy bean oil	Olive oil	Maple syrup	Oils extracted
Sugar	Honey	Maple sugar	from nuts, grains
Macaroni	Salad oil		and other seeds

Milk and its products, and eggs, are listed in the foregoing table as "suitable foods"—as a part of what is called the "lacto-ovovegetarian diet" which is by many good authorities accepted as the most desirable diet program; but the author wishes to maintain the distinction between them as "secondary" foods and those classed as "primary" foods earlier in this book, namely grains, vegetables, legumes, fruits, and nuts. This distinction will be discussed more fully in this book.

No meat, fish, or fowl appear in this list. While they may be found in certain lists of foods in the book, they are strictly excluded from all of the menus and are not recommended to those who want the best foods and the best possible health. Those who prefer to eat meat should use it in place of one of the protein foods listed in the Automatic Menu Planner.

Sugar and various syrups are included in this list of natural foods. The unrefined are the most desirable, but even they should be used in great moderation, and in certain conditions should be entirely discarded. Honey and sweet fruits are nature's sweets.

Balanced Meals

The foregoing pages have revealed that natural foods contain (with water, air, and sunlight) every element of life needed for the cells and their functions, and a list of them precedes this page.

However, it is one thing to have all these foods in the house, and quite another matter to arrange them in balanced meals three times a day. The perpetual problem in the home or at the public eating place is, What will we have for dinner today? This situation makes it necessary to provide some simple method of planning the meals so that the rations for the day are approximately balanced. The amounts of foods needed vary with individuals, but it is important that a sufficient number of kinds of food be eaten daily to secure the variety which is necessary to obtain a balance of all the elements. To meet these needs the following Automatic Menu Planner is provided.

AUTOMATIC MENU PLANNER

A Guide to Balanced Rations for Average Persons
Select one order from each group for each meal.

BREAKFAST

(1) A half hour or more before breakfast a glass of water or fruit juice. Grape and prune and apple juices are laxatives; otherwise orange juice is ideal.

(2)

Any whole grain cereal Wheat and oats are best

Add cream or milk from dairy or soybean and some kind of sweet fruit, if desired, such as banana, d a t e s, figs, raisins, etc., but no sugar.

Cereal may be omitted and use only the bread in group No. 3 if desired.

(3)

All-of-the-wheat bread or zwieback, with butter.

(4)

Laxative Fruits— Prunes, Figs, Pears, Apricots, Avocados. Ripe Olives.

(5)

Any other fruit as desired. Part of it to be raw.

(6)

If a serving of protein food is desired in the breakfast, it may be selected from the list in the dinner menu.

(7)

Drinks—

For adults, no drink unless milk is indicated.

For children, only milk, and to be taken at the close of the meal.

Soy bean milk agrees with some people better than cow's milk and may be substituted by any person.

Cereal coffee may be used if it does not hinder digestion.

Any drink should be taken by itself and not used to hasten food through the mouth.

DINNER

It is better to have dinner at noon instead of at night when it is possible.

(1) Potato
Irish or sweet; baked is best.

(2)

A cooked coarse Vegetable—
Swiss chard or other Greens
Brussels sprouts
String beans
Onions
Cauliflower
Kohl-rabi
Asparagus
Artichokes
Broccoli
Squash
Eggplant

(3)

A root—
Carrots
Beets
Turnips
Parsnips

(4)

A Protein—
Beans, (soy beans are especially fine)
Peas, Lentils
Nuts, Eggs
Cottage Cheese
Soy Cheese
Prepared meat substitutes by reliable manufacturers.

(5)

A raw vegetable or salad—
Lettuce
Celery
Radish
Cabbage
Carrots
Turnips

Cucumbers
Watercress
Any others obtainable

(6)

Drinks—
Milk
Buttermilk
Soy bean milk
Vegetable juice

(7)

Optional—
Bread
Corn, green or canned
Ripe olives
Tomatoes
Melons
Honey

Groups 2 and 5 are the most neglected and the most important.

Groups 1 and 3 may be combined before selecting, if desired. If it is desired to still further lessen the variety in one meal, groups 1, 2, and 3 may be combined before selecting one.

It is well to change selections until all have been used. This helps to secure a balance of all elements.

SUPPER

(1)	Ripe olives	See list in breakfast.
Whole-grain bread, if needed	(2)	(3)
(Many do well with only fruit at night.)	At least one laxative fruit	Any other fruits. Some of them to be raw.

Nothing is to be eaten between meals or after the evening meal.

Meals should be at least five hours apart. All food must be thoroughly masticated.

Drink water freely two or three hours after meals and until a half hour of the next meal.

Take six to eight glasses of liquid daily, and more if needed.

A glass of fruit juice may be taken at bedtime.

The essentials of a correct ration have been incorporated in this Menu Planner—protein, fat, carbohydrate, minerals, the alkaline balance, the vitamins, and the proper combinations. It provides for a normal ration, which is the basis of all diets. For modifications of this ration for special conditions, see the chapters in the book where those conditions are discussed.

BIBLIOGRAPHY

(1) "Ministry of Healing," page 295.

(2) Dr. E. V. McCollum, quoted in "Life and Health,' 'March, 1937, page 29.

(3) "Counsels on Diet and Foods," page 349, Review and Herald Publishing Association, Takoma Park, Washington, D. C.

(4) M. Hindhede, quoted in "Vegetarian News" March 1943.

(5) H. C. Sherman, "Principles of Nutrition and Nutritive Values of Food," U. S. Department of Agriculture, Miscellaneous Publication No. 546, June 1944, page 13.

(6) Fredrick J. Stare, M.D., Harvard School of Public Health, "Nutrition Review," January 1950.

(7) Michigan Public Health, March 1941.

How the Body Uses Food

A food may be defined as any substance which, when absorbed into the blood, will nourish the tissues, repair waste, furnish force and heat to the body, without causing injury to any of its parts or loss of functional activity, or calling for constantly increasing quantities of itself.

It is now in order that we consider how the body uses food. In this field of study we will discover something concerning the amounts the body uses of various foods, and that will reveal which foods are eaten to excess, and those of which we are usually deficient, and so we will get directly at the most common cause of disease. The uses of foods in the body have been separated into three classes to make the study easy to understand.

Classification of Foods

Class 1

Heat and Energy Foods

Carbonaceous: 90 per cent of total, exclusive of water

STARCH	Sago	Honey	Vegetable shortenings
Cereals	Legumes	Sweet fruits	Nuts
Breads	SUGAR	FAT	Milk
Macaroni	Sugar	Olives	Cream
Certain vegetables	Maple sugar	Vegetable oils	Butter
Tapioca	Sorghum	Salad oils	Soy beans

Class 2

Building and Repair Food, Protein:

Nitrogenous: 10 per cent of total

PROTEIN	Soy bean and	Lentils	Soy Cheese
Grains	products	Nuts	Milk
Beans	Peas	Cottage Cheese	Eggs

25

Class 3
Regulators of Body Processes

WATER	MINERALS	CELLULOSE	VITAMINS
Beverages	Bran and embryo	Indigestible matter	The vital spark
Fruits	of cereals	Bran	which activates the
Vegetables	Vegetables	Framework of	other food ele-
Soups	Legumes	vegetables	ments, w i t h o u t
(60% of the aver-	Fruits	Framework of	which growth can-
age diet is water.)	Nuts	fruits	not occur or life
	Milk and Eggs	Agar-Agar	continue.

Concerning Class 1. It is a matter of common knowledge that as a rule people overeat of sugar and starch; and that more people are overweight than underweight.

Class 2 is the tissue-repairing substance—protein. In the preceding chapter the daily need of protein was set at 2½ oz. From this it is apparent that an excess of protein is more common than a deficiency. Vegetarians might be an exception.

With Class 3 it is quite different; the average person does not take enough water, uses refined foods deficient in minerals, cellulose, and vitamins, besides using methods of cooking which destroy vitamins and remove minerals.

The result is that the system is filled with sugar, starch, fat, and protein, none of which can be used without the water, minerals, cellulose and vitamins; and so the former become a burden to the system.

The above unbalance of the average ration is cause number one of disease. No health program or medical procedure will ever cope with the resulting diseases. There is but one remedy—a proper balance of these elements. We must reduce our average consumption of sugar, starch, fat, and protein, and increase very markedly the use of water, minerals, cellulose, and vitamins—the elements which carry on the life processes which run low because we fail to supply the elements that would make their continuance possible.

There is no substitute for a balanced ration. This will become more and more evident as we proceed.

WHAT WATER DOES IN THE BODY

About three-fourths of the body is water. The blood fluid, of which a person weighing 150 pounds has about 10 pounds or 5 quarts, is 92 per cent water. The red corpuscles are 65 per cent water, the white corpuscles 70 per cent, the body cells 80 per cent, protoplasm 75 per cent, the saliva (about three pints daily) 99 per cent, the gastric juice (one to two quarts daily) 99 per cent, the pancreatic juice (three pints daily) 98 per cent, the liver bile (nearly two quarts daily) 99 per cent, skin perspiration (from one pint up to five pounds daily) 99 per cent, moisture in breath exhaled daily, one quart, the kidneys daily excrete from one to two quarts (one quart of water is required to eliminate 45 grams of waste in the urine); the brain is 85 per cent water, the nerves 75 per cent, the heart 70 per cent, the lungs 75 per cent, the liver 70 per cent, the kidneys 80 per cent.

Water is the body's solvent. In cooperation with chemicals it breaks down the food and prepares it for absorption and use in the cells. It is the medium of chemical activities in the body, which are legion. (1)

It is the medium of exchange of all life-giving supplies from one point to another until they reach the cells, and of all wastes from one point to another until they are excreted; without it the blood could not move. It is the agent in osmosis, which will be mentioned again a few pages later in this book.

Water is the medium in which all living matter functions.

It is the lubricant of all moving parts.

It is the regulator of body temperature. The body cells are "water cooled." Violent effort continued for twenty minutes would generate enough heat to coagulate the albuminous substances in the body, as you cook the white of an egg, unless this heat were promptly dissipated. The cells are surrounded with water and so are "water cooled." (2)

Water drinking gives the body an "internal bath" and purifies the medium in which the cells live and work and so quickens their work.

The storage of water in the body is largely in the skin and muscles.

When there is a deficiency of water, the processes of elimination will continue, but to do so the blood and tissues will be robbed of some of their water content, which will hinder their normal processes. If this continues, it may lower the blood pressure; headache, malaise, and other conditions may develop. Constipation may develop. Kidneys, lungs and pores will be hindered in eliminating wastes from the body and so the wastes will accumulate all the way back to each cell, and the inside of the body becomes like a stagnant pool.

When the loss becomes severe enough, the blood thickens so that its circulation becomes difficult and the corpuscles stick in the minute capillaries and the blood fails to return to the heart as it should, the blood pressure falls, and a state similar to shock may arise.

If by fasting one loses all of the stored glycogen, all of the reserves of fat, and even half of the body protein, the life is not in danger; but the loss of 10 per cent of the body's water is serious and a loss of 20 to 22 per cent is fatal. (3)

A person deprived of water will die in 60 to 80 hours.

Can the reader not see the importance of supplying the body with at least six glasses of water daily in addition to the moisture in the foods? The body is losing from two to four quarts of water daily, and this loss must be made good or the life processes will be hindered. The natural thirst of persons of sedentary occupation is not a sure guide to the amount of water they need, as they may need more water than their sense of thirst demands. They should establish a drinking schedule. Copious drinking early in the morning, and from one to two hours before the other meals, and at bedtime, should become a part of their daily program.

The Ministry of Minerals

A grain of wheat contains protein, fat, and starch, which are to be used in the body as explained in "The Classification of Food"; but these elements cannot digest themselves. They must first be prepared for absorption into the blood and use in the cells. They must pass through four digestive juices—the saliva, gastric juice, pancreatic juice, and the bile. It is at least as important that they be prepared for use as that they be eaten. If they are eaten and not prepared for use, the eater is worse off with them than without them. That was the point made in explaining cause number one of disease. These digestive juices contain substances which break down the starch, protein, and fat, and prepare them for use. These substances are groups and combinations of mineral salts.

The Saliva

Following is the chemists' analysis of the saliva of the mouth.

	Frerichs	Berzelius	Hammerbacher
Water	994.1	992.9	994.2
Total solids	5.9	7.1	5.8
Minerals	2.19	1.9	2.2

The analysis below is calculated for 1,000 parts by weight of Mineral Salts:

Potassium	457.2
Sodium	95.9
Iron Oxide	50.11
Magnesium Oxide	1.55
Sulphur	63.8
Phosphorus	188.48
Chlorine	183.52

The Gastric Juice

Below is the same sort of an analysis of the gastric juice of the stomach by C. Schmidt:

Water	994.40
Total solids	5.60
Mineral salts	2.19
Sodium chloride	1.46
Calcium chloride	0.06
Potassium chloride	0.55
Magnesium phosphate	....
Iron	0.12
Calcium phosphate	....

The Pancreatic Juice

And this is the analysis of the pancreatic juice calculated on 1,000 parts, as made by Schmidt and Kruger:

	Schmidt	Kruger
Water	900.8	980.44
Solids	99.2	19.60
Mineral salts	8.3	3.57
Sodium chloride	7.35	0.93
Potassium chloride	0.02	0.07
Calcium phosphate	0.41	0.01
Magnesium phosphate	0.12	0.02

The Bile

The analysis of the bile by Jocobson and Hoppe Sayler, based on 100 parts by weight of salts:

Sodium chloride	65.16
Potassium chloride	3.39
Sodium carbonate	11.16
Tricalcium phosphate	4.44
Trisodium phosphate	15.90
Calcium carbonate	Traces
Potassium sulphate	"
Sodium sulphate	"
Iron, silica	"
Magnesium	"

These mineral salts, then, are as important to life as are the protein, fat, starch, and sugar. These mineral salts are largely deficient in refined foods, and this deficiency must sooner or later hamper the digestive and other processes.

How Disease Is Produced

When there are not enough minerals to supply all of the life processes, the blood gives preference to the digestive juices because digestion must go on to maintain life. Therefore the nerves, tissues, teeth and bones will suffer from mineral deficiency first, and the lowering of their mineral supply and content lessens the processes of life in their cells and results in abnormal conditions which are interpreted as such and such diseases.

With mineral deficiency conditions increasing all through the body, and finally, with digestion hindered so that the foods eaten cannot be properly converted into nourishment for the body but lie around until they ferment and decay and so become poisonous instead of nutritious, the well-being of the body slowly diminishes and disease slowly develops. As these conditions continue year after year, disease becomes deep-seated and stubborn.

The blood serum and the blood cells, both red and white, each require their particular combinations of minerals to make it possible for them to perform their parts in maintaining life and health. Minerals regulate the intricate chemical reactions of the blood, upon which life depends. The chemist's analyses of the blood serum and red corpuscles are given here, showing the lists of minerals they must contain in order to carry on their work. If these minerals are not provided in the food, they will not be in the blood, and then the blood will be "poor" and cannot properly function as the life-giving current.

The Blood Serum

Here is the analysis of the blood serum as made by Cavazzani, calculated on 100 parts of fluid:

Potassium oxide	0.387
Sodium oxide	4.290
Chlorine	3.565
Calcium oxide	0.155
Magnesium oxide	0.101

There are five to six quarts of this liquid in the body and every drop requires all these minerals in these proportions.

The Red Blood Cell

And here is the same for the red cell of the blood as analyzed by S. Schmidt, calculated on 100 parts of the moist substance of the corpuscles:

Potassium chloride	3.68
Sodium chloride	Traces
Potassium phosphate	2.34
Sodium phosphate	0.63
Calcium phosphate	0.09
Magnesium phosphate	0.06
Iron oxide	0.47
Potassium sulphate	0.13

These mineral salts must be supplied in the food. They are automatically contained in a balanced ration of natural foods.

The Importance of Iron

Iron is a part of the structure of every body cell. It is also the chief mineral constituent of the hemoglobin of the red blood corpuscle which carries oxygen from the lungs to all body cells. When iron is deficient the body cannot be fully supplied with oxygen and then the "fires" of the body will diminish and the body will be lacking in heat and energy. In this way a deficiency of iron contributes to anemia. Iron also seems to help in the use of oxygen in the body as well as in its transportation.

The body's natural source of iron is in natural foods. When a balanced ration is employed, a normal amount of iron is automatically secured.

The Lymph

The chemical analysis of lymph, according to Bodansky's "Introduction to Physiological Chemistry," page 243, is as follows:

Water	93.99
Solids	6.01
Fibrin	.05
Other proteins	4.27
Fat, cholesterol, lecithin	.38
Extractive bodies	.57
Salts	.73

The lymph is the fluid which separates from the blood and is the medium of interchange of food supplies from the blood to the body cells, and of the cell wastes back to the blood for elimination.

To do its work it is dependent upon these mineral salts, which must be supplied in the daily rations.

Metabolism and Iodine

The rate of metabolism is set by the thyroid gland, which depends upon iodine to regulate this function. Although the quantity needed is very minute, it is necessary to health and life.

Only one part in three million of the body by weight is iodine, and yet it is essential to life—to the function of the thyroid gland. A person needs only 5 milligrams in a year. When there is a deficiency of iodine the thyroid gland enlarges. Other deficiency results may be poor quality of skin, hair, and nails, and faulty use of fats and calcium.

Muscular Movements

The contraction and relaxation of muscles (all muscular movements), depend upon the presence of calcium, sodium, and potassium in correct proportions. As an example: With a deficiency of sodium and potassium and an excess of calcium, the heart muscle may "go into rigor"—remain contracted and refuse to relax. Contrariwise, if there be an excess of sodium and potassium and a deficiency of calcium, the muscle may relax and refuse to function. When these minerals are in correct balance they interact upon the muscle cells in such a way as to bring about "alternate contraction and relaxation," and so maintain the normal rhythm of the heartbeat. (4) The correct balance of these minerals will automatically be obtained from a balanced ration, so that the individual need never give thought to the beating of the heart.

Putrefaction

Minerals influence the preservation of all tissue from disorganization and putrefaction.

Nerves

Minerals are an important part of nerve cells. When there is a deficiency of them in the nerve cells, the nerves become irritable, and nervousness and nervous diseases develop.

Teeth and Bones

Minerals constitute a large part of the teeth and bones, and are continually needed to maintain these parts of the anatomy. They are needed in much larger amounts by growing children than by adults.

Phosphorus

Phosphorus is necessary to the normal function of the brain and nerves. It is used in teeth and bones. It forms a part of every cell of the body. It is necessary to the vigor of the white blood cells which are the "soldiers" of the body, destroying enemy germs.

Osmosis

Minerals are a factor in the regulation of "osmosis," a word signifying the passing of fluids through permeable membrane. This is the process by which the lungs pass oxygen into the blood and receive wastes from the blood; by which food passes from the digestive tract into the blood, and by which every cell in the body receives its fresh supplies and sends out its waste products.

The Glands

Some of the most important and mysterious parts of the body are the various glands. These select their required substances from which they synthesize new compounds. Upon the work of these secretions which the glands send forth into the body depend digestion, absorption and utilization of all foods elements, and the very existence of cells. No physiological or mental activity is possible without them. In their absence the body and its activities would cease to be. Manifestly the glands cannot pick their required elements from the blood unless their progenitors were previously taken in the foods eaten.

It is impossible to describe and number the intricate processes of life in which mineral salts are a factor. Their work is fast becoming one of the wonders of modern science. Their importance is only beginning to be understood. Manifestly if they are continuously deficient in the body abnormal conditions must arise which will be known as "disease."

Calcium and Tuberculosis

An interesting example of how minerals protect from disease is seen in the case of tuberculosis of the lungs. Nature calls on the blood for calcium and builds a calcium deposit around the germ, walling it off and preventing its activity and ultimately causing its death, and the person's life is saved because the blood had plenty of calcium. But we take two-thirds of the calcium out of the "staff of life"—throw away one of our defenses against tuberculosis and then wonder why we and our children suffer with it. Space does not permit us to give other details of how minerals protect from disease.

Loss of Minerals from Foods

Damaged Foods Versus Natural Foods

This lesson takes on large proportions when it is realized that over half of the food eaten in the United States has been more or less depleted of the mineral content placed there by nature.

Let us be specific about this. When wheat is made into fine white flour, it loses two-thirds of its calcium, four-fifths of its iron, and five-sixth of its phosphorus, and the other minerals in similar proportions. And white flour is the food of the masses. It is made into bread, rolls, buns, biscuits, doughnuts, cake, cookies, crackers; pancakes, pies, and about everything. Bread should be the "staff of life," but it has become a broken staff. This has been going on since white flour was invented. Its loss of minerals makes it impossible for it to contribute as it should to all of the processes of life recently mentioned and those we cannot name. As a rule, whole grain flours should be used.

Similar mineral losses are found in certain breakfast cereals, in corn meal, polished rice, and refined sugar. The cereals regularly used should be whole grain ones. Some of these are named in the list of Natural Foods appearing on a previous page in this book; others can be found on the shelves of stores, particularly health food stores, in most cities.

When Dr. Harvey W. Wiley, the "father" of our pure food laws, was living, he was so concerned over the health hazards in the use of white flour and denatured cereals that he made this statement before the New York Academy of Medicine:

"Our bread-stuff is dead food. It has no soul. . . . I say this with all the earnestness of my soul. . . . Woe to this nation unless it re-establish the fundamentals of nutrition which white flour and other denatured cereal foods have broken down."

Vegetables are often cooked in water and the water discarded. This causes losses of minerals all the way from ten to seventy per cent. They should be cooked without lying in water. "Water-less" cooking utensils are on sale in every city. Select those made of the right kind of material. Another section of this book will discuss this matter further. Potatoes, as a rule, should be baked and the skins eaten; there is an abundance of minerals close to the skin. The eyes should not be removed as they are rich in vitamins. Dry beans should not be soaked in water and the water discarded. A good cookbook is needed in every place where food is prepared, which will explain how foods should be prepared so those losses will not occur.

The unnecessary losses of minerals and vitamins from foods by refining processes and by improper cooking methods are so common and so serious that "not more than a third of the calories of the average American diet carry with them any significant share of the vitamins and minerals which robust health demands." (7)

There are sections where the soil is more or less depleted of minerals and is not able to impart to vegetation the proper supply of minerals, but this loss is not usually as serious as that which is deliberately caused by those who process and handle foods.

There are writers who consent that one half of the grains eaten may be demineralized in the normal diet. The author of this book does not believe that to be safe. Our bodies need all of the minerals God has placed in natural foods; any loss is serious; and knowing that foods grown in some sections are deficient any way, it becomes very important that nothing be lost in processing and preparing foods.

When you review the list of life processes which depend upon these minerals and then note how great and constant are the losses, you will understand why this daily loss of minerals is cause number one of disease, as stated below.

The Primary Cause of Disease

"From a purely physical standpoint mineral starvation is usually the primary cause of disease. Loss of mineral bodies impairs the food value of foodstuffs, and moreover tends to make them poisonous. Mineral starvation, regardless of the caloric value of the food ingested, is followed by disturbances in the vital processes and activities of the human organism, a reduced supply of vital energy, pollution of the blood, body tissues and juices, and the preparation of a tissue soil in which parasites thrive and multiply without hindrance." (5)

The following diseases are among those which are believed by some writers to be in part at least caused by mineral starvation; there are probably others:

Anemia	Dysentery	Neuralgia	Rickets
Acid conditions	Heart disease	Neurasthenia	Sciatica
(Auto-intoxica-	Infantile	Neuritis	Scurvy
tion)	scorbutus	Paralysis	Sprue
Appendicitis	Intestinal	Pellagra	Tetany
Beriberi	diseases	Pleurisy	Thrush
Cancer	Malnutrition	Pneumonia	Tuberculosis
Colitis	Menstruation	Poly-neuritis	Xerophthalmia
Constipation	disorders	Rheumatoid	(Sore eyes)
Convulsions	"Nerves"	arthritis	And other diseases
Diabetes	(disorders of)	Rheumatism	

Although the life processes of the body are dependent upon the presence of mineral salts, we deliberately throw away two-thirds of one from this food, four-fifths of this and five-sixths of that as the case may be, and go merrily on as if all will be well; and when calamity befalls, we blame some particular organ or gland for it, or the weather, or the neighbors, or say we inherited it, or think we got it by accident—or it just had to be. We place the blame in every place except the right place—upon ourselves, for it is our fault.

Sources of Minerals

To aid the reader in restoring his depleted supply of minerals and hereafter maintaining it, he is directed to natural foods. Following is a list of foods which contain the largest amounts of minerals most needed. The use of vegetable and fruit juices to supplement these foods will be helpful in some cases.

Foods Rich in Calcium

The unstarred foods contain 45 milligrams or more of calcium in an ordinary serving of food.

The starred foods contain 100 milligrams or more in an ordinary serving of food.

The minimum daily requirement of an adult is about .45 gram, or 450 milligrams. During growth, pregnancy, and lactation, .90 gram or 900 milligrams are needed.

Almonds	*Chard	*Milk, soy, average
Artichoke, globe or	Cheese, cottage	brand (.49 gram
French	Chick-peas, whole	per quart)
Beans, common or	seeds	*Molasses
kidney, dry or fresh	*Collards	*Mustard greens
shelled; also snap or	Cottonseed flour	Okra
string	Cream	Parsnips
Beans, lima, fresh	*Cress, garden	Rutabagas
shelled	*Dandelion greens	*Sesame seed, whole
*Broccoli	Eggs, whole	Sorghum, syrup
Burdock, roots	Eggs, yolk	Soy beans, dry or as
*Buttermilk	Endive or escarole	green vegetables
Cabbage, headed, es-	Figs	Soy bean flour
pecially green	*Kale	Sweet potato tops
*Cabbage, Savoy and	Kohl-rabi	Tender greens, See
non-headed	Leeks	cabbage
*Cabbage, Chinese, non-	Lettuce, head or leaf	Turnips
headed varieties in-	Maple syrup	*Turnip greens
cluding tender greens	*Milk, whole or	Vegetable oyster or
Carrots	skimmed, evaporated,	salsify
Celery	condensed and dried	*Watercress

The above figures are taken from United States Department of Agriculture Bureau of Home Economics, and other sources.

Foods Rich in Phosphorus

The unstarred foods contain 65 milligrams or more of phosphorus in an ordinary serving of food.

The starred foods contain 130 milligrams or more in an ordinary serving of food.

The daily minimum requirement of an adult is about .88 gram or 880 milligrams. During growth, pregnancy, and lactation, about 1.00 gram or 1000 milligrams are required.

Almonds
Artichokes, globe or French
Bamboo shoots
*Barley, whole
Barley, pearled
*Beans, common or kidney, dry shelled
*Beans, lima, fresh or dry shelled
Beans, mung, dry
*Brazil nuts
Broccoli
Brussels sprouts
Buckwheat flour
*Buttermilk
Cashew nuts
Cheese, cottage
Chick-peas
Collards
Corn, green, sweet
Corn meal, whole

ground
*Cottonseed flour
*Cowpeas, or black-eyed peas, dry or fresh shelled
Cress, garden
Dasheens or taros
*Eggs, whole
*Egg yolk
Hazelnuts and filberts
Kohl-rabi
Lentils, dry
*Milk, whole or skimmed; evaporated, condensed, and dried
*Milk, soy, average brand (.98 gram per quart)
Millets
Oatmeal or rolled oats
Parsnips

Peanuts
Peas
Pecans
Pistachio nuts
Rice, brown
*Rice, bran
*Rice, polished
Rye flour
*Sesame seed
*Soy beans, dry or as green vegetable
*Soy bean flour
Walnuts
*Water chestnuts
Wheat flour, graham or whole wheat
Wheat, shredded or puffed
Wheat, whole; grain, meal, or cereals
Wheat bran
Wheat germ

The above figures are taken from the United States Department of Agriculture Bureau of Home Economics Bulletin, and other sources.

Foods Rich in Iron

The unstarred foods contain one milligram or more of iron in an ordinary serving of food.

The starred foods contain two milligrams or more of iron in an ordinary serving of food.

The daily minimum requirement of an adult is from .006 to .016 gram. Sixteen-thousandths of a gram equals 16 milligrams, the daily requirement.

*Apricots, dried
Barley, whole
*Beans, common or kidney, dry shelled
*Beans, lima, fresh or dry shelled
Beans, snap or string
*Beet greens
Broccoli
*Broccoli leaves

Brussels sprouts
Cabbage greens or outer leaves
Cane syrup
*Chard
Collards
Corn meal, whole ground
*Cowpeas, or black-eyed peas, dry or fresh

shelled
*Dandelion greens
Dates
Dock or sorrel
*Eggs, whole
*Egg yolk
Endive or escarole
Figs, dried
*Kale
*Lentils, dry

Lettuce, leaf lettuce
   only
*Milk, soy, average
   brand (.0104 gram
   per quart)
*Molasses
*Mustard greens
*New Zealand spinach
   Oatmeal or rolled oats

*Peaches, dried,
   Peas, fresh or dried,
   whole seeds
   Prunes, dried
   Raisins, seedless, in-
   cluding currants
   Rye flour, whole
*Sorghum syrup
*Soy beans, dry or as
   green vegetable

*Spinach
*Turnip greens
   Vegetable oyster or
   salsify
*Watercress
   Wheat flour, graham or
   whole wheat
   Wheat, whole; grain,
   meal or cereals
*Wheat bran

The above figures are taken from the United States Department of Agriculture Bureau of Home Economics Bulletin, and other sources.

Foods Rich in Iodine

The iodine content of foods has not been tabulated in as great detail as has been done with calcium, phosphorus, and iron, and therefore it is possible only to give a list of the foods known to contain it. The iodine content of foods varies according to the locality where they are grown. A physician can determine whether or not a person needs more iodine. If so, the following foods may be emphasized, or iodized salt, or sea kelp may be added if necessary. In some sections goiter has nearly disappeared through the use of iodized salt.

Agar agar, rich
   source
Apples
Asparagus
Barley
Beans, kidney,
   green
Beans, string
Beets
Butter
Cabbage

Carrots
Cherries, bing
Corn
Garlic
Irish moss, rich
   source
Kelp
Leeks
Lettuce
Loganberries
Melons

Milk, cow's
Milk, goat's
Oats
Peas, green
Pears
Pineapple
Prunes
Radishes
Rice, whole
Rye
Sea salt

Spinach
Shorts
Strawberries
Tomatoes
Turnips
Water
Wheat
Wheat Bran

This list of foods has been made from information gathered from a number of authorities including Sherman, McCollum, Kellogg, and Sansum.

Lists of foods containing other minerals are not given because the foods which contain calcium, phosphorus, iron, and iodine also contain all of the other minerals the body needs, and therefore if proper amounts of these four are obtained, all of the other required minerals will also be secured.

The following tables taken from the bulletin number 975 of the United States Department of Agriculture show how far one pound of each of the grains named will go toward supplying the daily need of one person for the minerals named. For instance, one pound of graham flour will yield about one-fourth of the calcium one person need in one day, and more than enough phosphorus and iron. And so on down the list. It should be noted that wheat and oats are very rich in mineral salts.

WHEAT FLOUR	per cent
Calcium	26
Phosphorus	125
Iron	112

OATMEAL	per cent
Calcium	46
Phosphorus	135
Iron	115

WHOLE RICE	per cent
Calcium	6
Phosphorus	33
Iron	27

WALNUTS	per cent
Calcium	59
Phosphorus	123
Iron	63

CORNMEAL	per cent
Calcium	12
Phosphorus	65
Iron	27

BEANS	per cent
Calcium	107
Phosphorus	162
Iron	212

SPINACH	per cent
Calcium	29
Phosphorus	23
Iron	109

TURNIPS	per cent
Calcium	29
Phosphorus	11
Iron	9

LETTUCE	per cent
Calcium	25
Phosphorus	12
Iron	18

TOMATOES	per cent
Calcium	9
Phosphorus	8
Iron	12

Death Without Minerals

"Unless food contains sufficient mineral matter, no matter how well-balanced the ration may be in the ternary food elements, nor how large quantities are ingested, nor how high the caloric value, there will be malnutrition. In Foster's experiments, dogs and pigeons fed on demineralized foods died earlier than those that were entirely deprived of food." (6)

Persons who have been using foods more or less depleted in minerals should take liberal servings of the suitable mineral-high foods in this list, but should remember to work them into balanced meals as organized by the Automatic Menu Planner.

Do not accept the theory sometimes heard that it is all right to eat demineralized grains and seek to make up that deficiency by using more vegetables and milk. The Creator put these minerals into both cereals and vegetables because we need the full supply, not merely part of it.

Examples of a Mineral-high Vegetable Dinner

Baked potato with vegetable butter and cream
Lettuce and tomato salad   100-per-cent-entire-wheat bread
Buttered beets   Spinach   Lima beans
Ripe olives   Almonds

A BALANCED RATION

In establishing a balanced ration we begin with the foods which provide heat, energy and repair substances. These are the protein, fat, and carbohydrate. Some years ago Dr. Russell H. Chittenden, after much experimental and research work, concluded these foods should be used in the following proportions: protein, 10 per cent; fats, 25 per cent; carbohydrate, 65 per cent. This standard has been quite widely accepted as an approximate balance.

This book has made it plain that these food elements cannot be used in the body without mineral salts and that the average diet is alarmingly deficient in minerals.

We have now laid the foundation of a balanced ration. The following sections of this book will complete it.

BIBLIOGRAPHY

(1) "The Wisdom of the Body," by Walter B. Cannon, M.D., page 77.

(2) "The Wisdom of the Body," by Walter B. Cannon, M.D., page 22.

(3) "The Wisdom of the Body," by Walter B. Cannon, M.D., pages 78, 79.

(4) "Home Physician," 1931, page 387.

(5) Herman Hille, at the Fifth Annual Meeting of the American Association of Clinical Research.

(6) William E. Fitch, Major, Medical Reserve Corps, U.S.A., in his "Dietotherapy," Volume 1, page 260.

(7) Russell M. Wilder, M.D., Rochester, Minn. in "American Journal of Digestive Diseases" July 1941, page 243.

How Acids and Alkalies Affect the Health

A BALANCED RATION

In the preceding pages brief information has been given concerning the use the body makes of protein, fat, carbohydrate and mineral salts. A balanced ration has been partly explained and its foundations have been laid.

We must continue our study of the body and its processes to discover what other food elements are needed to cause the organs of the body to function normally. In this way we shall ultimately learn what is required to make a complete ration.

In the study of the body the chemist finds that all of its contents fall into one or the other of two classes—acid or alkaline. Alkaline is also termed base-forming.

The Blood Plasma

The analysis of the blood fluid shows it contains the following:

Analysis of Mineral Salts of Blood Serum by Cavazzani, calculated on 100 parts of fluid:

Potassium oxide	0.387
Sodium oxide	4.290
Chlorine	3.565
Calcium oxide	0.155
Magnesium oxide	0.101

The chemist says that the first two and the last two minerals are alkaline, and that the chlorine (a gas) is acid-forming. Inasmuch as the alkaline substances slightly exceed the acid, the fluid or blood plasma is said to be slightly alkaline.

The Red Blood Corpuscles

A similar examination of the red blood corpuscles reveals their mineral content to be as follows:

Analysis of Mineral Salts of Red Corpuscles by C. Schmidt, calculated on 100 parts of the moist corpuscles:

Potassium chloride	3.68
Sodium chloride	Traces
Potassium phosphate	2.34
Sodium phosphate	0.63
Calcium phosphate	0.09
Magnesium phosphate	0.06
Iron oxide	0.47
Potassium sulphate	0.13

The chemist says these minerals are all alkaline. Therefore, the blood as a whole must be alkaline. This is normal, and in the body, normal means healthy. This slightly alkaline condition of the blood must be maintained; if it varies a little from normal, disease must result.

The Life Range

The chemist measures the acids and alkalies of the blood and other fluids by the following scale known as the pH.

Alkalinity of the Blood

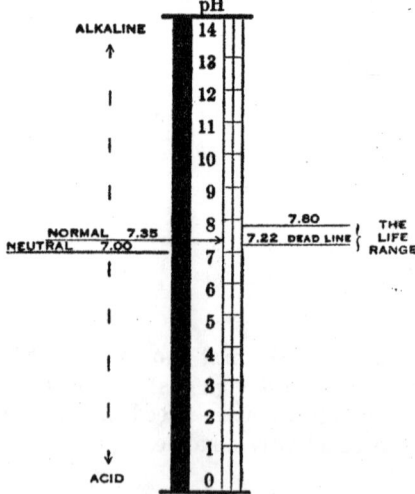

A descent of one degree on this scale means the alkalinity has diminished ten-fold, and an ascent of one degree means the acidity has decreased ten-fold.

Alkalinity or acidity can be raised to the seventh power, and the other will be correspondingly reduced.

The "H" means the hydrogen ion which is the name the chemist gives to the particular element which constitutes "acid." The "p" means the potency, power, or amount in which the acid is present. The reverse end of the scale measures the potency of the alkalies present.

The scale is 14 degrees from end to end. Seven in the middle is neutral—it is neither acid nor alkaline.

Note with care that normal blood is a very little above neutral —at 7.35. That slight elevation above neutral is called "slightly alkaline." On the right side of the scale you see 7.22 which is called the "dead line." In other words if the alkalinity of the blood lowers from 7.35 a condition known as "acidosis" exists and grows more severe as the alkalinity lowers toward 7.22. Between 7.35 and 7.22 many diseases develop, as will soon be explained.

Look again at the right side of the scale and you will see 7.80 forming the upper side of the "life range." This means that if the alkalinity of the blood rises above 7.80 death occurs from "alkalosis." In a state of health, the blood is always between these two points. This provides a "life range" of only about .6 of a degree of variation. The right alkaline balance of the blood is maintained by (a) foods, (b) the kidneys, pores and lungs which eliminate acids, and (c) an arrangement called the "buffer system" which works automatically within certain limits.

The important factor is the food intake. To raise the alkalinity of the blood above normal with food is difficult and rare and therefore this presents very little practical danger. It can be raised by taking soda. It might be raised by excluding all acid-forming foods and using only those of an alkaline balance, but that cannot occur while one lives on average foods and certainly cannot happen while living on a balanced ration. The constant danger is that the alkalinity of the blood will lower toward the acid line—death.

The nicety to which the Creator has arranged the body processes to maintain this alkaline balance is revealed by the chemist in this statement:

"Very considerable amounts of acid are constantly being produced in the body during the processes of normal metabolism. These acids, like all others, owe their activity to the hydrogen ions liberated in solution, and the hydrogen ion is capable of bringing about marked physiologic changes, or even death. Fortunately, the body processes are very effective mechanisms for rendering the hydrogen ions ineffective. So efficient are the mechanisms that under all ordinary conditions of life the chemical reaction, that is, the hydrogen ion concentration of the blood and the fluids bathing the body cells, remain practically constant."

"Some idea of the delicacy of the regulation may be obtained from a consideration of the fact that a reaction of the blood as acid as distilled water, on the one hand, or as alkaline as ordinary tap water, on the other, is incompatible with life."

"The degree of acidity or alkalinity within the various cells of the body differs slightly from that of the blood, but the blood reflects the reaction throughout the body." (1)

The Alkaline Fluids

There are other important fluids in the body which are alkaline. Note this complete list with care:

Pancreatic juice	Joint lubricant	Saliva
Succus entericus	Tears	Bile
Colon secretion	Lymph	
Muscle lubricant	Blood	

None of these alkaline juices are body wastes, though the bile contains wastes, but are all used to aid in carrying on its life processes.

Acid Fluids

Now note the list of body fluids which are acids:

Gastric juice		Perspiration
Fatigue wastes		Respiration
	Urine	

Only one of these fluids contributes to any life process—the gastric juice—the other four all being wastes.

It is very important at this point that the reader recognize that the body fluids which contribute to life processes are all alkaline except one (the gastric juice), and that the wastes are all acid. Therefore the body wastes are usually expressed in terms of acid. The acid products must be promptly eliminated because the healthy state of the body is one of alkalinity.

The Body Must Be Alkaline

This has been plainly stated by Doctor Sansum:

"The living body is always slightly alkaline. If the tissues of the body become acid to the slightest degree, death occurs, and serious illness results long before the alkalinity of the body has been reduced to the neutral point." (2)

Inasmuch as the wastes of the body are acid and they must be quickly eliminated or they will cause death, our danger, insofar as they are concerned, is that they will accumulate in the body and so menace health and life. The danger is from an excess of acid.

On the other hand, there are more processes of life which are aided by fluids that are alkaline than there are which are aided by acids; both are necessary. That life may continue, the alkalies are continually being consumed and the supply depleted. Therefore, concerning the alkalies, the danger is not from an excess but from a deficiency. The alkalies are like your bank account—continually being consumed so that the danger is that the supply will be exhausted. When the alkalies are deficient, life ceases; and when the acids are in excess, life ceases. A definite balance between these two is necessary, and that is called the acid-base balance.

From this simple chemistry of the body it is very plain that if foods will influence the alkalinity and acidity of the body we need to eat abundantly of those which will keep the alkalinity of the body high, and eat sparingly of foods which will increase its acidity.

Reputable authorities have stated that a normal diet for the average person should contain, in volume, about 75 per cent alkaline foods and 25 per cent acid-forming foods. The reasons for this high preponderance of alkaline foods have already been made plain.

Symptoms and Diseases Caused by Acidosis

No doubt the reader by this time is desiring to know how the health is affected by the lowering of alkalinity and increase of acidity. We have consulted a wide range of authors, many of whom have had much experience in caring for the sick. Their reports have been condensed and combined into the following summary of abnormal conditions which may arise in which "acidosis" is often a factor:

Colds — a tendency toward taking cold easily
Constipation
Nervousness
Headache
Migraine headaches
Malaise
Drowsiness in the daytime
Mental confusion
Mental fatigue
Mental depression
Sleeplessness
Convulsions

Nausea, vomiting, loss of appetite
Gastric juice too acid
Perspiration abnormally acid
Urine abnormally acid
"Acid disposition"
Kidney "stones." see Note No. 1
Partial blindness
Lowered immunity to disease and bacteria. See Note No. 2.
Calcium excreted by the intestine instead

of being absorbed into the blood. See Note No. 3.
Teeth and bones degenerate, and waste. See Note No. 4.
"That tired feeling"—lassitude, chronic fatigue
Excess lactic acid. See Note No. 5.
Muscle aches
Weakness

Muscular movements handicapped. See Note No. 6.
Oxygen consumption diminished. See Note No. 7.
Breathlessness. See Note No. 8.

Electric forces of cells diminished. See Note No. 9.
Arteriosclerosis. Increases impregnation of artery walls by cholesterol.
High blood pressure

Kidney damage
Heart disease
Heart arteries injured
Apoplexy
Gangrene
Coma
Death. See Note No. 10

Note No. 1

Kidney "stones" are sometimes concretions of uric acid crystals which are more apt to form when the urine is too acid. A more alkaline urine tends to dissolve them. The alkalies of potatoes have been found to be helpful in dissolving such formations. (3)

Note No. 2

The more acid the fluids and tissues of the body become the more subject they are to the growth of bacteria and disease germs and the less able they are to combat them.

The acid wastes of the body favor the growth of bacteria and predispose to infection. (4)

The pH of the human body has a life range from 7.80 down to 7.22.

In the laboratory about 99 per cent of the pathogenic bacteria sometimes called "unfriendly" to human life, grow best at a pH of 6.90, which is acid. See the pH scale on previous page.

A few examples are given below of certain important pathogenic bacteria which grow in alkaline media, but most of them grow best in media which is less alkaline than the body when it is normal.

The pH at which they grow	Name of the bacteria
7.0	Tuberculosis
7.2	Diptheria
7.0 to 7.4	Tetanus, Welchii, and Botulinum
7.2 to 7.5	Syphilis
7.2 to 7.6	Actinomycosis
7.4	Relapsing fever
7.4 to 7.6	Typhoid fever and Meningitis
7.5	Gonococcus
7.5 to 7.8	Anthrax
8.4	Asiatic Cholera

Note that a few of these thrive at about the same pH as the normal body.

Certain pathogenic bacteria thrive in acid media.

The foregoing means that when the alkalinity of the body falls below normal the majority of the "unfriendly" germs grow more readily and the body fights them with greater difficulty.

Therefore high immunity to disease is materially aided by normal alkalinity of the blood and tissues. See "Medical Bacteriology" by R. W. Fairbrother.

"It is generally known to observing physicians that a state of high resistance to infection is associated with a pronounced alkalinity of the blood, by the lowering of which resistance is diminished." (5)

Note No. 3

It is now known that acid-forming foods increase the excretion of calcium and phosphorus from the intestine, and that alkaline foods tend toward a greater retention of these mineral salts in the body. This matter has an important bearing on several conditions which will be mentioned later in this book. (6)

Note No. 4

A dog fed one month on a meat diet, short of alkaline phosphates, will show a thinning of the bones because he has used up the alkalies counteracting the acids of the diet. The same might cause bone and teeth destruction in humans. (7)

"When acidosis is threatened, lime is taken from the bones to neutralize the excess acids." (8)

Note No. 5

Extreme muscular exertion produces lactic acid in the muscles so fast that it would neutralize all the alkalies of the blood if other agencies did not operate to prevent such a disaster. (9)

Note No. 6

In an acid fluid the heart will relax and stop beating. In a more alkaline fluid it will go into rigor and stop beating in its contracted phase. While this refers to an exaggerated degree of acidity or alkalinity, it shows that a proper proportion of these two opposites is necessary to the normal activity or function of the heart and all automatic muscles, organs, and glands. (10)

Note No. 7

When there is an increase in acidity, the oxygen consumption decreases. At pH 2.6 oxygen consumption of experimental cells ceases and death occurs. (11)

A reserve of alkalies in the blood is necessary to aid the blood corpuscles to carry carbon dioxide to the lungs for elimination. A lowering of this reserve is very common, and is a condition of acidosis." (27)

Note No. 8

If breathing ceases for a few minutes, death occurs from carbonic acid acidosis. This carbonic acid results from the burning or metabolism of our ordinary foods—sugar, starch, fat, and some of the protein.

In order for the blood to carry carbon dioxide to the lungs to be exhaled it must carry a certain concentration of alkalies.

In violent exercise so much food is oxidized to provide energy that a large amount of carbonic acid is produced. Then we feel weary. When the blood-carrying capacity for taking this to the lungs for elimination is exceeded we want more air. This causes breathlessness. The extra breathing removes the carbonic acid and we feel rested and the fatigue is relieved.

Note No. 9

The acid-forming elements are phosphorus, sulphur, silicon, and iodine, which are solids but not metals, and chlorine and fluorine which are gases. They become acid-forming in solution when combined with hydrogen. These acid-forming elements take on a positive charge of electricity.

The base-forming elements are the following metals—potassium, sodium, calcium, magnesium, iron, manganese, copper, zinc. They become base-forming in solution when combined with oxygen and hydrogen. These base-forming elements take on a negative charge of electricity.

It is now taught that the exterior of body cells is alkaline and therefore carries a negative electrical charge, and the inner section or nucleus is acid and therefore carries a positive charge, and that this arrangement makes the cell a bi-polar mechanism like a common battery. It is said that the inner and outer parts are separated by a permeable membrane, that the electric charges are generated by oxidation, which is greater in the inner acid portion than in the outer alkaline portion, so that an electric tension is produced causing a positive current to pass intermittently through the membrane to the outer section as it is generated within; and that this electric factor is responsible for the existence of the cell, for its activity, and its resistance to disease; that this electric "potential" is essential to life and furnishes the immediate driving energy of the living process itself; that when the current ceases to discharge from the inner to the outer part of the cell (when the electric tension of the two are equal), that is zero hour and the cell dies. It is said that the protoplasm in the outer alkaline section

of the cell ceases to function if it becomes too acid or too alkaline—
that the right balance of these extremes is necessary to its function. (12)

From the foregoing it is evident that the body's intake of oxygen and its use of acid and alkaline foods, and the processes of
elimination, must be balanced to a very fine degree to make life
possible.

This is deep science and is getting down close to the secret mystery of life in the body. It does not solve the mystery but leaves
us confronted with the mystery of electricity which no one understands. It brings us face to face with the Author of electricity
who maintains its mystic behavior in all matter and throughout all
nature. It reveals that there are fixed laws which govern every
minutia within the body, and that the continuance of life depends
primarily upon living in harmony with those laws. These principles call loudly upon man to know his Maker's will and observe it.

Note No. 10

"Every year not less than 500,000 persons in this country die of
chronic disorders in which chronic acidosis may be an active or
predisposing factor." (13)

"Practically the whole American nation is suffering seriously
from the excessive use of acid-ash foods."

"The disastrous results of a national endemic of acidosis are becoming more and more evident in the yearly increase of the mortality rates of heart affections, Bright's disease and other degenerative diseases." (14)

This formidable list of conditions which arise more or less from
the excess of acids and deficiency of alkalies in the body should
place sufficient emphasis upon the importance of a ration with a
preponderance of alkaline foods to cause every reader to want to
know how to properly balance his rations and to carefully do so.

Before studying further the subject of foods we need to give a
little more thought to the physiological processes within the body
wherein these acids and bases are involved.

The Lungs

Both food and oxygen are taken by the blood to the cells and
are there converted into heat and energy by a process similar to
combustion. When common fuel is burned a by-product is formed
—a gas or smoke which must be removed from the furnace by a
stack and not allowed to pass into the house or automobile because

it is deadly. In like manner the burning of food and oxygen in the body cells produces a carbonic acid gas which is taken by lymph and blood to the lungs to be exhaled, thus saving the body from harm. If this elimination should cease for a few minutes, life would cease. (It is released as carbon dioxide and water.) About thirty quarts of carbonic acid gas are exhaled per hour by one person. About one-third of the body wastes, which are poisons, go out from the lungs. We should always so arrange our ventilation that these wastes will quickly go out-of-doors rather than accumulate in the room, and so that the lungs will always have a good supply of fresh, clean air. We should breathe deeply, maintain a good posture to assist in proper breathing, and refrain from any practice which may hinder the lungs in putting oxygen into the blood and receiving its waste products.

The Kidneys

The processes which consume the food and convert it into heat and energy and tissue produce other by-products which are acid, but being "ash" they cannot be exhaled by the lungs. These are taken by the blood to the kidneys for elimination. The urine is slightly acid. When "acidosis" is developing, the urine may become so acid that it causes a burning sensation. That is nature's warning that trouble is brewing. It is not necessary to take soda for this, as it can be corrected within a few hours with foods which will be named presently. The kidneys are removing acid waste so rapidly that if they should cease for twenty-four hours, death would occur in a short time. They of necessity use much water to keep the blood pure because it is by water that they remove these wastes from the blood. The kidneys will be more fully explained in a later chapter of this book.

The Pores and the Perspiration

The skin is provided with approximately 1,500,000 sweat glands which excrete the perspiration which is acid unless it is very profuse. The perspiration is nearly all water, the evaporation of which is an important part of the cooling system of the body. About one quart of water comes out of the pores in twenty-four hours as insensible perspiration; during exercise or hot weather it is much more—it may be a quart per hour. If the pores should cease to function for a day, more or less, life would cease in the body.

It is very important that the skin be washed often to remove this waste or some of it may be absorbed into the body again.

The Total Elimination

The body is producing these acid wastes by converting food and oxygen into heat and energy and food into tissue. The wastes of the cells as they wear out are also acid. Exercise increases this waste, and therefore fatigue is partly an increase of acidity, which means that we become rested by decreasing our acidity and increasing our alkalies.

In addition to these poisons which are naturally produced within the body, some people deliberately but unnecessarily put extra acids and poisons into the body and so overwork the pores, lungs, and kidneys—especially the kidneys. The faster the total of all acids accumulates in the blood the faster they will be passed to the kidneys, and so a test of the acidity of the urine is a good index of the general condition throughout the body.

The Remedy

The correction of "acidosis" is not taking soda or other medicines, but in lessening the intake and increasing the output of the body acids, and increasing its supply of alkalies; if given this help, nature will take care of the matter. Manifestly drinking copiously of water will help much to speed the processes of elimination through the pores and the kidneys—especially the kidneys. The pH of the urine can be changed in a few hours with food. (15)

THE STUDY OF FOODS, ACIDS AND ALKALIES
What Does "Acid-Forming" Mean?

Harmless Acids

The presence of some kind of acid in food does not make it an acid-forming food. The citric acids in grapefruit, lemons, oranges, and most other acid fruits; the malic acid in apples; and the tartaric acid in grapes, are all oxidized in the cells of the body to the respirable carbonic acid which is exhaled by the lungs so that these sour fruits leave behind in the body an ash that is alkaline. These acids by oxidation become sources of energy. Lactic acid in sour milk appears to be used by the body.

Harmful Acids

On the other hand, acetic acid in vinegar hinders digestion, and has the same effect on the liver as does gin. It cannot be used in the body and must be excreted by the kidneys.

Oxalic acid in rhubarb is still more harmful and must be excreted. It can easily contribute to stone in the kidneys or bladder and to a group of distressing nervous symptoms. It should be excluded from the diet. (6) Used as greens, rhubarb leaves have in several cases caused death from oxalic acid poisoning. There is a small amount of this acid in spinach, but this may be removed by parboiling it before cooking. The small amounts which occur in other foods are excreted by the kidneys.

Tannic acid is found in large amounts in tea and coffee, and a smaller amount in cocoa. It is an astringent drug and should not be used in large quantities, especially as found in tea and coffee.

Benzoic acid is an antiseptic and used as a food preservative and should be avoided as far as possible. It is found in small amounts in cranberries, cherries, prunes, and plums. (17) As it cannot be oxidized in the body, it must be excreted by the kidneys. (18) Persons with a tendency toward acidosis or stone in bladder or kidney may do well to avoid these fruits. Some authorities say they do not increase the acidity of the body but only of the urine, while others class them as acid-forming foods. They appear to be handled by the kidneys without harm except in cases where all acids not readily oxidized in the body have to be excluded.

Uric acid is one of the waste products of the cells, and is the acid under consideration when we were discussing the work of the kidneys.

The foregoing "harmful acids," together with the four mineral acids mentioned in Note 9, of which phosphorus, sulphur, silicon, and iodine are the sources, make up the acids which we have to deal with when considering the acid conditions in the body. Some of them are necessary, others are injurious, still others are developed in the body by its normal processes. With this information before us, we are ready to discuss foods more intelligently.

ACID-FORMING FOODS

Meats, fish and fowl head the list. They are acid-forming from two standpoints. (a) They contain their own cell wastes so they already contain uric acid before they become human food. (b) They also contain considerable amounts of phosphorus and sulphur which are acid-forming.

Eggs, lentils, peanuts, and all cereals contain elements which become acid-forming when used in the body.

All foods contain base-forming elements, sodium and potassium, and nearly all foods contain acid-forming elements, and the class that predominates in a given food determines in which list that food will be placed. The list of acid-forming foods stands as follows as compiled from all available sources:

Barley	Corn meal	Lentils	Salmon
Beef, all kinds	Crackers, soda	Liver	Sardines
Beef juice	Cranberries	Lobster	Shredded **Wheat**
Bluefish	Eggs, whole	Macaroni	Shrimp
Bread, white	Egg yolks	Mackeral	Turkey
Bread, whole	Fowl	Mutton	Veal
wheat	Frog legs	Oatmeal	Walnuts
Buckwheat	Gelatin	Oysters	Wheat flour,
Cheese, Cheddar	Goose	Peanuts	entire
Cherries	Haddock	Perch	Wheat flour,
Chicken	Halibut	Plums	patent
Codfish	Ham	Pork	Whitefish
Corn, canned,	Hominy	Prunes	
green	Lamb	Rice	

ALKALINE OR BASE-FORMING FOODS
Compiled from all available sources

Acidophilus, dairy	Carrots	Kale	Pineapple
and soy	Cauliflower	Kohl-rabi	Potatoes, Irish
Almonds	Celery	Leek	Potatoes, sweet
Apples	Chard	Lemons	Pumpkin
Apricots	Chestnuts, **fresh**	Lemon juice	Radishes
Artichoke, globe	Cherry juice	Lettuce	Raisins
Asparagus	Citron	Loganberries	Raspberries, red
Avocados	Cocoanuts	Mangoes	and black
Bamboo shoots	Collards	Maple syrup	Raspberry juice
Bananas	Cream	Milk, soy	Rhubarb
Beans, dried	Cucumbers	Milk, dairy	Rutabagas
Beans, dried lima	Currants	Molasses	Sauerkraut
Beans, fresh lima	Dandelion	Mushrooms	Soy bean flour
Beans, soy	Dates	Muskmelons	Spinach
Beans, string	Eggplant	Olives	Squash, Hubbard
Beets, fresh	Endive	Onions	Squash, summer
Beet greens	Figs	Oranges	Strawberries
Blackberries	Garbanzos	Orange juice	Tomatoes
Brazil nuts	Grapes	Parsnips	Tomato juice
Broccoli	Grape juice	Peaches	Turnips
Brussels sprouts	Grapefruit	Peas, dried	Turnip tops
Buttermilk	Guava	Peas, fresh	Watercress
Cabbage	Honey	Pears	Watermelon
Cantaloupe	Honeydew melons	Peppers, **green**	

Brussels sprouts are classed as acid-forming by one authority. (19)

Although rhubarb contains the harmful oxalic acid, as previously stated, it also contains base-forming elements in excess of the amount of oxalic acid present and therefore must be classed among the base-forming foods. This does not lessen the harmfulness of the oxalic acid any more than the danger of a pound of dynamite would be less when surrounded by four pounds of beans.

Milk is only slightly alkaline.

Milk made from the soy bean is highly alkaline.

The most highly alkaline food known is the soy bean. Dried lima beans come next to the soy bean.

Foods which are very potent to reduce the acidity of the urine quickly are: soy beans, lima beans, all other dried beans, apples, bananas, muskmelon, oranges, potatoes.

NEUTRAL FOODS

Pure starch, sugar, and fats (both animal and vegetable) are classed as neutral. When used in the body they form carbonic acid which is exhaled. Tapioca is in this class.

If carbohydrates are deficient in the diet, the fats cannot then be completely burned and will in that case produce an acid.

Plan the Meals

Every food has now been classified, and it remains for us to arrange them into meals in which the alkaline foods will be at least 75 per cent.

The reader may not yet sense the fact that his meals need reorganizing, but if he will examine them he will find that, if he eats as most people do, the alkaline foods are not nearly up to 75 per cent of the whole.

The Average American Diet

The typical American diet has been estimated in the Home Economics Bureau of the U. S. Department of Agriculture, based on the distribution of calories, to be as follows:

	Per cent
Grain products	27
Milk	14
Vegetables and fruits	13
Fats, including butter, cooking oils, bacon, and salt pork	14
Sugar	15
Lean meat, fish and eggs	17

Examination of this report reveals that only 27 per cent of the calories in the average American diet is alkaline, whereas of the total amount of food eaten at least 75 per cent should be alkaline. When the long list of diseases which arise from "acidosis" is recalled, the reason for all of this sickness is clearly seen. This unbalance is cause number two of disease. It is not that people are not getting enough food but that they are eating the wrong foods;

that they are not getting enough of the vegetables and fruits is immediately manifest. That is the first adjustment to make. When this is done it will be found that there is no room for meat, fish or fowl. It will also be found that to bring the amount of acid-forming and neutral foods within 25 per cent there will have to be, in many cases, a marked reduction in the amount of cereals eaten as well as the elimination of all meats. In many instances it will call for a reduction in the use of eggs.

ALKALIES ECONOMIZE PROTEIN; A BALANCE EMPHASIZED

When considering reducing the amount of meats eaten, one should know that when the total diet contains the right proportion of alkaline foods he does not need as much protein as formerly because the abundance of alkalies causes a saving of protein (20) so that a smaller amount of protein will accomplish as much work as the larger amount formerly did when the ration was too strongly acid-forming. This is a very important point. It illustrates the principle that foods must be rightly balanced with each other to secure the greatest efficiency. Foods which are all right will not produce right results if unbalanced. For instance, everyone knows that gasoline and oxygen must enter the automobile carburetor in the right proportions or combustion is impossible and the car is "dead."

Eat More Vegetables and Fruits

A very common mistake made by those who reduce their consumption of meats is to eat more eggs and bread and so fail to make any reduction in the total amount of acid-forming foods. Instead, we should adopt the rule given in 1868 by a noted health educator who said, "Eat largely of fruits and vegetables." (21)

Let the reader keep a record of his meals for a few days and he, if he be an average man, will be astonished to discover how seriously out of balance they are. Refer now to the Automatic Menu Planner and see how meals are planned to bring them into balance.

Strength—Always Rested Versus "That Tired Feeling"

Some people are alarmed when the suggestion is made that they eat no meat because many people have said, "We have to eat meat to give us strength." A little very simple thinking will reveal a fallacy there. We have already shown that the accumulation of the acid wastes of cells and their processes is the thing that makes us tired. All meats carry within them their own waste products of fatigue which were on their way to the organs of excretion when the animal was killed, so that the eater of meat gets the acid wastes of the animal which made it weary and so adds the animal's weariness to his own and gets a double dose. There is no escape from that conclusion when physiology is understood. Furthermore, meat is not necessary to provide "strength"; the draft horse and the mighty elephant are both vegetarians. The cow which man thinks he must eat to be strong makes her strong meat out of vegetation. Man is but getting vegetation secondhand when he eats her, and gets only secondhand benefit. By going direct to the vegetation himself for all of his food he can make just as good meat as the cow can and so avoid her fatigue wastes and her diseases and pay less money for his food. One physiologist put the matter in these simple terms, when speaking of fatigue:

"Fatigue is the result of chemical changes which occur within the tissues and organs of the body and which give rise to certain toxic products that act to depress these tissues or organs. . . . The constitution of the blood is altered by the absorption of these acid products of fatigue, in consequence of which its alkalinity is greatly diminished, a condition which results in serious disorders." (22)

These acid fatigue wastes in the body constitute weariness. Alkalies are required to neutralize and eliminate the acids, and therefore alkaline foods (fruits and vegetables) will rest the weary person as acid-forming foods cannot do. Furthermore, a liberal supply of these alkaline foods will aid much in preventing weariness.

Dr. J. H. Kellogg has said:

"Running at top speed, a sprinter makes a dram of lactic acid every second, half a pound in one minute. This acid must be instantly neutralized. If it accumulates, the runner becomes exhausted and his muscles refuse to act. To neutralize this acid, the blood is made alkaline. The more alkaline the blood, the longer the athlete can run or wrestle or row." (23) And the blood is kept alkaline by alkaline foods.

A very widely recognized authority has made this statement about the cause of everyday fatigue:

"The widespread custom of eating diets which are too acid is the cause of much of the chronic fatigue of the tired business man and woman which is attributed to overwork. Even the hardest physical work does not make one chronically tired. A couple of nights of sleep and a day of rest between is sufficient to refresh one who is tired from muscular work. The tiredness from which one cannot rest, the inability to concentrate on mental work or to apply one's self to the day's task is in many cases due to poisoning the nerve cells because of pollution of the body fluids which bathe them.

"The accumulation of fatigue products, mainly acid in nature, is probably the primary cause in most cases. In the laboratory it is found very difficult to fatigue a nerve. Eminent physicians have gradually come to believe that nerve-drugging through over-production of acid products which require alkali to neutralize them so that they can be excreted, with consequent reduction of the 'alkali reserve' of the blood accounts for the injury observed." (24)

Note: McCollum also states that the use of fruits and vegetables in the diet tends to maintain a normal acid-base equilibrium in the fluids of the body. (28)

The Best Diet the U. S. Government Can Suggest

Still another opinion from a high source is here offered the reader to make sure he is convinced that at least 75 per cent of our daily foods should be alkaline.

The U. S. Department of Agriculture issued a bulletin describing the foods comprising four types of diets for one man for one year. The "Liberal Diet"—the one which was offered as the best of the four—is given below. More than 75 per cent of the total foods are alkaline. Here it is:

YEARLY FOOD RATION

Liberal Diet

	Pounds	Alkaline	Acid	Neutral
Flour, cereals	100		100	
Milk, or equivalent, 305 qts.	610	610		
Potatoes, sweet potatoes	155	155		
Dried beans, peas, nuts	7	7		
Tomatoes, citrus fruits	110	110		
Vegetables, leafy, green, and yellow	135	135		
Dried fruits	20	20		
Other vegetables and fruits	325	325		
Fats (butter, oils, bacon, salt pork)	52		27	25
Sugars	60			60
Lean meat, poultry, fish	165		165	
Eggs, 30 dozen	40		40	
Total	1,779	1,362	332	85 (25)

We are now taking a very important step in establishing a balanced ration. We began by adopting the Chittenden standard of calories—protein 10 per cent, fat 25 per cent, and carbohydrate 65 per cent. To these we added the mineral salts. Now we added to these items the rule of getting 75 per cent of each day's food from among the alkaline foods.

A most marvelous thing about the proper alkaline balance of food is that it automatically brings all other food essentials into balance. The important alkaline foods are the fruits and vegetables, and it is now recognized that an increase in their use will improve almost any diet which needs improvement from any standpoint. (26) Almost any person who will follow this way of living very carefully will find a marked improvement in his feelings and health, and very likely an improvement in mental alertness. This change in food selection will be the greatest single step that can be taken to establish a normal daily balanced ration.

ALKALINE MEALS

A Balanced Ration for One Day

Breakfast

Shredded Wheat with cream
100-per-cent-entire-wheat bread, toasted crisp, two slices; with vegetable butter

Ripe Olives, one dozen, medium size
Prunes, five
Cottage cheese, 4 tablespoons
Banana, one

Dinner

Baked potato with vegetable butter
Carrots with vegetable oil, creamed (See Note)
Celery and cabbage salad with mayonnaise

Ripe olives
Spinach with lemon
Bread, 100 per cent entire-wheat, 1 slice with vegetable butter
Kidney beans, creamed
Honey

(Note: A small amount of vegetable oil may be added when vegetables are put on to cook.) All vegetables to be cooked by the waterless method.

Supper

100-per-cent entire-wheat bread, 2 slices, with vegetable butter

Figs, four
Peach sauce, one serving
Orange, one

One meal alone is not balanced, but the three meals together will give an approximately balanced ration for one day.

In properly planned meals, fruits will occupy a large place in the breakfast, a still larger proportion of the supper, while vegetables will be the bulk of the dinner.

Consult the Automatic Menu Planner daily to keep all meals in proper balance.

BIBLIOGRAPHY

(1) "Hand Book of Blood Chemistry," LaMotte Chemical Company, page 53.

(2) "The Normal Diet," W. D. Sansum, M.D., page 29.

(3) "Chemistry of Food and Nutrition," by H. C. Sherman, pages 273-280.

(4) "High Blood Pressure," G. K. Abbott, M. D., page 55.

(5) "Good Health," J. H. Kellogg, M. D., February, 1937.

(6) Alfred T. Shohl, Boston, in "Journal American Medical Association," August 13, 1938, page 617.

(7) "The Normal Diet," W. D. Sansum, M. D., page 74.

(8) J. H. Kellogg, M.D., in "Good Health," May, 1934.

(9) "The Wisdom of the Body," by Walter B. Cannon, M.D., page 22.

(10) "The Wisdom of the Body," by Walter B. Cannon, M.D., page 170; and "Home Physician," page 355, 1923.

(11) "The Phenomena of Life," by George Crile, M.D., page 300.

(12) "The Phenomena of Life," by George Crile, pages 25, 34, 35, 48, 49.

(13) J. H. Kellogg, M.D., in "Good Health," April, 1936.

(14) J. H. Kellogg, M.D., in "Good Health," July, 1936.

(15) LaMotte Chemical Company Bulletin.

(16) "Food, Nutrition and Health," by McCollum and Becker, pages 111-115.

(17) "New Dietetics," page 237, by J. H. Kellogg, M.D.,; "Food, Nutrition and Health," pages 111-115, by McCollum and Becker; U. S. Department of Agriculture Bulletin 411-R, 1-22-35.

(18) "Food, Nutrition and Health," pages 111-115, by McCollum and Becker; "High Blood Pressure," by G. K. Abbott, M.D., page 178.

(19) U. S. Department of Agriculture Home Economics Bulletin, 411-R, 1-22-35.

(20) "American Journal of Digestive Diseases," Volume 5, No. 3, article by A. A. Horvath.

(21) Mrs. E. G. White, Vol. 2, page 63.

(22) Eugene Lyman Fisk, M.D.

(23) "Should an Athlete Eat Meat?"—pamphlet.

(24) "Food Products and Health," page 115, by McCollum and Becker. By permission of the Macmillan Company, publishers.

(25) U. S. Department of Agriculture Circular No. 296, November, 1933. "Diets at Four Levels of Nutritive Content and Cost."

(26) "Food and Health," by H. C. Sherman, page 175.

(27) See "Newer Knowledge of Nutrition," page 146.

(28) E. V. McCollum, "Newer Knowledge of Nutrition," Third Edition, page 146.

The Mysteries of Life

The secret of life is not in an elixir from some far-off clime, in a mysterious potion, package, or bottle; it is right at your door, in your back yard, in the garden, on the farm. Life comes from food, water, air, and sunshine; but we must get the food without the life having been removed from it. Here is where mischief has entered.

COMPLETE THE RATION

In seeking sustenance for the body we have already seen the necessity for protein, fat, carbohydrate, mineral salts, and a preponderance of alkaline foods; but these are not enough; something more must be added to them; if these are all we get, we will die inside of ninety days; the ration is not yet complete; one more thing is necessary, and that is the vital thing, the secret of life itself.

The sixteen primary elements of life of which the body is constructed, while necessary to life, do not contain life; there is no life in them; they are inert, lifeless, dead. They are but chemical elements which can be put into bottles and kept for a thousand years, and no life will appear among them; if it would, evolution might be true. The chemist can even put them together in the shape of a man, but he cannot make a living man out of them, nor can he put life into them. He can watch them till doomsday, but no life will appear there. They cannot give life though they are necessary to life. They are only dirt like that in your back yard or garden—they are the same elements as in your garden—but are without life. Here are the elements as listed by science:

THE BODY'S ELEMENTS

	Per Cent in Human Body	Per Cent in Earth
Oxygen	66.0	49.85
Carbon	17.5	.19
Hydrogen	10.2	.97

Nitrogen	2.4	Trace
Calcium	1.6	3.18
Phosphorus	.9	Trace
Potassium	.4	2.33
Sodium	.3	2.33
Chlorine	.3	.20
Sulphur	.2	Trace
Magnesium	.05	2.11
Iron	.005	4.12
Iodine	Trace	Trace
Fluorine	Trace	Trace
Other elements	Trace	1.00
Silicon	.....	26.03
Aluminum	.....	7.28
Titanium	.....	.41 (1)

If life is to be present, something must be added to these to give life. Life itself must be put in among them and associated with them to make them move and go to work and construct cells, tissues, nerves, bone, and all the organs, and to supervise all of the life processes of the body.

One of the forces which constitute the difference between living and dead matter science has named the "vitamin." Without it no food can be utilized by the body. Without it no activity will take place in the body. All of the primary elements are dependent upon the vitamin to get them going—to make them work. This diagram visualizes this thought.

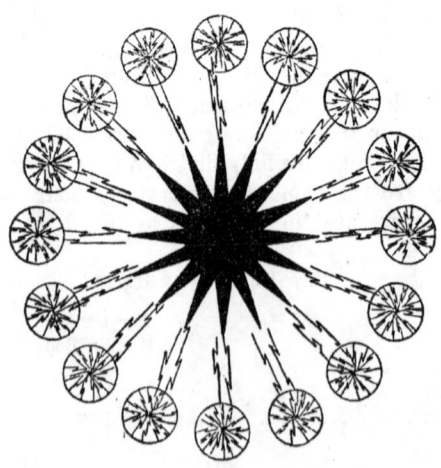

THE VITAL SPARK

The vitamin is the vital spark which vitalizes all the food elements and sets them at work. Without this they are inert.

It is like building a fire in your fireplace. You may lay all of the materials ever so carefully but there will be no fire until you apply the spark—the match; no amount of wishing will take the place of that vital spark.

MYSTERIOUS FORCES

In nature there are mysterious forces at work that cause action, another name for growth, which is one manifestation of life. The plants are composed of elements in the soil, but the soil has no power or ability to assemble itself into forms of potatoes, cabbages, strawberries, peaches, corn, apples, beans, or nuts. Other powers and forces not found in the soil must be associated with its elements to cause them to work and arrange them into the various forms of vegetation which will aid in sustaining the life which is within humans and animals. Among these mysterious forces is the vitamin.

To explain: Plant a bean, which is last year's dirt (it grew from dirt last year), and beside it plant a pebble, another lump of dirt. Water both and watch. Soon the insides of the bean begin to move, then the interior will move so much that it bursts the shell, cracks the soil, sends up leaves, blossoms, and soon you have more beans. But nothing will ever happen inside that pebble! It will never grow! If it would, evolution might be true. The bean contained something which the pebble did not—it contained every earthly element, *plus vitamins.*

Likewise, not one of these elements will ever stir in your body to cause growth or activity any more than in a bottle or in the dirt of your garden unless that mysterious vitamin and other forces be associated with them to make them move and go to work.

The vitamin is necessary to the growth of all plants. It also makes boys and girls grow. Without it all food is as dead as the dirt in your garden; and to eat food without vitamins is almost comparable to eating dirt. You may make sure of an ample supply of calcium in the rations, but if vitamins are not present no bones or teeth will ever be made. And thus it is with all of the other elements.

VITAMINS—WHERE?

The vitamins are present in all seeds—the grains, legumes, and nuts. They are in the fruits, leaves, and roots. They are in all vegetation. They are one of the essential factors of growth.

As in all plants, so in animals. The life and growth of all animals depend upon the vitamins found in seeds, fruits, leaves, and roots. The vitamins function in some way as an activating principle which sets going the processes that develop energy, power and activity. All animals are dependent upon this life principle to sustain their lives. A monkey fed a good ration but with vitamins removed, died in ninety days.

As in plants and animals, so in man. His life and growth depend upon the vitamins found in all vegetation. They are as necessary to the daily food as any other element.

When vitamins were discovered they were designated by the letters of the alphabet—A, B, C, and so on. The number of vitamin factors discovered has grown until names as well as letters are used to designate them. Knowledge of them is developing rapidly. The chemical nature of several vitamins is now known; others are being studied, and no one knows how many more will be found in the years to come. Fifteen are now known and others are postulated. Advance in knowledge concerning them is developing so rapidly that any book written today about them is out of date tomorrow.

The number of them known, and the variety of their functions and their sources, constitute a field of study so broad that a library of books is required to cover it. To try to cover this field in this book would only confuse the reader, and we shall not attempt to do so.

We Always Had Them in Natural Foods

However the reader may rest assured that he will lose nothing that is necessary to protect the health because of the brevity of this chapter. It is all as simple as this: No vitamin has been discovered or ever will be found that has not been in natural foods since the dawn of time; no scientist can discover anything which God did not set in operation thousands of years ago. When He made man and commanded his rations to grow out of the earth, He provided for all of man's necessities. My confidence in my Creator is complete, and I am free to say that scientists will never find a nutritional need of the human body that is not met by natural foods—whole grains, vegetables, fruits, legumes, and nuts.

What Vitamins Do

It appears that vitamins assist in the maintenance of every life process and the normal conditions of every cell in the body. This, then, includes every organ, gland, tissue, nerve, bone, and tooth; the eyes, skin, hair, blood, digestive juices and all other fluids—everything that can be named in the body.

Certain ones promote growth; some contribute to the health of the skin and mucous membrane and glands throughout the body; others maintain nerve vitality; some sustain the health of the capillaries; still others assist in building bones, or aid digestion, or reproduction, or coagulation, and so on at length. This is marvelous indeed.

The chemical composition of several vitamins is now known, but how they work to accomplish the marvels attributed to them is as far beyond the ken of man as are the other mysteries of which the human body is so full.

Several vitamins have been photographed. Vitamin A crystals are said to consist of one molecule of oxygen, twenty of carbon, and thirty of hydrogen. It seems wonderful that the composition of a vitamin can be caught by the camera, but even that does not help to solve the mysteries of their functions. How can oxygen, carbon, and hydrogen do the things that are attributed to vitamin A? The mystery is as deep as ever! We are no nearer the solution of the mystery of life than we were before the vitamins were known.

DEEP MYSTERIES IN NATURE

These manifestations of the functions of vitamins are still as deep a mystery as is electricity. You may ask any eminent electrician what electricity is and to explain the reasons for its behavior, and he will not proudly proceed to tell you, but will meekly say, "I do not know."

"This attitude is illustrated by an interview with Dr. Willis R. Whitney, vice-president of the General Electric Company and director of its research department. This interview appeared in the *New York Times Magazine,* November 2, 1930, cited by George McCready Price.

"In the course of this interview, mention was made of electricity and magnetism, and the scientist illustrated his meaning by bringing a bar magnet into action, remarking that nobody knows why a magnetized body acts as it does. 'We speak of lines of force,' he said. 'We draw a diagram of the magnetic field. We know there are no lines there, and "field" is just a word to cover our ignorance.'

"Dr. Whitney then adjusted the bar magnet above another and larger magnet, with the result that the smaller one was held suspended above the larger one, an experiment often repeated in the laboratory. 'What supports it?' he asked. 'Sir Oliver Lodge says it is the all-pervading ether. But Einstein denies that there is any ether. Which is right? I say that the magnet floats in space by the will of God. The magnet repels another magnet by the will of God. And no man today can give a more precise answer.'

"He was asked what he meant by this expression, 'the will of God.'

" 'What do you mean by light?' was his retort. 'A beam of light comes speeding from a star, traveling hundreds of years, and finally it reaches your optic nerve, and you see the star. How does it do that? We have our corpuscular theory of light, our wave theory, and now our quantum theory, but they are all just educated guesses. About as good an explanation as any is to say that light travels by the will of God. The best scientists have to recognize that they are just kindergarten fellows playing with mysteries— our ancestors were and our descendants will be.' " (2)

The Literary Digest of November 22, 1930, quoted Dr. Whitney on this point as follows:

"No cut-and-dried bundles of words made up into a scientific formula will suit; they simply cover up the investigator's ignorance. In the last analysis, everything operates by the will of God."

Price continues:

"Very similar to those of Whitney were the sentiments expressed by Dr. Arthur H. Compton, then head of the Physics Department of the University of Chicago, a man known all over the world for his discoveries connected with the scattering of X-rays. I give some excerpts from the published accounts of an address given by him recently in South Bend, Indiana:

" 'The world is beautiful to the scientist, who is opening new vistas continually. The molecules made from atoms, the atoms made from electrons and protons, show the universe within a universe. And a God who can control a universe like that is mighty beyond imagination.

" 'If a scientist is to have a God, he must take the God of Newton. He must understand that the mechanical laws believed by other and earlier scientists to be sufficient in themselves are but expressions of His desires. . . .

" 'We have had this world of nature presented before us, and its Ruler must be great beyond our comprehension. The present-day scientist is rapidly coming to the point of view that there is a God and a creative Intelligence back of the world. . . .

" 'The physicists' problem of reconstructing the atom points to a tremendous Intelligence back of creation. We cannot ascribe the properties of the atom to chance. Chance could not create the atom any more than it could a salad. " (3)

Dr. Whitney took us into the field of electricity and light which pervade the universe. Dr. Compton directed our attention to the composition of matter all around and within us. I shall now let a medical man speak of the forces of life within us.

A MEDICAL SCIENTIST SPEAKS OF GOD

Dr. Richard C. Cabot, dean of Boston physicians, is another celebrated scientist who believes that the mysterious processes going on within the body are the work of God. At a meeting of the Massachusetts Medical Society, speaking of "the healing power of nature," he said:

"But what is Nature? What are the characteristics of this power? The first is that it has superhuman wisdom. . . . Where does this force come from? Where do we get the healing substances in our tissues? . . . I do not see why we should not call it by its natural name. . . . It is perfectly obvious that it is God; it is the power of God on which each one here depends today for the fact that he is here instead of being underneath the earth. . . . There is no reason, then, so far as I can see, why doctors should be afraid of the simple old-fashioned word, God. The medical profession has learned in studying disease more about the meaning of this word than the vast majority of the so-called religious people. Why not tell this truth, because it is true?" (4)

Inasmuch as these great scientists thus recognize God in their respective fields and attribute every unexplainable phenomenon to a great infinite living Creator, I feel free to say that these partially understood vitamins are in some way associated with life and are used by the Almighty to maintain it.

LIFE COMES ONLY FROM LIFE

Let us pursue this study of life a little further. We behold the bean and watch the mysteries of the growth of the sprout and the plant and blossom and on to the development of another crop of beans. As I hold an apparently lifeless bean in my hand I say,

Give me the mystery of the life within you. Where did you get it? If the bean could talk it would say, I got it from my mother bean which you planted lasted year! But whence the life that was in that bean of a year ago? Oh, from the generation before. And so on and on until I go back to a day in remote antiquity when someone made the first bean and put within it that mysterious thing we call "life" and gave it power to continue to impart that life to succeeding generations of beans as long as time should last, if to all eternity!

And thus it is in all animals. Go out on the farm and ask the frisky calf, Where did you get that life that makes you so blithe and gay? He says, From my mother cow. But where did mother cow get her life? Oh, from her mother. And, as with the bean, so with the cow, we will go back and back through many generations of cows until we come to the time when the first cow and her mate were made and life was put into them and they were commanded to reproduce themselves and pass on that life to countless succeeding generations as long as time should last. And that life can be sustained only by the constant partaking of a fresh supply of the life principles which that same Creator maintains in all vegetation.

And thus it is with man. I take a babe in my arms and say, Where did you get your life? He will say, From my mother. But where did mother get her life? Oh, from her mother. And so again we must go back through all the generations of man until we reach the day when the Creator made the first man and woman and placed life within them and commanded them to pass it on to the succeeding countless generations as long as time should last. And the continuance of that life has been made to depend in a great degree upon a constant fresh supply of that life principle in plants which the scientist has called the Vitamin. Since when was it thus? Let the evolutionist tell if he can. Thus it has been since the world began. Life comes only from life.

Therefore the secret of life is life, the ceaseless gift of God! Please understand that these things we are saying are not remote from the study of foods because the Creator has placed minute quantities of certain elements vital to life within our food, and these are a part of His plan to sustain life in animals and human beings. It is necessary that we secure them.

Although I would direct your attention first to the fact that all vitamins are found in natural foods, I must not neglect to give you some specific information about certain ones and their functions and sources, that the proper emphasis may be placed upon them and you make sure that you secure them.

As the chemical composition of some of the vitamins has been learned, there is a growing tendency to discontinue designating them by letters and to name them somewhat according to their elements so that today we find both methods of designation in use.

A very good summary of the subject of vitamins was published by the United States Department of Agriculture in the Year Book, "Food for Life." The quotations we reproduce here are from pages 115-120 and 228-291. Other material has been gathered from a wide variety of sources. Certain foods not endorsed in this book are listed in some of the tables because some readers may wish to know the vitamin content of those foods.

VITAMIN A

"Vitamin A is essential for life, health, and growth. It is indispensable for the maintenance of normal epithelium." The epithelial cells have been explained by Dr. G. K. Abbott in the next paragraph.

"The parts of the body which are built of epithelial tissues are the skin and its appendages, the hair and the nails, the sweat glands and the oil glands, the mucous membranes of the nose, mouth, sinuses, throat, trachea, bronchial tubes, and air sacs of the lungs. The enamel of the teeth, the salivary glands, the mucosa of the esophagus, the stomach and all its glands, the liver, the pancreas, the tubules of the kidney, the kidney pelvis, the ureters and bladder, all the ductless glands of the body, the nervous system, the brain and spinal cord, are also governed in their development, structure, and function by vitamin A. For these reasons a deficiency of vitamin A produces a host of diseases—over ninety main types with many more subtypes, and many infections which are enabled to gain entrance to the body because of the breakdown of the entrance barrier presented by the skin and the mucous membranes." (7)

Cells Degenerate

When vitamin A is deficient the cells flatten, become hard and horny with a tendency to slough off. They then of course lose all power of normal function. As an example, tear gland cells cannot produce tears and the eyes will be dry. Again, the mucous membrane in all the places mentioned above will be unable to secrete its accustomed fluid.

Bacteria Find an Open Road

Furthermore, healthy mucous membrane does not allow bacteria to pass through into the blood, but as this deficiency of vitamin A continues these cells slowly lose their power to stop bacteria and then may follow infections of many kinds like those of the respiratory tract, broncho-pneumonia, inflammation of the intestine, infection of the kidneys, gall-bladder, reproductive glands, and so on throughout the body. (8)

Fifty-three per cent of a certain group of tubercular patients were found to be deficient in vitamin A. (9)

Infection in the kidney is understood to be a factor in the formation of kidney "stones." One authority contends that the formation of these stones can be prevented by vitamin A, and that after such stones have formed they will disappear in 50 to 107 days by giving sufficient vitamin A. (10)

Full protection against pneumonia has been worked out upon mice in the laboratory. (11) One hundred-fifty thousand Americans die annually of pneumonia to which man might be more nearly immune if he lived as he ought to live.

Sinusitis

The same thing has been done with sinusitis in rats in the laboratory.

"The work of Shurley and Daniels is revolutionizing our conception of what constitutes sinusitis. The control rat in the same cage and exposed to the same organisms as the rat on a deficient diet does not develop sinusitis. Daniels has shown that every rat fed on a diet deficient in vitamin A developed sinus suppuration.

"Wolbach of Harvard and Smith of Yale have shown that with a diet deficient in Vitamin A there is Hyperplasia (too rapid increase) of epithelial cells and a metaplasia (change to another kind of tissue) of these cells in different parts of the body, such as at the base of the tongue, in the submaxillary gland, and in the pelvis of the kidney. These changes precede infection.

"It is not unreasonable to suppose a deficient diet does not cause infection of the sinuses; it changes the integrity of the epithelium membrane, which leads to stagnation of the sinuses and subsequent infection. A similar pathology might be produced in allergy (produced by reaction to a foreign protein)."

"Shurley has shown that gram negative organisms in the nose and throat other than meningococcus become pathogenic when injected into animals fed on diets deficient in Vitamin A, and that the control rat is not affected. He has also shown that virulence of organism plus resistance of cells determine the degree of infection." (12)

The Glands

Vitamin A helps to maintain the health and function of all of the glands—the life activators—of the body. Note the processes of life which depend upon them.

Duct Glands

Eye	Lacrimal glands secrete tears.
Eye-lids	Meiboman glands secrete oily substance of liquid.
Ear	Ceruminous glands secrete a waxy oily substance which protects the eardrum.
Mouth	Salivary glands secrete saliva.
Liver	Secretes bile, a digestive juice.
Stomach	Gastric glands secrete gastric juices, pepsin, rennin, and hydrochloric acid.
Duodenum	Glands of Brunner are a continuation of the pyloric glands of the stomach.
Pancreas	Behind the stomach, delivers a digestive secretion into the duodenum.
Small intestine	Glands of Leiberkuhn, between the villi, secrete digestive juices containing enzymes.
Mucous membrane	In the colon and many places in the body like stomach, mouth, throat, nose, etc., secretes mucus. Colon mucus membrane secretes no enzymes.
Skin	Sweat glands excrete perspiration.

Ductless Glands

Pituitary	Between base of brain and roof of the mouth. Influence growth in height; stimulate certain muscles and organs.
Pineal	At the roof of the interbrain. Influences growth and digestion.
Thyroid	Neck. Secretion stimulates metabolism.
Parathyroids	Back of thyroid. Secretion assists in the elimination of toxic substances accruing from metabolism and favors coagulation of the blood aids in the use of calcium.

Thymus	At base of the heart, behind sternum. Disappears at about age twenty. Has to do with the development of sex characteristics and with the growth of the bones.
Islands of Langerhans	In pancreas, give a secretion directly into the blood which influences the metabolism of carbohydrates—the oxidation of carbohydrates in the tissue.
Suprarenals	As caps on the upper ends of the kidneys. Are closely related to the nervous system, classed by some as an accessory organ to the nervous system. Their secretion influences the tone of the blood vessels; increases the rapidity and force of the heart. They have to do with involuntary impulses.
Reproductive glands	Male and Female, including mammary glands. They function, certain of them, as duct glands, and some are classed in the ductless glands.

We have heard much about glands for a number of years, but we are now learning more about how to maintain their vitality for more years. But to do so, we cannot wait until their vitality is gone. Vitamins are pre-eminently necessary.

Thus we could go up and down within the body and at every turn find marvelous activities upon which life depends, and which cannot continue without the various vitamins. These elements are not here by accident. They have all been planned and provided by a Master Mind. If we would know the plan and use the elements which the Creator has provided for us, it would help us to have the health He intended us to have.

But here is the mischief; the vitamins have been removed from ever so many of our staple foods upon which we live from youth up, and this is one of the reasons why men and women are going to pieces so often after age forty.

For Optimum Health No Damaged Foods

For optimum health we need four times the quantity of vitamin A as is required to support life (13), and therefore we cannot with safety destroy it from any natural food where the Creator placed it for our sustenance.

Important Sources of Vitamin A

The chief sources of vitamin A have been given, but the reader's attention is now directed to the recently discovered fact that vitamin A in carrots and spinach is more potent than in cod liver oil; that 100 units of it from dried spinach will do as much work as 4,000 units in cod liver oil (14) (15).

Food sources of vitamin A and provitamin A

Type of food	Excellent sources	Good sources
Vegetables	Kale, spinach, dandelion greens, dock, escarole, chard, lambs quarters, turnip tops, green lettuce, collards, water cress, Chinese cabbage, broccoli, mustard greens, beet greens, carrots, sweet potatoes, yellow squash, sweet peppers, red tomatoes, green peas, green beans.	Green asparagus, okra, Brussels sprouts, globe artichokes, yellow tomatoes.
Fruits	Apricots, papayas, mangoes, prunes, yellow peaches.	Avocados, guavas, cantaloupes, blackberries, black currants, blueberries, bananas, pineapples, green and ripe olives, dates, deep-yellow juice oranges.
Cereal		Yellow corn meal.
Animal products	Fish-liver oils, liver, fish roe, egg yolk, butter, cheese.	Cream, kidney, oysters, whole milk, red salmon.

Vitamin A is easily destroyed by heat or boiling if oxidation takes place at the same time. It is well retained in frozen foods until they are removed. Drying may cause some loss. Shredding or dicing will cause a loss if the food stands afterward.

VITAMIN B COMPLEX

This is now known to consist of a group of vitamins some of which have been named thiamin (formerly B-1), riboflavin (formerly B-2), niacin or nicotinic acid, pyriddoxine or B-6, and pantothenic acid. Several others are being studied which may belong to this complex.

It is now understood that vitamin B complex is an important factor in metabolism, and that the need for it is in proportion to the amount of carbohydrate taken. An important source of this B complex is in the germs of the grains which are removed by the modern processing methods, including rice. The bulk of grain is carbohydrate which must have the B complex in order for it to be used in the body. Thus a serious deficiency of these vitamins closes the door to the use of carbohydrate even though plenty of it is eaten. This is an example of the dependence of one element upon another, and emphasizes the importance of having a balance of all the elements used by the body. One lesson easy to understand is that to use the parts of refined grains and discard the germ and bran is against the law of life.

Thiamin

"A lack of thiamin causes a marked loss of appetite, a loss of tone in the muscles of the intestines, loss in weight, impaired functioning of the nervous system, occurrence of pains and weakness in the limbs, a lowered body temperature, edema, and a slowing of the heart rate."

Brain and Nerves

When vitamin B1 is deficient, the chief injury caused is to the nervous system and brain; nerve degeneration is the end product, and that is known as beriberi. Some workers believe that the spinal cord is affected with a paralysis in pernicious anemia because this vitamin is lacking. (16)

When nerve vitality is lowered, then come "nerves," neuritis, polyneuritis, irritability, impatience, fits of temper, and—last of all—a suit for divorce.

If the preacher does not know his vitamins, he may try to patch up with advice, preaching and prayers, situations which can be patched only with vitamins which have been provided by the same God to whom he prays but whose plans for maintaining good nerves have been ignored and violated. One writer said, "There is more religion in a loaf of good bread than many think." (17) The loaf of "good" bread contains all of the elements God put into the wheat kernel and is a protection against nerve degeneracy.

Another serious consequence of deficiency of this vitamin is that the muscles of the stomach and intestines lose their power to cause the peristaltic waves which knead the food and pass it along the tract, and constipation results. (18)

There is a wide variety of foods from which to secure this vitamin, but the whole grains are of first importance. It is not a good plan to indulge in the use of devitalized grains and then expect to make up the loss by taking vitamin concentrates. Rice polishings and wheat germ are rich in this vitamin and will help one to quickly make up his loss. (19)

Food sources of thiamin:

Type of food	Excellent sources	Good sources	Fair sources
Vegetables	Green peas, green lima beans.	Potatoes, sweet corn, sweet potatoes, Brussels sprouts, cauliflower, cabbage, mushrooms, spinach, turnip greens, water cress, garden cress, lettuce, collards, kale, onions, leeks, tomatoes, wax and green beans, parsnips, beets, corrots.	Turnips, broccoli, kohl-rabi, eggplant.
Fruits		Prunes, avocados, pineapples, oranges, grapefruit, tangerines, dates, figs, plums, pears, apples, cantaloupes.	Bananas, watermelons, raspberries, blackberries.
Seeds	Wheat germ, corn germ, rye germ, rice polishings, wheat bran, oats, whole-grain wheat, rye, barley, brown rice, peanuts, soy beans, cowpeas, navy beans, dried peas.	Hazelnuts, chestnuts, Brazil nuts, walnuts, almonds, pecans.	
Animal products	Lean pork, chicken, kidney, liver.	Egg yolks, brains, lean beef, lean mutton, fish roe, codfish, sardines, whiting.	Fresh milk (whole or skim).

If the medium is acid thiamin will stand a high temperature.

Riboflavin

"A deficiency of riboflavin in animals is characterized by cessation of growth, marked loss of hair, nutritional cataract, appearance of a skin disorder, and a general failure in physical wellbeing. Riboflavin is widely distributed in natural foods. It seems unlikely that a deficiency would often be encountered without the appearance of other deficiencies at the same time."

Food sources of riboflavin:

Type of food	Excellent sources	Good sources	Fair sources
Vegetables	Turnip tops, beet tops, kale, mustard greens.	Peas, lima beans, spinach, water cress, collards, endive, broccoli, green lettuce, cabbage, cauliflower, carrots, beets.	
Fruits		Pears, avocados, prunes, mangoes, peaches.	Bananas, cured figs, grapefruit, oranges, apricots, guavas, papayas. muskmelons, apples.
Seeds	Germ portion of wheat, rice polishings, peanuts, soy beans.	Whole-grain wheat, dried legumes.	
Animal products	Liver, kidney, heart, lean muscle meats, eggs, cheese, dried (whole or skim), condensed and evaporated milk.	Fresh (whole or skim) milk, buttermilk, whey.	

Niacin (Nicotinic Acid)

"Lack of nicotinic acid or of certain very closely related chemical substances which occur in many natural foods would seem to be the deficiency of first importance in pellagra, though this disease may be the result of several dietary deficiencies. Chronic alcoholism often results in the development of a condition very similar to, if not identical with, pellagra. In these cases, it is believed that bad food habits and poor condition of the digestive tract account for the dietary deficiency, or for the inadequate utilization of food, or both. . . .

"Pellagra is characterized by a certain type of skin eruption affecting especially the backs of the hands and forearms, the face and neck, feet, and genitalia. The severity of the disease is increased by exposure to sunshine. The disease is also accompanied by digestive disturbances and nervous disorders. About two per cent of pellagrins develop mental disturbances requiring institutional care. . . .

A list of good to fair sources of nicotinic acid follows:

"Vegetables: Green peas, collards, turnip greens, kale, tomato juice, cowpeas, soy beans, green cabbage, spinach, and mustard greens.

Seeds: Wheat germ, peanut meal, and green (dried) peas.

Animal products: Liver, salmon, rabbit, fresh and corned beef, lean pork, chicken, buttermilk, egg yolk, skim milk (fresh and dried), evaporated milk, and haddock."
This vitamin can withstand boiling.

PYRIDOXINE

Not very much is known as yet about this vitamin, but it is understood to be concerned with the metabolism of protein and fat. Good food sources are the cereals and legumes.

PANTOTHENIC ACID

This vitamin is believed to have a part in the metabolism of protein and fat, and to increase longevity.

FOLIC ACID

A deficiency of this vitamin is associated with some forms of anemia. There may also be inflammation of the mouth and other parts of the food tract. A lack of it is part of the cause of sprue. Food sources are green vegetables, egg yolk, yeast, and liver.

VITAMIN C (*Ascorbic Acid*)

"The nutrition and structure of the teeth are affected very early in the absence of vitamin C intake. Later the tiny capillary blood vessels become weakened and cause hemorrhages throughout the body, bleeding of the gums takes place, the teeth loosen, the joints become swollen, and the bones become porous and fragile. These symptoms are characteristic of the vitamin C deficiency disease known as scurvy, which has been known for hundreds of years. . . ."

Another authority says:

Scurvy—injury to the capillary blood vessels with tendency to hemorrhage, bleeding gums, loose teeth, tooth decay, are chief among the results of deficiency of vitamin C. In some cases the skin becomes discolored from a slight bruise which would not harm a healthy skin.

Many Americans are suffering from scurvy in mild forms and do not recognize it.

To protect from tooth decay requires twice as much vitamin C as to protect from scurvy. (20)

"Liberal amounts of vitamin C in the body increase its ability to resist toxins formed by certain species of bacteria." (40)

Because vitamin C is easily destroyed by cooking, it is important that liberal amounts of raw fruits and vegetables be used every day. Sherman has said that to protect one from scurvy he should at least have one of the following daily—one ounce of orange juice, grapefruit juice, or tomato juice, or a pint of milk, or an ounce of raw cabbage (21). Sprouting seeds are an excellent source.

Food sources of vitamin C:

Type of food	Excellent sources	Good sources
Vegetables	Collards, turnips greens, mustard greens, kale, water cress, spinach, dandelion greens, sweet peppers, kohl-rabi, rutabagas, turnips, Brussels sprouts, cauliflower, cabbage, broccoli, asparagus, fresh and canned tomatoes, green peas, corn salad, radishes.	Endive, cucumbers, potatoes, sweet potatoes, green beans, parsnips, rhubarb, leeks, onions, globe artichokes.
Fruits	Guavas, mangoes, oranges, lemons, grapefruit, tangerines, currants, strawberries, gooseberries, raspberries, cantaloupes.	Pineapples, cherries, cranberries, papayas, bananas, peaches, apples, avocados, watermelon.
Seeds	Sprouted seeds.	
Animal products	Liver, brain.	Kidney.

Food and Life

Vitamin C is easily destroyed by cooking.

"Tomatoes canned in glass jars and stored, lost from 30 - 50% while commercially canned tomato juice showed no significant loss in ascorbic acid value." (41)

There is some loss when vegetables stand for days or weeks at room temperature.

Vitamin D

"In order that growing children may develop normal teeth and bones it is essential, first of all, that their diets contain liberal amounts of mineral bone-building materials—chiefly calcium and phosphorus. Vitamin D is a further essential, for it aids in the absorption of calcium and phosphorus from the food. If the food is none too rich in calcium and phosphorus, vitamin D enables the body to make the best use of what there is. Vitamin D also corrects or offsets certain unbalanced portions of calcium and phosphorus in the food which are not the best for purposes of bone-building.

"The exposure of the body to the rays of the sun creates some vitamin D from a substance present in the skin, but under modern conditions of living this means of providing vitamin D is not always reliable.

"In the absence of Vitamin D, growing bones do not deposit normal amounts of calcium and phosphorus, and as a result they are easily deformed. The Vitamin D deficiency disease known as rickets is often associated with marked deformities of the limbs, chest, and head. . . . In addition to liberal amounts of both calcium and phosphorus, the diets of all children should include suitable amounts of vitamin D from a very early age. Pregnant and lactating women also should receive vitamin D regularly.

"Vitamin D does not seem to be so important for the ordinary adult as for growing children and for pregnant or lactating women.

"Good sources: Salmon, sardines, eggs, butter.

"Small amount: Liver, cream, whole milk, and oysters."

Note the importance of being out of doors, especially children. The sunshine seems to be nature's best provision for this vitamin.

The main action of vitamin D is to prevent excretion of calcium and phosphorus from the intestine, increase their absorption and mobilize them for activity. Its action is also associated with the acid-base balance. (22)

The most popular sources have been fish liver oils. However, there is a growing desire to avoid their use and to secure from non-animal sources the help this vitamin gives. One reason for this is that every now and then unfavorable effects are reported about cod liver oil. For instance, it is more or less toxic and sometimes causes fatty degeneration of muscle, including the heart, producing heart lesions. (23)

Vitamin D From Non-Animal Sources

To those who wish to secure the benefit vitamin D gives without the use of animal products, the following information is offered.

First, General Sources

The various tables extant on vitamins when searched for sources of vitamin D give the following, which of course includes the fish oils as all tables do:

Beans, string, canned	Present
Spinach, raw	"
Carrots, young, raw	"
Corn germ	"
Wheat, whole	"
Cocoanut oil	"
Cabbage, green leaves	Fair
Potatoes, sweet	"
Oranges, fresh	"
Butter	"
Eggs	"
Milk, whole, condensed, dried, evaporated	"
Egg yolks	Good
Fish oils	Excellent

Inasmuch as this vitamin is needed only in small amounts, the first step to take is to see that as much as possible is secured from natural foods suited to the age of the individual.

Second, Natural Foods Help Each Other

It should be understood that when a ration consists of natural foods and is in perfect balance, one part helps the other parts to function perfectly. An example of this is seen in the fact that when the ration is high in alkaline foods the vitamin D is more efficient and therefore less of it is needed.

Third, Soy Beans

It should be remembered that the Chinese people down through the centuries have not used cod liver oil, but soybeans have been a staple food, and they have been well protected from rickets. We Americans are only beginning to realize the phenomenal food value of this legume.

Manifestly we will benefit by using the soybeans and the soybean oil freely in our food. There are many ways of doing this, some of which will be discussed in a later chapter. A new type of cook book is now needed.

Fourth, Viosterol

When more vitamin D is needed, it is now available from a vegetable source in viosterol, which is irradiated ergosterol, a yeast product. This is 150,000 times more potent than is cod liver oil and therefore must be used with discretion under the advice of a physician (24). One preparation is put up in corn oil, one drop of which contains 166 units of vitamin D, which is 100 times stronger than cod liver oil. A day's requirement is 400 units (25).

Fifth, the Same Help from Citrus Fruits

It is not believed that vitamin D acts directly upon calcium and phosphorus to cause calcification, but that it retards excretion and increases absorption as already stated in the beginning of this section. Manifestly, any other food which has the same action on calcium and phosphorus will do the same work as vitamin D does. (26) It has now been learned that the citric acid and alkalies in citrus fruits perform this function.

Dr. G. K. Abbott in commenting on the foregoing statement says: "In brief, and with a simple statement of fact, grape juice and orange juice, in their end-effects and even in their manner of effect, act precisely as does vitamin D upon calcium and phosphorus in correcting the harmfulness of a diet unbalanced by an excess of cereal food. . . . The use of lemon juice on spinach and various other greens, and on all salads, is a most highly beneficial practice. It makes a maximal calcium ration available to the body from vegetables by increasing its absorption from these sources, and, of course, decreasing also the excretion of calcium by the kidneys and the intestinal mucosa. . . . Hitherto it has been considered that an adequate calcium ration could be obtained only or principally from milk, of which many adults take but little. This vitamin D-like action of the acid-organic salts of fruits, if carried out by the free use of salads with lemon juice, would serve to provide the larger calcium ration which could otherwise be obtained only from an entire quart of milk daily." (27)

The juices of these fruits and vegetables are highly suitable for use with babies and children, as well as the whole foods with adults.

A two-year experiment was made on 341 children in one school. The first year they all had a standard ration which included one quart of milk daily; 78 per cent of them developed new cavities in the teeth. The second year the same diet was given but with the addition of 16 ounces of orange juice and the juice of half a lemon daily. With this one addition during the second year, the number of new cavities was reduced 57 per cent, gum troubles reduced 83 per cent, and growth rate increased 75 per cent. (28)

Conclusion Concerning Vitamin D

A minimum amount of calcium will accomplish a maximum amount of work if the diet contains the other necessary factors to make this possible. Those facts are explained in the foregoing. From among the five suggestions here given, it is easily possible and practical for any person of any age to secure the needed elements from non-animal sources to protect the teeth and bones. It must be remembered, however, that for a child to have normal teeth in youth and adult life it is necessary that the mother have a proper prenatal ration. (29)

Vitamin E

It is said that this vitamin aids in growth and in heart muscle function, and in the function of the reproductive cells.

"It appears to occur in a great many foods, at least in small quantities. The germ portion of the wheat grain is an especially rich source, while vegetable oils, green leaves, and eggs contain considerable amounts."

Vitamin K

This is in some way associated with liver function and the proper clotting of blood. It abounds in alfalfa and various greens, and smaller amounts in roots and seeds.

VITAMINS IN GENERAL

Col. Robert McCarrison, M.D., in "Studies in Deficiency Diseases," gave this summary of the results of the deficiency of vitamins in general, as follows:

> Degeneration of digestive tract
> Colitis of hidden cause—a cardinal sign
> Hemorrhagic lesions
> Inflammatory changes in mucous membrane
> Degenerative changes in the neuro-muscular mechanism of tract
> Degenerative changes in secretory glands of tract
> Derangement of digestive assimilative processes
> Impairment of protective resources against infection
> Toxic absorption from diseased bowel
> Infection of mucous membrane
> Production of juices impaired
> Ulcers of stomach and duodenum
> Obstinate constipation
> Degeneration of nervous tissues throughout the body
> Insanity
> Death

From this you can see that—

Without the constant intake of this life principle in our foods, life constantly, gradually ebbs away; the tissues and nerves and cells slowly lose their life and vitality and degenerate and prepare for disintegration. The entire body begins to decay and go to pieces a little at a time.

This slow departure of life manifests itself in many forms and various unhealthy conditions known as diseases which are given the medical names common to us although the cause has seemed like a mystery to us. I could not possibly give you a more important lesson than this one on vitamins.

The Sources of All Vitamins

Perhaps the number of vitamins, the multiplicity of conditions which grow out of deficiencies and the large number of foods from which the various vitamins are to be obtained, are causing the reader to feel that it is not possible to comprehend the whole subject in a way to put this information to a practical use, but that is not true.

In Natural Foods

"The vitamins are always present in natural foodstuffs as instinctively consumed by men and animals. There is evidence to suggest that they are formed only in the tissues of plants. . . . Their distribution in the tissues of either plants or animals may be partial or irregular, but broadly speaking it is safe to say that the individual always finds a sufficient supply of vitamins in his food so long as that food is reasonably varied and has received no artificial or accidental separation into parts, and so long as no destructive influence has been applied to it." (30)

Note the three points which secure the vitamins:

(1) Foods reasonably varied; the Automatic Menu Planner calls for a good variety at each meal and for a change in variety from day to day.

(2) No food is to be separated into parts; the grains are to be entire grains, and other foods to be eaten in as nearly their natural wholeness as possible.

A Government Warning

"Removal of the germ and seed coats or bran of cereals also removes practically all of the vitamins. Consequently, polished rice, patent white flour and degerminated corn meal are practically devoid of vitamins." (31)

Dr. Wiley on Milled Grains

"Our breadstuff is dead food. It has no soul. . . . I say this with all the earnestness of my soul. . . . Woe to this nation unless it re-establishes the fundamentals of nutrition which white flour and other denatured cereal foods have broken down." (32)

(3) "No destructive influence applied to it." On this third point it is necessary to mention heat, soda, and baking powder. Concerning the last two items the reader is asked to consider statements of authorities which follow.

Destruction of Vitamins

Soda and Baking Powder Destructive to Vitamins

From bulletin of the Indiana State Board of Health of June, 1916, we read: "Another disease, called pellagra, which frequently ends in insanity and death, is also produced by eating devitamined foods. It is found that soda kills vitamins, therefore we must not put soda in our foods. Biscuits made light with bicarbonate of soda, and which always have a 'soda taste,' are very unwholesome. Cooks should not use bicarbonate of soda in cooking dried peas, dried corn, dried beans, and the like, even if it does shorten the process."

"Green vegetables are made a deeper green by adding a little bicarbonate of soda to the water in which they are cooked. . . . It is well established that the alkalies are very harmful to vitamins if they are added to the foods during cooking. For this reason, even if the green color is deepened, this alkaline product should not be used." (33)

Dr. I. P. Pavlov, Professor of the Imperial Academy of Medicine of Leningrad, in his book, "Work of the Digestive Glands," says on this point: "Concerning the effects of a continued addition of sodium bicarbonate to the food—such an addition for a length of time markedly depresses the secretory activity of the pancreas." (The pancreas secretes digestive juice for protein, fat and carbohydrate, and is perhaps the most important organ of digestion.)

"All baking powders leave residues in the food. The alum baking powders leave a residue consisting of Glauber's salts (sulphate of soda) and aluminum hydrate. The cream of tartar baking powders leave a residue of tartrate of soda in potash—Rochelle salts. The phosphoric baking powders leave a residue of phosphate of lime and soda. My advice to housekeepers is to use as little baking powder as possible. Serve unleavened bread or that which is leavened with yeast." (34)

Fitch (35), in speaking of the residual salts left in bread when chemical leavening agents are being used, makes the following statement: "Rochelle salts and many other chemicals in food are not food, and cannot be used by the body, and must be eliminated. This puts extra and uncalled for work upon the organs of elimination, especially those whose function it is to destroy poisons. All of these chemicals interfere with the digestion and with the life processes of the body, and affect those who are not vigorous, and who, from their vocations, are kept indoors."

From the book, "Foods and Their Adulteration," by Harvey W. Wiley, chemist and food expert, on page 253, appears the following: "It would be better, evidently, if all people used more yeast breads and less baking powder rolls. My advice to housekeepers is to use as little baking powder as possible. Serve unleavened bread, or that which is leavened with yeast. The man who will invent a pure carbon dioxide in a compressed form which can be liberated in bread without leaving any residue, will be a benefactor to the race."

"The use of soda or baking powder in bread-making is harmful and unnecessary. Soda causes inflammation of the stomach and often poisons the entire system. Many housewives think that they cannot make good bread without soda, but this is an error. If they would take the trouble to learn better methods, their bread would be more wholesome, and to a natural taste, it would be more palatable." (36)

"Salaratus in any form should not be introduced into the stomach; for the effect is fearful. It eats the coatings of the stomach, causes inflammation, and frequently poisons the entire system." (37)

Now that you are to abandon the use of soda and baking powder, you will need a new cook book which makes the health way of cooking food very easy and at the same time provides the most satisfying flavors.

While discussing the harmful effects of soda, it is well to take notice that it cannot be an ideal medicine. Besides destroying vitamins, it alkalinizes the gastric juice, and an excess of it can cause alkalosis.

But, you say, what shall we take for sour stomach? Answer: The correction of sour stomach and indigestion will be explained in the next chapter of this book, after which there should be no reason for taking soda.

BEWARE OF LOSSES

Some individuals are inclined to be careless about the use of devitamined foods, or feel that they can make up such losses in other ways. A common error is to use white flour and then expect to make up for lost vitamins by using fruits and vegetables. But he who indulges in the use of any depleted food is by that much deficient, because the Creator who knows our needs placed the right amount in each food and did not plan that we would remove any of them. The fullest possible quota is necessary to our defense against disease.

Others feel that they can make up deficiencies by using vitamin concentrates. While this may be true to some extent, it is not the ideal plan.

"Authorities agree that all the vitamins a normal person needs can be obtained from a proper balanced diet, and that it is far better to have a proper diet than it is to have a diet which needs to be supplemented by vitamins from the drugstore in order to maintain health. Therefore, what the ordinary person needs to know about vitamins is very simple. He only needs to know what his diet should be in order to supply all the needs of his body for vitamins."

"There is one general principle to be kept in mind, and that is that the more nearly we take our food in the form that nature supplies it, the more certain we are to get sufficient vitamins. When it is highly refined or altered by mechanical or chemical processes we may lose many or all of the vitamins." (38)

It is estimated that one-third of the average American diet consists of foods from which the vitamins have been largely removed. (6) This must be a serious hazard to the health of millions of our people and the welfare of the nation. Certainly this is an important chapter in this book.

"Country" Vitamins

"Vitamins have come into significance through their absence." (42)

In other words, if we had always lived on natural foods, unspoiled by modern processing, grown on healthy soil, no one would ever have known there were any vitamins, and all would have secured their quotas of them in proper balance unconsciously without knowing anything about them. This is the way it should have been and even now should be, and the nearer we can come to that ideal the better it will be for us.

All of the technical, scientific knowledge we now have of the vitamins should not forever be used to operate mammoth laboratories to manufacture artificial ones to be consumed in pills, capsules, and shots, at enormous cost to the people, but that money and knowledge should be devoted to the return to nature's way of raising food and serving balanced rations of natural foods whereby all of the vitamins will again be unconsciously eaten with knife and fork. May God hasten the day.

Some people will say that it is not possible to raise by the compost gardening process the enormous quantities of food in the country to feed the countless millions of city dwellers who can have no gardens of their own. Right, of course! But let those families who read this book move to the country where they can grow much of their own food on healthy soil and take it fresh to the table and so escape from the commercial artificial vitamins business, and incidentally escape from a host of other artificial conditions and influences of the cities which are even a greater curse than are the deficient foods. That is possible. "Where there is a will there is a way."

Vitamins Where? Natural or Synthetic?

Bread: "Enriched" or Naturally Rich?

The long-standing controversy over white vs. whole grain breadstuffs took a new turn during the second world war.

The functions of minerals and vitamins had become so well understood, and were known to be so important, that the advocates of white flour could no longer stand their ground. Consequently a wide-spread campaign was inaugurated to enrich the white flour by adding to it synthetic vitamins and one mineral. This was seen by the advocates of white flour as a way out of their dilemma.

Every argument used in favor of so-called enriched bread was an admission that the white bread, which has been popular so long, is a deficiency food. The enrichment program was a graceful, much belated retreat from the untenable position which the proponents of white bread tried so long and desperately to defend, even contending at times, that for human nutrition it was more healthful than bread made of the whole grain flour.

If it were not so serious a matter it would be a ludicrous spectacle,—the millers and bakers taking out the vitality of the wheat kernel, then admitting the robbery, and stingily restoring a portion of that which they have removed, and still trying to make us believe that it is "just as good" as the whole grain flour. Of course they must keep out of the flour the food elements which make it of interest to bugs and worms, (which elements are also good for humans), or they will lose money in handling it. For this reason we may be sure they will never restore the full original food value of the wheat; if they were to do so they might better cease robbing and restoring, and so save two processes. Here is the story in brief.

The physical examination of the young men drafted into the U. S. army revealed conditions which were said to be "because of vitamin and mineral deficiencies in their diets." (43)

These discoveries led the authorities to realize that they were confronted "with a nation-wide problem" which "affected every man, woman, and child in the country. If an answer to the problem was to follow, all interested agencies were aware of the fact that it must include a simple, direct approach through some item of daily food accepted and used at each meal by everyone."

"Only by such procedure could every individual in the country have his average daily intake, particularly of the B vitamins and of iron, raised to the point where the nation's ability to resist disease, and its vulnerability to getting a bad case of the 'jitters,' be noticeably improved."

"It is an interesting fact that if everybody ate only whole wheat bread their daily intake of these same vitamins would approximate desired levels . . . If you eat enough whole wheat bread, your requirements of B vitamins and minerals would be pretty well taken care of." (44)

"The enrichment program rests upon the following basic considerations:

(1) Research has shown that many millions of Americans do not get, in their ordinary diet, enough vitamins and minerals to maintain health and vigor.

(2) Since these elements are present in important amounts in natural whole wheat, flour is a logical carrier for them.

(3) Since bread is one of the most widely used and most economical of foods, enrichment of bread, makes additional vitamins and minerals available to the great mass of the population without upsetting their budgets, or their food preference, or eating habits." (45)

Therefore it was agreed that thiamin, niacin, riboflavin, and iron be added to the white flour of which the bread of the nation would be made.

In the United States nation-wide publicity and advertising appeared in papers and magazines of all kinds, informing the public of the benefits they would receive from eating the new enriched white bread. It was even claimed by some writers that all the elements removed by milling and refining were restored by the enriching of the flour, and some extra.
(This was not true.)

Nutritionists, great and small, dietitians, doctors, and editors, even, of some of the health magazines, hailed the plan as a lifesaver, and dinned into the ears of the public, young and old, that a wonderful advance step had been taken which would improve the health of all of the people.

Their efforts were two-fold. While they extolled white bread they spared no pains to attack and undermine the value of whole wheat bread as if it were their mortal enemy. Their arguments against the bread were:

(1) People do not like bread of a dark color but insist on having "white" bread. This was their leading and strongest point.

(2) It is too coarse and rough for the human digestive tract.

Their most caustic statements were not directed at the bread, but at its advocates, who, at the present time are called "faddists," and Sylvester Graham after whom graham flour was named about one hundred years ago, was a "charlatan."

When the enrichment plan was put into operation, rejoicing

knew no bounds, and shouts of victory were sounded among the bakers.

It was declared that "a century of controversy between white bread and brown has come to a happy end in complete co-operation between nutritionists, government bureaucrats, flour millers and commercial bakers toward making white bread better by adding to it certain vitamins and minerals, deemed now to be essential to public health in the light of nutritional knowledge that had not illuminated the problem a generation ago." (46)

Widespread joy was revealed in statements like these: "Our white breads are now virtually equivalent in nutritive properties to 100 per cent whole wheat." (47)

"Enriched white bread is one step and a vital one on the road to the national goal of a richer, fuller life for all." (48)

"The new turn of affairs now promises to restore the staff of life to the place it once held at the head of the table." (49)

Mind you, every word uttered and printed in favor of the "enriched" flour contradicted their former claims about the value of white flour, and yet, the same voices that sang the old song, vociferously took up the new song with lusty vigor.

However, warnings were sounded by certain scientists and by health education teachers here and there who dared brave the popular trend, and they continued to advocate, as of yore, the use of bread made of the old fashioned flour containing all of the wheat kernel.

Stubborn Facts

The enrichment program being followed adds thiamin, niacin, riboflavin, and iron to the white flour, which are said to be "natural to the whole wheat." This sounds very good, but here are some facts.

Whole wheat contains 10 to 12 vitamins from 50% to 95% of which are removed in milling. Enrichment returns only three of them. It also contains 15 to 20 minerals, depending upon the soil where it is grown, and the enriching calls only for the restoration of part of the iron. (50)

There is still another serious failure in the enrichment plan. It is now understood that the protein of wheat germ is superior to the protein of meat, and that one ounce of it gives as much protein as two-thirds of an ounce of meat, or four ounces of milk. Two ounces daily will make meat, eggs, and milk unnecessary as a source of protein. (39) In making white flour this germ is removed which seriously impairs the protein of the wheat. Enrichment does nothing to restore this loss.

And so the controversy continues, but the voices calling to the good old ways are almost drowned by the din of acclaim in favor of the wonderful "improved" flour.

In the United States since world war second the matter of bread enrichment is being left, since October 18, 1946, to the individual states, many of whom have adopted approximately the same plan as was enforced during the war.

One editor made this comment:

"Converting wheat into flour usually involves the loss of certain vitamins. In an effort to replace them, vitamins are added to the flour, and the bread baked from it is called **vitamin enriched;** certainly a misnomer which misleads the public. This bread, made of white flour, is not in reality enriched at all, but has had added to it synthetic vitamins, the value of which in comparison with those manufactured by Mother Nature is still a moot question. It is almost analogous to stealing a man's purse which is bulging with bills and then enriching him by returning enough money for carfare home." (51)

Trusting In a Broken Staff

The sad feature of this entire piece of mercenary business is that the people are led to innocently and unwittingly trust to a false source for good health and therefore they will not seek for and obtain the superior "staff of life" as nature has enriched it. Once more the health of the nation has become the toy of commercialism. The Book says, "The love of money is the root of all evil."

Canada and England

Food authorities in the Dominion of Canada did not see fit to join in the artificial enrichment plan, but proceeded to include a larger portion (78%) of the wheat kernel in the flour. This enriched the flour with an extra amount of nature's own elements which she put in the wheat for good reasons. The flour was branded "Canada Approved." Since the war the millers and bakers have been allowed to resume their former practices. (52)

In the British Isles the government was determined to retain even more of the life-giving elements nature placed in the wheat, and their process kept 85% of the wheat kernel in the flour. They called it "85% extraction." Since the war England still requires 83% extraction as the minimum. (53)

The attitude in Great Britain, and that of certain leaders in the United States, is revealed by the following:

Prof. A. J. Carlson, Department of Physiology, University of Chicago, during the graduating exercises of the University of Texas Medical School in December, 1942, said: "The germ and the outer coats of the grain hold valuable proteins, vitamins, and minerals. Human dietary safety on this front would seem to be: go back to first principles, putting the whole grain into the flour of the bread. This can be done. We can learn to like it. If Great Britain . . . can take an important step in that direction, why can't we? Fortunately, we still eat oatmeal, a whole grain food, having among other valuable nutrients, proteins of high biologic value.

"I believe we could learn to prevent the oxidative rancidity of whole grain flour . . . Until we have that problem licked, what is the matter with storing the wheat and milling the flour as we need it? I do not see any essential economic principle in storing the flour in place of the wheat. In my judgment, the recent addition of a little of the vitamins and minerals now milled out of the grain, and singing peans of dietary salvation over this 'enriched' flour and bread, is not a sound policy, either for today or tomorrow. Let us go back to first dietary principles on this front. The whole wheat, rye, oat, barley, corn and rice grain are among our most valuable and least expensive protective foods. This is nothing new. We are told in the Book of Genesis: 'Behold I have given you every herb —to you it shall be for meat.'

"On the whole, we can trust nature further than the chemist and his synthetic vitamins. Recently Prof. J. C. Drummond, the

scientific adviser to the British Ministry of Food, voiced his reluc-
tance to put the dietary safety of a nation on synthetic vitamins,
as a long range policy. He thinks we must and should provide the
natural vitamins in the natural foods. I stand on that platform,
until we know a great deal more than we do today about foods and
human nutrition." (54)

Nature Still Makes Wheat

In the United States there still are those, both scientists and
laymen, who believe and teach that the Creator, who continues
to be responsible for the operation of the laws of nature, which
have not changed in thousands of years, is infinitely superior to
the human chemist whose work is so imperfect that he has to
change his position every few years, or oftener. Such people, while
they recognize that certain individuals cannot tolerate whole
grains, are continuing to advocate that the rank and file of the people would benefit from the use of the naturally "rich" whole grain
flour. The writer of these lines is one of those advocates. The
masses may continue to use an inferior food and receive their
punishment "after many days," but it is hoped that the reader of
these lines will follow the laws fixed by the Creator, and receive
His reward.

Bread Made of "Bleached" Flour

While we are discussing bread there is one other matter which
should be mentioned. Most of the white flour used has been
"bleached" with materials called "improvers." The reasons do not
appear to be in favor of the consumers, but of the breadmakers. It
is said that the process makes the bread whiter to meet the demand of the consumers. But there appear to be other reasons,—
that the flour will take up more water and so make a heavier loaf
with less flour, and that the loaves will extend more and make
larger, well-rounded loaves without using more flour.

It is difficult to find any white flour in the market which has
not been bleached so that the public is practically compelled to use
it or go without. We have never heard of whole wheat flour being
bleached.

Warnings are now and then given from various sources but the
practice continues. It seems that the effects of long time use of

bleaching agents are not determined before those agents are used. One of them has been found to produce hysteria in dogs and a government order to cease using it went into effect August 7, 1949, after it had been used for 25 years on the unsuspecting public. Other ingredients are now being used which the baking industry fears will sooner or later be forbidden. We hope the reader will be able to find unbleached flour in the market.

A COMPLETE RATION

All of the vitamins are necessary to sustain all of the functions of life in the body, and they all are to be found in a balanced ration of natural foods.

Some raw fruits and vegetables should be taken every day. The Automatic Menu Planner indicates how to plan all of your meals.

You have now been taught how to secure a complete ration. The formula is this:

Protein 10 per cent, fat 25 per cent, carbohydrate 65 per cent, plus all of the minerals placed in natural foods, with an alkaline proportion of 75 per cent to 25 per cent of acid-forming foods, and the vitamins without any loss.

BIBLIOGRAPHY

(1) "Home Physician," page 257 (1930).

(2) George McCready Price, in "Signs of the Times," February 24, 1931.

(3) George McCready Price, in "Signs of the Times," February 24, 1931,

(4) June 1, 1937, and reported in "New England Journal of Medicine," November 18, 1937.

(5) "Food and Life," published by United States Department of Agriculture, 1939, pages 115-120, 288-291.

(6) "Good Health," October, 1935, quoting Dr. Llewellyn R. Lewis in "American Journal of Obstretics Gynecology."

(7) G. K. Abbott, M.D., in "Life and Health," May, 1940, page 17.

(8) "Food, Nutrition, and Health," by McCollum and Becker, pages 19-21.

(9) "Journal American Medical Association," April 8, 1939, page 1308.

(10) Cleveland Clinic, report in "Journal American Medical Association"; "Journal American Dietetic Association," June-July, 1939.

(11) "Man the Unknown," by Alex Carrell, M.D., page 207.

(12) Harveian Society Abstracts, "Medical Evangelist," October 2, 1930.

(13) "Food and Health," H. C. Sherman, pages 110-120.

(14) Doctors C. Friderichsen and C. Edmund of Copenhagen, Denmark, tests on 106 children, reported in "Good Health," May, 1937.

(15) Published also in "American Journal of Diseases of Children."

(16) "Food, Nutrition, and Health," by McCollum and Becker, pages 24-26.

(17) "Ministry of Healing," page 302.

(18) "Food, Nutrition, and Health," McCollum and Becker, page 24; "Food and Health," by H. C. Sherman, pages 121-130.

(19) "Food and Health," by H. C. Sherman, pages 121-130.

(20) "Food and Health," by H. C. Sherman, pages 131-140.

(21) "Food and Health," by H. C. Sherman, pages 131-140.

(22) "Food and Health," by H. C. Sherman, pages 141-149; Alfred T. Shohl, M.D., Boston in "Journal American Medical Association," August 13, 1938, page 614; "Food, Nutrition, and Health," by McCollum and Becker, pages 30-35.

(23) Dr. A. A. Horvath, in "The American Journal of Digestive Diseases," on "The Nutritional Value of the Soy Bean," Vol. 5, No. 3.

(24) "Food, Nutrition, and Health," by McCollum and Becker, pages 30-35; Edward A. Park, M.D., in "Journal American Medical Association," Vol. III, No. 13.

(25) Edward A. Park, M. D., in "Journal American Medical Association," Vol. III, No. 13.

(26) "The Vitamins," by American Medical Association, pages 462, 474.

(27) "The Ministry," August, 1940, page 31.

(28) "World's New Dental Story."

(29) "Newer Knowledge of Nutrition," by McCollum, pages 472, 481; "The Wheel of Health," by G. T. French, London, page 42.

(30) Report of Committee appointed by Lister Institute and Medical Research Committee, London, pages 1 and 2.

(31) U. S. Department of Agriculture Bulletin, Bureau of Chemistry, Washington, D. C.

(32) Dr. Harvey W. Wiley, formerly Chief Chemist U. S. Department of Agriculture.

(33) Dr. Harvey W. Wiley in "Good Housekeeping," June, 1925, page 96.

(34) Dr. Harvey W. Wiley, in "Good Housekeeping," May, 1914.

(35) "Dietotherapy," Fitch, Vol. 1, page 386.

(36) "Ministry of Healing," pages 300, 301.

(37) Same author, Vol. 2, page 537.

(38) "Health Bulletin," June, 1939, Brookline, Massachusetts Board of Health.

(39) Reported in "Good Health," June, 1943, page 84.

(40) Henry C. Sherman in "Principles of Nutrition and Nutritive Balance of Food," U.S.D.A. Misc. Pub. No. 546, June, 1944.

(41) Journal of the "American Dietetic Association" October, 1939, page 693.

(42) Johnathan Foreman, B.A., M.D., Editor of Ohio State Medical Journal, Columbus, Ohio. "The Doctor's Attitude Toward Fertilizers," page 94, The Roadale Press, Emmaus, Pennsylvania.

(43) Dr. J. L. K. Snyder of Merck and Co., Address to Associated Retail Bakers of America, Chicago, Ill., June 8, 1942.

(44) Ibid.

(45) "What Enriched Bread Means to America," an address by Dr. J. L. K. Snyder of Merck and Co., Inc., before the Convention of Associated Retail Bakers of America, Chicago, Ill., June 8, 1942.

(46) Carroll K. Michener, Managing Editor of "The Northwestern Miller," in issue of February 19, 1941.

(47) James A. Tobey, "Hygeia," February, 1942.

(48) Dr. J. L. K. Snyder of Merck and Co.

(49) Carroll K. Michener.

(50) Dr. J. A. LeClerc, Senior Chemist, U. S. Dept. Agriculture (since retired). American Soybean Association, Reprint.

(51) "Good Health," August, 1946, page 119.

(52) Letter July 1, 1949, by C. C. Fifield, Senior Baking Technologist, U. S. Dept. of Agriculture.

(53) Ibid.

(54) "Meals for Millions." Final report of the N. Y. State Legislative Committee on Nutrition, 1947, pages 37, 38.

Twenty-seven Varieties
of Indigestion

Good digestion is at least as important as good food. If one's food is perfect but ferments in the stomach and decays in the intestine, it enters the blood stream as poison. Spoiled food is deadly, and that which spoils within the tract is as poisonous as that which spoils without the body. A poor ration well-digested will do the body more good than good food if it is not well-digested. Thus it may be that this chapter is of even more importance than any which have preceded it.

Good Digestion

As a rule nature has provided each person with digestive forces which will function normally provided proper food is properly eaten and nothing is done to interfere with the digestive processes. Our troubles usually come from practices which retard digestion and therefore the correction is automatic when these practices are abandoned.

The proper food has been described in the preceding chapters. We will now explain correct and incorrect eating habits and other matters which aid or hinder digestion.

The Causes of Indigestion

1. *Eating too Fast*

The food should be prepared for the stomach by thorough mastication and salivation in the mouth. Many people bolt in ten minutes the food which should have forty-five minutes of chewing. Digestion should begin in the mouth, but these people give it no time to begin here, and the work that is not done here must be done, if done, farther down. This is a very common cause of indigestion.

Time to eat must be provided in the day's schedule. Food should be taken in small portions and it will then be easy to eat slowly. He who does not take time to eat properly will some day take time to go to the doctor and the hospital and perhaps to the undertaker.

2. *Overeating*

A very common cause of indigestion is eating too much. There is a limit to the amount, even of good food, which the stomach can successfully handle at one time. The ordinary healthy person should stop eating while he still has an appetite.

3. *Meals too Close Together*

Time is required by the stomach to do its work. (See Digestion "Time Table.") A few foods will digest in an hour or two; others require four hours and some five hours. Raw cabbage digests in two hours and thirty minutes, while boiled cabbage requires four hours. The average person should allow five hours between the meals. This provides time for digestion and for the stomach to have a short period of rest before undertaking the work of digesting the next meal. The rest is necessary for two reasons. First, a tired stomach cannot digest the next meal even if it be of perfect food. After the gastric glands have been strongly stimulated to produce gastric juice, they will not respond again until after four hours. They must rest to prepare for further activity. (1) A rested and ravenous stomach is quite sure to take good care of the next meal if it is properly eaten. Many people never stop to think that the stomach must have rest. They think it is like the heart—can work always. But the heart rests more time than it works—it rests between beats. The stomach must have rest between meals. Making it work continuously will bring disaster. Many people are afraid to be hungry a short while, but that is a fine experience for then you know the stomach will take good care of the next meal. Again, if the stomach is asked to work continuously without rest, it will be short-lived. You cannot work without rest and continue to work very long.

The day's schedule should provide for eating hours spaced at least five hours apart, and as far as possible should be at the same hours every day. Regularity is the word.

4. *Eating Between Meals*

Eating between meals is a constant hindrance to digestion because it does not allow the stomach to complete any of its work, and that means indigestion. It also results in a ruined stomach at about age forty.

Dr. Stephen Smith, founder of the American Public Health Association, at the age of ninety-nine stood before a body of eight or nine hundred professional men and delivered an unusual address, and among other things said, when asked to explain the secret of his long life, "Take care of your stomach the first fifty years of your life, and the next fifty your stomach will take care of you." (2) But most people have worn out their stomachs at fifty and after that their prospect is poor and life is painful.

The following experiment is very revealing.

Washington Sanitarium Experiment

Four nurses were given a standard meal consisting of a cereal with cream, bread and butter, a cooked fruit, one egg, and a glass of barium buttermilk in order to make it possible to take the X-ray pictures. In every case the stomach was empty or nearly so at the end of four hours. Later the same nurses were given a duplicate meal, and two hours later were given additional food with the following results—

Eating Between Meals, X-ray Findings

Nurse		
No. 1	2 hours later ate one ice cream cone	6 hours after the meal the stomach was still at work.
No. 2	ate nut butter sandwich	9 hours after the meal the food was still in the stomach
No. 3	ate one piece of pumpkin pie, glass of milk	9 hours after the meal some food was still in the stomach.
No. 4	ate one banana	8 hours after the meal some food was still in the stomach. (3)

MORAL—NEVER EAT BETWEEN MEALS

Please note that the things that caused these stomach contents to sour are considered by almost everyone as very little sins, and yet how dire are the consequences.

New England Sanitarium Experiment

A healthy nurse was given an ordinary breakfast at 7:30 a.m.

with barium included in order to make it possible to take an X-ray picture. Four pieces of fudge were given during the day, one at 9:00 a.m., one at 11 a.m., one at 2:00 p.m. and one at 4:00 p.m. Dinner was eaten at twelve o'clock, and supper at six. Nine hours after the breakfast was eaten the X-ray showed the breakfast was still there. Thirteen and one-half hours after breakfast the X-ray showed the breakfast was still there. The day before this the same stomach digested the same sort of a breakfast without the fudge in four hours.

If we would have the best digestion, nothing should be eaten between meals, not even fruit, candy, or ice cream.

Many people have never learned the true purpose in eating— that it is to sustain the body. They seem to think it is to gratify the taste. Socrates said, "Bad men live that they may eat and drink, whereas good men eat and drink that they may live." To which class does the reader belong?

5. *Eating Late at Night*

The evening meal should be eaten long enough before retiring so that the work of digestion will be nearly complete, and no food should be eaten again until breakfast time. The stomach should be empty while we sleep. (4) The work of digestion proceeds at only half the pace when we are asleep as when we are awake and active. Therefore if we partake of food in the late evening or just before retiring, the stomach which has worked all day will work all night. If you follow that plan from youth up, your stomach will go on a "strike" by the time you are forty, and too late, you will bitterly repent of your mistakes of earlier years. You will likely go to a sanitarium.

Social ethics and habit have established an almost universal practice of eating late at night. Yet health is of first importance. Custom should change. When entertaining guests in the evening, a serving of a mixture of fresh fruit juices, or even of a single juice, will very effectively take the place of food so far as social ethics are concerned.

WHEN TO EAT THE HEAVY MEALS

"For thrifty use of food, eat most heartily early in the day. A nourishing breakfast is not only important for health and morals; it also means most efficient use of food.

"Food eaten early in the day is digested and absorbed largely during the most active daytime hours, studies at the University of Chicago have shown. Therefore the body is likely to get the most good from food eaten at breakfast and at noon. In contrast, food eaten at night shortly before going to bed, is digested and absorbed largely during the period when the body needs it least and when the excess is likely to be deposited as fat.

"It means that any one who goes shy on breakfast, slights lunch, and then loads up on a heavy meal in the evening may actually be wasting food, because he cannot use it to best advantage. Nutritionists of the U. S. Department of Agriculture say that children who go with little or no breakfast, are likely to be undernourished, because they cannot take a large enough quantity of food at the other two meals to supply their daily needs. The forgotten or hasty breakfast, and the skimpy lunch, may be responsible for Junior's drowsiness and low grades at school, Jane's poor appetite and loss of weight, father's morning temper, mother's overweight, and even grandma's edginess or hurt feelings."—Review & Herald, p. 14, Feb. 5, 1948.

6. *Eating When Tired*

When the body is exhausted the stomach shares in that condition and is not prepared to take on digestive work. Take water or fruit juices and rest before eating a regular meal.

7. *Loss of Sleep*

When one has lost considerable sleep, it is of more importance than food. One should get the needed sleep first.

8. *Nervousness*

Just plain "nervousness" is a very common cause of disturbed digestion. Help for this should be found in this book.

9. *Mental Depression*

When one is worried or mentally disturbed over some matter which has arisen, the stomach will not secrete its juices and cannot digest food. Take water or fruit juices, but do not eat until the mind has had time to become composed and adjusted.

10. *Unripe Fruit*

Eating unripe fruit can cause very serious indigestion.

11. *Spoiled Food*

Eating spoiled food can not only cause indigestion, but may endanger the life.

12. *Condiments*

Condiments—mustard, pepper, etc.—are very irritating to the stomach and contribute to indigestion.

13. *Bread Not Well Done*

Bread should be well done all the way through—well baked. Too often the interior of a loaf of bread can be squeezed into a ball of dough. Such bread easily ferments in the stomach.

14. *Fresh Bread*

Yeast bread is not ready to eat until it is at least twenty-four hours old. Most people do not know this and have become accustomed to the taste of fresh bread, and it may require a little time to change their tastes, but it can be done. The reward will be added length of life.

Since reading the chapter on "The Mysteries of Life," you will not use soda or baking powder, and those fresh breads will not appear in your menus hereafter. However, there are ways of making delicious small breads which may be eaten hot.

15. *Vinegar*

It is claimed by some that the acetic acid in vinegar prevents the action of the saliva, and that one teaspoonful can stop the starch digestion of an ordinary meal; that it also hinders the digestion of protein.

16. *Fried Foods*

Fried foods are difficult to digest and should not be eaten.

17. *Complex Mixtures*

Simple foods simply compounded are easier to digest than are complex mixtures and a great variety. The cooking should be simplified. We do not need so much to know how to put ingredients together as we do how to keep them apart. The more we learn about healthful living the less cooking there is to do and the simpler it becomes.

18. *Combination of Fruits and Vegetables*

Fruits and vegetables should not be eaten in the same meal by people with weak digestion; they may cause fermentation. The Automatic Menu Planner suggests fruits in the breakfast and supper and vegetables in the dinner. This is ideal. Many people, however, seem to be able to combine them without trouble. This is a caution to those with feeble digestion. See the lists of fruits and vegetables on another page of this book.

Cereals, grains, legumes, dairy products, nuts, olives, squash, melons, pumpkins, mushrooms, and tomatoes all combine well with either fruits or vegetables. I have never found any scientific reason to indicate that starches and proteins should not be combined, and the menus in this book approve of that combination.

Protein and Starch Can Combine

Every now and then you read or hear that protein and starch should not be combined in the same meal. There are several ways to interpret this. First, it might apply to protein in animal flesh which vegetarians do not use and therefore we do not need to consider it here. Second, protein in eggs and milk which lacto-ovo-vegetarians often do use. In that case, such vegetarians should not henceforth eat bread and milk or eggs on toast. We do not believe that. Third, protein in natural foods where it is sometimes more abundant than in animal flesh. Inasmuch as nature combines protein and carbohydrate in very many foods as they grow, we cannot take exception to her arrangement.

19. *Combination of Milk and Sugar*

The combination of milk and sugar or milk and honey is one which favors fermentation, and therefore it is better not to use much sugar in connection with a quantity of milk. This applies to eating of cereals, to ice cream, custards, puddings, and similar foods. To be sure, they taste good for a little while, but we suffer from them a long while—many for a life-time. In many instances sweet fruits can be used in place of sugar. Change your habits and you will soon learn to enjoy correct simple foods as much as you ever did the others, and you will save money on the sugar bill.

20. *Too Much Sugar*

Sugar ferments rapidly. Most people of today far overeat their sugar requirement, beginning in childhood. It is the undoing of many. Sugar is also an irritant in the digestive tract. Refrain from eating candy; put less sugar into your foods; discover and learn to enjoy the wonderful flavors residing in natural foods. You are not getting as much joy out of life as is waiting for you.

"Far too much sugar is ordinarily used in food. Cakes, sweet puddings, pastries, jellies, jams, are active causes of indigestion. Especially harmful are the custards and puddings in which milk, eggs, and sugar are the chief ingredients. The free use of milk and sugar taken together should be avoided." (5)

The quantity of sugar eaten by most people should be reduced. Then too, some sugars are more injurious than others. Concerning sugars of various kinds see a later chapter in this book. While it is true that refined sugars have lost certain minerals which are beneficial, yet it is also true that the unrefined sugars are just as irritating and will ferment as quickly as the refined. Whatever sugar you use, cut down the amount to a low minimum. Honey is more healthful than sugar or molasses, but even it should be used with discretion especially when combined with milk.

21. *Tea, Coffee, Cocoa*

Tea, coffee, cocoa, chocolate, and colas and similar drinks all hinder digestion. Usually cocoa hinders more than tea or coffee, although they are more injurious than cocoa in other ways. Their use is a bad habit and for many reasons should be discontinued. Other reasons will be given later in this book.

22. *Too Much Liquid Food*

The use of an abundance of liquid food—soups, stews, bouillon, etc.—often contributes to indigestion because this excess liquid dilutes the stomach juice and hinders it from beginning its work. Most people can safely take some liquid food, but many overdo it. In certain conditions, none should be used.

23. *Drinking With the Meals*

Worse still is the practice of drinking with the meals.

"The more liquid there is taken with the meals the more difficult it is for the food to digest; for the liquid must be absorbed before digestion can begin. . . . Soft or liquid foods are less wholesome than dry foods which require thorough mastication." (6)

Their use is only a habit. Cease to do so and soon you will enjoy your meals more than before and will have better digestion and better health.

The times to drink are any time between two hours after eating and one hour before the next meal. Early in the morning, an hour before dinner and supper, and at bed time, are good drinking times.

Those who drink milk should do so at the close of the meal and not use it to wash down the food.

A normal person can use a cup of cereal coffee in the breakfast.

A normal person who does not take a glass of milk or cup of cereal coffee might take a glass of water before or at the close of the meal. There is no hard and fast rule which can be applied to all alike, but the fact is, most people drink too much liquid with their meals and would have better digestion if they would cease to do so. Let the reader experiment and see what method gives him the best digestion, remembering that moderation is the better plan.

24. *"Soft Drinks"*

"Soft drinks" are a very common cause of indigestion. They often contain sweetening agents some of which are very irritating as well as easy to ferment. Their flavors are unnatural and often not healthful. They are harmful in many other ways, but at this time we are stressing good digestion. Do not indulge. Save your health and your money.

25. *Chewing Gum*

Dr. J. H. Kellogg says, "The habit of chewing gum is likely to produce sour stomach by interfering with the digestion of starch through lessening the activity of saliva." (7)

26. *Loss of Minerals*

In an earlier chapter the mineral content of the four digestive juices was given. Their ability to digest food depends upon these minerals, which are picked out of the blood by the glands which supply the juices to the digestive tract; but they cannot get them from the blood unless they were in the foods previously eaten. Therefore, he who uses foods which have lost more or less of their natural mineral content may rightfully expect that sooner or later his digestive juices will be too weak to do their work. Result, indigestion. It is said that half of the food eaten in the United States has lost more or less of its minerals. This, then, is not an imaginary menace to good digestion.

27. *Aluminum*

Many people have become convinced that the use of aluminum utensils for food and drink is the source of very serious digestive disturbances. The number of such people is rapidly increasing. Doctors in many parts of the country are beginning to recognize this, and such recognition by doctors is growing rapidly. See the chapter on this subject.

Beside those habits which people deliberately or unwittingly practice, there may be pathological conditions present and causing fermentation which can be determined only by a physician. As an example: When the hydrochloric acid in the stomach is deficient it is not able to destroy the bacteria which enter the stomach as it should do, and these will pass into the small intestine and cause fermentation and gas there.

SOUR STOMACH AND CATARRH

An eminent nose and throat specialist has made the following statements:

"Any habit of eating which deranges the stomach, causing increase of mucous, also stimulates the same glands in the nasal mucosa, and thus, if continued, makes a 'catarrhal condition.' This chronically inflamed mucous membrane makes a favorable soil for bacterial invasion." (8)

Therefore, you can see a very direct relation between stomach conditions and catarrhal conditions.

Sour Stomach and Sour "Disposition"

It is impossible to have a sweet disposition over a sour stomach. Why does not the gospel minister investigate this field of human experience in his work of leading mortals to higher levels of Christian living? If he does not know the laws revealed in physiology and the effects of health habits on disposition and character, he will at times be sure to undertake to correct mental and social conditions by religious means while ignoring the cause which is physiological. While following such a course he expects God to ignore His own laws and remove the results of their violation while the violation is continued, unreproved. This is the height of inconsistency.

High Acid in the Stomach

The stomach conditions already discussed were those of sour stomach where a meal, or a day's ration, had fermented. I want now to explain a condition entirely different, known as high acid. It is not a condition that comes and goes with the fermentation of one meal but rather a chronic state in which the millions of secretory glands which provide the gastric juice have been stimulated so that the gastric juice has too much hydrochloric acid. This acid is the element that digests protein, and if it becomes too strong it attacks the stomach itself which is made of protein, and this irritates and hurts the stomach. It makes one feel very nervous, perhaps giving a burning sensation, something akin to pain, quite distressing. The sensation called heartburn may be present.

This irritation by this excess of acid may continue until a spot becomes sore which, if continued and grows larger, will be called an ulcer. If the ulcer continues long enough it may sometimes become a cancer.

These conditions result from many years of wrong living during which the one violating nature's law cannot be convinced that he is doing wrong or that evil consequences are to follow.

That you may see that certain foods cause high acid and others do not, the following table of "total acids" of the stomach from eating certain foods is presented:

"Total Acids" of the Stomach

Cow's Milk	40
Vegetables	60
Bread and Cereals	70
Eggs	76
Pies, Puddings, Cakes	82
Nuts	90
Beef and Products	104
Pork and Products	110
Chicken	120
Fish	130
Lamb	134
Turkey	140
Veal	140 (9)

While it is true that the eating of meat gives immediate relief in cases of hyperacidity yet you can see that it also will increase the future acidity and therefore it is in no sense a remedy.

Normal gastric juice is .2 of 1 per cent hydrochloric acid. This digests protein. An excess of protein food calls for an excess of acid to digest it. When the acid is .3, .4, .5, or possibly .6 of 1 per cent (three times above normal) then we say we have hyperacidity and this excess acid works on the protein of the stomach and attempts to digest it and that produces an ulcer which may become a cancer.

The remedy for this condition is not in taking soda or in resorting to eating meat, but in correcting the living. The most important step is to cease eating the foods or doing the things which cause high acid. Here is the list gathered from the best sources.

Causes of Hyperacidity

Meat	Candy	Fried foods	Improperly
Fish	Jam	Excess of salt	cooked foods
Fowl	Jellies	Strong acid foods	Poorly baked
Tea	Preserves	Excess of starch	bread
Coffee	Pastries	Eating between	Soft drinks
Tobacco	Sweet desserts	meals	Cola drinks
Pepper	Soda	Eating late at	Overwork
Mustard	Baking powder	night	Worry
Spices	Hot cakes	Foods too hot or	
Vinegar	Hot breads	to cold	

Reflex irritation from bad teeth, constipation, pyorrhea, appendicitis, gallstones.

You may say, If I am not to eat those foods there is nothing left. In that case you have been living wholly wrong. You were offered two hundred delicious foods before this list of stomach destroyers was mentioned. Please refer to pages listing natural foods and see what you may still have to eat.

The Correction of High Acid in the Stomach

If you know that you have high acid the first thing to do is at once to totally discontinue every practice which helps to cause it. Then, live as you have been taught in this book but with certain modifications which follow.

It is of first importance that you have a highly alkaline diet.

Foods to Use

Practically all of the natural foods listed may be used except those named above as causes of your condition and excepting strong acid fruits like strawberries and tomatoes; but they must be prepared according to the following directions.

Liquid Foods

Gruels made of entire-grain cereals like whole wheat, whole oats, corn meal, or any whole grain. Wheat and oats are best. For the first few weeks, put them through a colander to remove the coarsest fibers. Use milk or cream in them, but no sugar or honey. Soy bean milk is preferred to dairy milk.

Eggnog if desired, gluten gruel, cream eggnog, malted nuts, buttermilk with cream or without.

Soft Foods

All thoroughly cooked whole-grain cereals. Soft eggs.

All kinds of vegetables that contain coarse particles or fibers, after being cooked must be put through a colander to take out the fibers. This makes a puree. This applies to corn, beans, peas, lentils, turnips, cabbage, cauliflower, and possibly some others, depending upon the severity of the case. The farther the condition has progressed toward ulcer the more roughage has to be removed. Use cream and olive oil or soy bean oil in these purees.

Fat Fools

All fat foods are good for acid stomach, and the quantity of them taken depends upon the weight of the patient. If up to weight, he can take more fats and oils by reducing the starchy foods like cereals and potatoes.

Walnuts, almonds, pecans, ripe olives, olive oil, soy bean oil, nut oils, butter or vegetable butter, egg yolk, and malted nuts are good.

Fruits

All of the mild fruits—pears, dates, bananas, figs, prunes, peaches, melons, oranges, will probably be all right—possibly every fruit in the list of natural foods can be used except strawberries and tomatoes; but experimenting will reveal any exception an individual must make.

Bananas, used freely with cream, have been found to be a boon to many cases of high acid in the stomach.

Miscellaneous

Entire-wheat bread made of very finely ground flour, only after it is twenty-four hours old. If this gives trouble, dry it into toast by drying it all the way through. Some may have to resort to white bread for a short time, but usually not.

Scrambled eggs, cream sauce and gravies, cottage cheese, soy cheese.

Make sure of one good vegetable meal daily, preferably at noon. A glass of milk, soy bean milk, or milk and cream, or buttermilk, or soy acidophilus, with the meals will be good, as the gastric juice is too strong and this will dilute it. Soybean milk is superior to cow's milk.

Drink freely one-half hour before meals. When the stomach hurts, take a glass of water or a sip of milk, or soy bean milk.

Take one or two teaspoonfuls of olive oil or soy bean oil before eating.

Avoid constipation. Consult the section of this book concerning it.

Remember your condition has resulted from years of wrong

living, and one must not expect to be cured at once. It will require persistent, painstaking care, for which one will be rewarded.

When the discomfort has entirely disappeared the purees may be discontinued. If the foods then give no distress the individual is well on the way to permanent recovery. But even after, he must very carefully avoid everything in the list of "causes" at the beginning of these rules.

These instructions also apply to cases of modified gastric or duodenal ulcer. However, one who suspects these conditions should consult a competent physician and have an examination and not experiment ignorantly with special diets. Know that these conditions exist before dieting for them.

Low Acid in the Stomach

This is a condition opposite to high acid and some of the symptoms are opposite. When food is eaten the meal may feel like a heavy load, very burdensome. When it is digested and gone the stomach feels much better and you may wish you never had to eat again. It feels best when empty, whereas in high acidity it feels better when something is in it.

A common cause of this condition is that of overworking the stomach glands, as in the case of high acidity, until they become exhausted and go on a strike and refuse to produce the required amount of acid.

Thus low acidity in the stomach may arise from the same causes as high acidity and therefore the same list of causes should be scanned and all violations abandoned.

Dr. J. H. Kellogg believes constipation to be one cause of low acid in the stomach.

In this condition liquids are useful but they should not be eaten with solid foods because they dilute the gastric juice which is already too weak to do its work. Fats should be eaten sparingly. Roughage must be taken out of the food by straining it the same as for high acid. Two ounces of lemon juice, or six ounces of either grapefruit juice or unsweetened pineapple juice taken with each meal will help to supplement the absent hydrochloric acid and so aid digestion. Rest after meals is helpful as is the application of a little exterior heat to the stomach after eating.

One should not guess at his condition but should have a medical examination to determine it. Do not experiment at random.

Low acidity often accompanies anemia. For information concerning the cause see the section on Anemia.

Two Kinds of People

You have observed that the conditions we have discussed in this chapter—sour stomach, high acid, low acid, ulcer—are caused by habits very commonly practiced and dearly loved. When you recognize the commonness of these habits you can understand why these afflictions are so common.

Manifestly, if we wish to avoid these ailments, or already have them and wish to correct them, there must be great changes made in our habits of living.

This lesson is hard to give and hard to take because it cuts squarely across so many cherished habits. However, you can change, and do it easily, and soon work a transformation in yourself if the injury has not become too great. Other people are doing it and find more joy than can be expressed in words. This is what I want to encourage you to do.

Two kinds of people will read this book. Some love the bad habits more than they do good health or the keeping of the laws of life which are the laws of God. Others wish to learn as much as possible and are willing to surrender every harmful practice for their own good, the good of their families, and in humble obedience to Him who doeth all things well.

Digestion Time-Table

Showing the length of time required for the digestion of various articles of food in the stomach, according to the observations of Dr. Beaumont on the stomach of Alexis St. Martin.

	Hrs.	Min.		Hrs.	Min.
Rice, boiled	1	00	Eggs, fresh, raw	2	00
Eggs, fresh, whipped	1	30	Codfish, cured, dry, boiled	2	00
Salmon trout, fresh, broiled	1	30	Barley, boiled	2	00
Soup, barley	1	30	Apples, mellow, raw	2	00
Apples, sweet, mellow, raw	1	30	Milk, boiled	2	00
Venison steak, broiled	1	35	Milk, raw	2	15
Sago, boiled	1	45	Turkey, domestic, boiled	2	25

Tapioca, boiled	2	00
Beans, pod, boiled	2	30
Turkey, domestic, roasted	2	30
Parsnips, boiled	2	30
Potatoes, Irish, baked	2	30
Cabbage, head, raw	2	30
Hash, meat and vegetables	2	30
Goose, roasted	2	30
Lamb, fresh, broiled	2	30
Custard, baked	2	45
Beef, with salt only, boiled	2	45
Apples, sour, hard, raw	2	50
Oysters, fresh, raw	2	55
Corn cake, baked	3	00
Apple dumplings, boiled	3	00
Soup, bean, boiled	3	00
Soup, mutton, boiled	3	00
Soup, chicken, boiled	3	00
Mutton, fresh, boiled	3	00
Mutton, fresh, broiled	3	00
Beef, fresh, lean, rare, roasted	3	00
Bass, fresh, stripped, boiled	3	00
Beefsteak, broiled	3	00
Eggs, fresh, soft boiled	3	00
Oysters, fresh, roasted	3	15
Pork, steak, broiled	3	15
Mutton, fresh, roasted	3	15
Carrots, boiled	3	15
Bread, corn, baked	3	15

Eggs, fresh, hard boiled	3	30
Eggs, fresh, fried	3	30
Oysters, fresh, stewed	3	30
Oyster soup, boiled	3	30
Beef, dry, roasted	3	30
Butter, melted	3	30
Beef with mustard, etc., roasted	3	30
Cheese, old, strong, raw	3	30
Bread, wheaten, fresh baked	3	30
Potatoes, fresh, boiled	3	30
Turnips, flat, boiled	3	30
Beets, boiled	3	45
Green corn and beans, boiled	3	45
Salmon, salted, boiled	4	00
Beef, fresh, lean, fried	4	00
Veal, fresh, broiled	4	00
Fowls, domestic, broiled	4	00
Fowls, domestic, roasted	4	00
Ducks, domestic, roasted	4	00
Beef, old, hard, salted, boiled	4	15
Pork, recently salted, fried	4	15
Soup, marrow bone	4	15
Veal, fresh, fried	4	30
Ducks, wild, roasted	4	30
Cabbage head, boiled	4	30
Pork, fat, lean, roasted	5	15

Soy flour sometimes digests in 80 minutes, but usually in two to three hours.

BIBLIOGRAPHY

(1) "Good Health," May, 1934, page 23, from Smith and Cowgill of Yale.
(2) Quoted by Dr. D. H. Kress, in "The Lifeboat."
(3) "Medical Papers," pages 211, 212.
(4) "How to Live," page 116, 1928.
(5) "Ministry of Healing," page 302.
(6) "Ministry of Healing," page 301, 305.
(7) "Question Box," page 550.
(8) Leslie D. Trott, M.D., Nose and Throat Specialist, "Medical Evangelist," November 20, 1930.
(9) Dr. Martin E. Rehfuss, Philadelphia, Pennsylvania.

Causes and Conquest
of Constipation

He who secures a good ration, enjoys good digestion, and has good daily elimination is usually blessed with good health. The most of our ill health comes from failures in these three realms.

Primitive people do not suffer from constipation, but among so-called "civilized" people it is the most common malady, and is the forerunner of a host of acute and chronic diseases.

Constipation cannot exist without a cause; it is not natural; there are inherent forces within the body which carry the food along the digestive tract and eliminate the residue so long as we provide the blood with the substances from which the glands elaborate their juices, with which to give tone to the muscles, and to provide stimuli to the nerves. A normal person living in a normal way will have normal elimination. He who has constipation usually is daily and deliberately producing it.

NATURAL FOODS CAUSE NATURAL ELIMINATION

In other words, in natural foods and drinks there are elements which cause elimination. On the other hand there are unnatural foods and drinks, and habits, which are constipating. Herein lies our trouble. There are two ways of living—right and wrong—and we get the results of the one we follow. "Whatsoever a man soweth, that shall he also reap." The two ways of living will be made very plain in this chapter.

First let me say that the plan of living as already presented in this book and crystallized in the Automatic Menu Planner, will correct almost any common case of constipation, and especially if the individual will adopt the higher of the two levels there, the one which excludes the use of not only meat, but all animal products.

115

The Travels of a Meal

The Mouth

The Creator gave us a keen sense of taste for a double purpose; first that we might derive very great pleasure from the experience of eating, which is an act necessary to existence. The only time food gives us any special pleasure is while it is in the mouth; when it is swallowed our joy is over. It would seem natural that we would desire to prolong this joy to its utmost, which would automatically fulfill the second purpose of the sense of taste by keeping the food in the mouth long enough so that it will be thoroughly masticated and salivated. This is necessary to normal digestion and elimination and is a part of the Creator's perfect plan for our existence.

Science has revealed that while we are chewing and tasting our food the peristaltic activity of the colon is four times as vigorous as at other times, and consequently if one chews and tastes his breakfast for ten minutes he gets but little of this extra help toward elimination, while if he chews and tastes the meal for forty minutes he receives four times as much help.

"When food is taken into the stomach, the movements of the tube become vigorous. Indeed, while the food is still in the mouth and being chewed, and before a morsel has been swallowed, the movements begin, and are four times as vigorous during the taking of a meal as at other times. This is a very excellent reason why constipated persons should eat deliberately, taking ample time at meals and chewing long and well. Food is the natural laxative. The act of eating starts the action of the muscular machinery by means of which first the food and later the food residues are transported along the alimentary canal, and so long as chewing continues new impulses are continually transmitted to the stomach and intestines which quicken the peristaltic movements and activity of the whole digestive machine. The observations of Hirsch, Case, and others have shown that the colon contents advance as far during the hour of eating as during four hours just before the meal." (1)

The Stomach

After the chewing is finished the food passes to the stomach and is mixed with the gastric juice which begins the digestion of protein. After about four hours the food should have passed out through the pylorus, which means "gate keeper," into the duodenum where it receives the juice from the pancreas and the bile from the liver, and thence it passes into the small intestine where digestion is completed by the combined work of the saliva, gastric, and pancreatic juices and the bile. Now it is ready for absorption into the blood and to be used in rebuilding the body.

The Intestine

The interior of the small intestine, which is about twenty feet long, is provided with many millions of villi which absorb the food into the blood. Mineral oil cannot be absorbed as it is only a lubricant, and so it smears over these villi and hinders them from passing the food into the blood. After about four hours in the small intestine, digestion should be completed and the nutrient passed into the blood and the residue into the colon for elimination.

Note: Four hours in the stomach and four in the small intestine. The residue should not take over sixteen hours to complete the journey so that no food would remain in the tract over twenty-four hours.

If foods move according to this schedule the ordinary cases of sour stomach, intestinal decay, gas, and constipation will disappear, for this is normal.

"A breakfast should reach the colon with all of the good already absorbed by the body about noon and it should pass through and out of the body not later than after breakfast time the next day, and if we are perfectly normal the lunch and supper residue may go along with it. Anything slower than this is constipation, and is a retention in the intestine of residue for too long a time.

"Under normal conditions there is an impulse to move the bowels after each meal. A well-trained set of organs in a well-managed body will react in this desirable fashion under perfectly normal conditions." (2)

But people do not live that way. If people secured an elimination for each meal, the majority of our ills would disappear; but most people believe that if there is one elimination each day they are doing well, and the majority do not succeed at that without taking some laxative or cathartic. (Americans spend fifty million dollars a year for seven hundred kinds of laxatives.) The X-ray has shown that most of the people who live on the one-a-day plan are holding the residue in the tract for fifty hours. Often there is delay in the stomach, producing fermentation. When fermented food reaches the small intestine and is held there overtime it decays; and when it remains in the colon for still more hours, its condition cannot be accurately described.

The natural foods recommended in this book will not ordinarily putrefy in the tract in twenty-four hours, so that if they remain in the stomach four hours, in the small intestine another four, they still have sixteen hours to pass through the twelve feet of the colon and yet be within the safety limit of twenty-five hours. But after twenty-five hours putrefaction begins, so that the people who live on the one-a-day plan and unknowingly carry the remains for fifty hours are allowing twenty-five hours for putrefaction for every meal, every day, year after year. Decayed food is passing into the blood and thence to every organ, gland, nerve, and cell day and night during every hour of life. That program makes health impossible and the coming of disease sure. On the other hand, if all residues leave the body inside of twenty-five hours, there can be no sour stomach, gas, and putrefaction, and life will be one continuous joy. Why not live on that high plane?

Many people do not know that an elimination for each meal is the health rule. They would know it if they but stopped to think. An untrained child often has to go to the toilet before the meal is finished. There is proof that the rule is right. Here is another. When your nose gets the aroma of delicious food, your mouth "waters." Why? Because the nose said to the mouth, "Something good is coming, get ready for it," and the mouth prepared the saliva. Likewise when the food is in the mouth an advance message goes to the stomach saying that food is coming, and it in turn prepares the gastric juice before the food arrives. In similar manner, when the food is in the mouth and also while it is in the stomach other advance messages go on to the intestine announcing that something is coming and that room should be prepared for it, and the only way room can be ready for it is for the intestine to pass its contents to the colon and the colon eliminate its contents. That is easy to understand once you think about it. Any rhythm slower than this is some degree of constipation. Establish this rule and follow what you are reading until you attain this ideal.

The Colon

The colon is not provided with villi to absorb food into the blood; its cells absorb water, but very little nutrient. It serves as a garbage can to catch the residue and pass it out of the body. It is a muscular organ, filled with sensitive sympathetic nerve-endings which carry reflex messages back to other parts of the body. Sometimes the source of these messages is recognized and sometimes it is not.

When the colon is filled with decayed matter and bacteria, these nerve-endings become irritated and inflamed. This causes them to send complaints to other parts of the body. One message goes to the head, but it does not say that there is trouble in the colon, it merely says, "Head, please ache," and the head promptly aches without the owner suspecting where the trouble lies. Everything is blamed except the right thing. Inasmuch as the colon is a bundle of nerves, a very common complaint is "nervousness."

THE CONSEQUENCES OF CONSTIPATION

I want to draw a very vivid picture of what constipation does to all parts of the body. It is called "The Mother of Disease." I here present to you a "family" of complaints engendered by her.

Medical authorities claim it may be a contributing factor to the following conditions. (The list has been gathered from various authors.):

Group One—General

Coated tongue	Acne	Delusions	Hemorrhoids
Foul breath	Insomnia	Dementia	High blood pressure
Indigestion	Nervousness	Epilepsy	sure
'Biliousness'	Neuritis	Headache	Apoplexy
Dizziness	Neuralgia	Migraine	Lowered resistance
Constant fatigue	Absent-mindedness	Asthma	tance
Physical depression	Inability to concentrate	Bed-wetting	Pernicious anemia by weakening
Loss of pep	centrate	Gallstones	ia by weakening
Muddy complexion	Melancholia	Arthritis	gastric glands
ion	Mental depression	Diabetes	Premature old
Pigmentation of skin	Mental prostration	Faulty metabolism	age
skin	tion	lism	Cancer*
		Colitis	

That is a terrible flock to rear in any home, but many people are daily doing it and do not realize the source of their troubles.

But after a few years along comes another "family." Here it is:

Group Two—Infection in These Organs

Colon	Gall-bladder	Tonsils	Lungs (Tuberculosis)
Appendix	Arteries	Teeth	losis)
Small intestine	Kidneys	Gums	
Pancreas	Liver	Sinuses	
Stomach	Bladder	Mastoids	

A noted clinician states the matter very plainly:

"To tolerate infection within the body is to court disaster. It is a menace, even when mild, and failure to eradicate it is to neglect a patient's health interests.

*See Note 1 at close of chapter.

"The gastrointestinal tract offers no exception to the application of this principle. When infected, it is a fertile source of toxin absorption and a point of focal infection, perhaps second to none. Infection travels from one part of this tract to another, e.g., from colon to appendix, to gall bladder, to liver, to pancreas, and to stomach. The peritoneum, the kidneys, the urinary bladder are near and they frequently fail to resist the spreading infection. On passing into the blood stream, it reaches the arterial walls, the heart, and other distant organs and tissues of the body." (3)

You no doubt think that this "Mother of Disease" has now reared her last brood; but no, the worst is yet to come. After living as has been described for a term of years, degenerative changes appear. Here is the list:

Group Three—Degenerative Changes in:

Thyroid glands	Nerves	Teeth	Lymphatic tissue
Adrenal glands	Eyes	Uterus	of nasopharynx
Ductless glands	Ears	Ovaries	Blood-making
Heart	Skin	Breasts	organs
Kidneys	Fat	Testes	Spinal cord ac-
Liver	Hair	Prostate	companying
Pancreas	Gums	Arteries	anemia

Think! If food ferments and decays in this tract it is absorbed by the villi into the blood and is carried everywhere so that poison is fed every day and hour to every organ, gland, muscle, tissue, nerve, and cell in the entire body. Under those conditions everything in the body must degenerate. No part of the body can be healthy. Almost every disease named in the doctor book can develop. Believe it or not, that is the truth. Read more from authorities on the question:

"The colon is a sewerage system, but by neglect and abuse it becomes a cesspool. When it is clean we are well and happy; let it stagnate, and it will distill the poisons of decay, fermentation and putrefaction into the blood, poisoning the brain and nervous system so that we become mentally depressed and melancholic, irritable and restless; it will poison the heart so that we are weak and listless; poison the lungs so that the breath is foul; poison the digestive organs so that we are bloated, belching and distressed with gas pains; poison the blood so that the skin is sallow, blotched, and unhealthy. In short, every organ of the body is poisoned; we age prematurely; we look and feel old; the joints are stiff and painful; neuritis, dull eyes and a sluggish brain overtake us. The pleasure of living is gone." (4)

"It is but a slight exaggeration to declare that every chronic disease is a symptom of chronic constipation. It is no exaggeration whatever to say that chronic constipation is at least a contributory cause in all chronic diseases. At the back of the microbe there is to be sought the cause of the microbe, and this cause in every case is the state of the soil which permits him to flourish.

"Such a state of soil is described as a chronic auto-intoxication, which is only another way of saying that the drainage system is defective. And when the drainage system is defective to the point of there being a cesspool under the floor of the gastric dining-room, the powers of resistance are so reduced that the microbe comes and takes possession with easy and stupefying assurance." (5)

"If we would keep the stomach and bowels clean we would avoid every ill known except those due to accident." (6)

The Health Trio

Let me remind you that he who secures a good ration, has good digestion, and prompt elimination is quite sure to have good health.

The Causes of Constipation

Surely you are now anxious to know the causes of these dreadful conditions, and I am ready to tell you. Barring some extraordinary condition like constrictions from adhesions, or some growth or conditions other than constipation, the causes are one or all of three:

1. Wrong habits.
2. Elements left out of the food which would cause action, or
3. Elements put in which hinder action.

I will explain each group.

1. Habits: failure to heed promptly the call of nature; sour stomach of which there are twenty-seven "varieties"; lack of exercise, poor posture.

2. Elements left out which would maintain normal muscles and nerves and cause action: cellulose, minerals, and vitamins and water as explained in previous chapters. There is a laxative program, which will be explained presently.

3. Elements which hinder action — a constipating program — which now follows:

Constipating Program

1. Refined grains, chief of which is white flour and all foods of

which it is an ingredient; polished rice and all other refined cereal foods; corn starch.

2. Faulty methods of cooking vegetables.

3. Meat, fish and fowl, eggs.

4. Dairy milk.

5. Chocolate, cocoa, tea, coffee.

6. Drinking with meals.

7. Cheese. "Ripened" cheeses are worse than cottage cheese and sweet cream cheese.

8. Indigestion from any of the twenty-seven causes.

9. Fried foods.

10. Highly seasoned foods.

11. Pepper, mustard, horseradish, and all irritating condiments.

12. Tobacco, alcohol, opium, sleep-producing drugs.

13. Hasty eating.

14. Alum and aluminum are astringents and so tend to lessen mucous secretions and are held to be potential causes of constipation.

A LAXATIVE PROGRAM

1. Use whole grains, flours, and cereals, rich in cellulose, minerals, and vitamins.

2. Cook all vegetables without loss of minerals and vitamins.

3. Eat freely of vegetables, especially the coarse, leafy ones.

4. Get a liberal order of raw vegetables daily.

5. Eat freely of fruit. Have some raw fruit daily. Most fruits are more or less laxative.

6. Use soy bean milk in place of cow's milk.

7. Use soy bean cheese in place of dairy cheese.

8. Have meals at regular hours and take time to eat them.

9. When it is possible to do so, dinner should be eaten at noon and a very light meal eaten at night. When this is not possible, the evening dinner should be eaten as early as can be done.

*10. Ripe olives are very helpful, and can be eaten at every meal with much benefit. A cupful during the day is not too many.

11. Zwieback is better than bread.

*See Note 2 at end of chapter before Bibliography.

12. Cereals eaten with milk, or mushy cereals, are not as well salivated as zwieback, and therefore the zwieback is more helpful.

13. Copious drinking of water early in the morning helps many people.

14. A glass of fruit juice early in the morning and late at night is good.

15. A little olive oil at bed-time helps.

Special Helps

Prunes	Pears	Raw celery	Fresh apple juice
Figs	All cooked greens	Prune juice	
Apricots	Raw cabbage	Grape juice	

An evening enema is a good treatment in an emergency.

Most people can get a thorough cleansing in this way: In the morning when the stomach is empty drink from one to three glasses of grape juice, depending on the severity of the case and the individual tolerance for grape juice. Sometimes one glass is enough. Some stomachs rebel against grape juice, but these people may succeed by sipping it slowly. There are those who cannot take it; for them, prune juice or fresh apple juice are suggested. With certain people these drinks are tolerated better if diluted with water. These fruit juices should work like a charm.

Another cleansing procedure is to take one to four glasses of lemonade sweetened with honey, on an empty stomach.

Still another, but not as good as the two above: drink, on an empty stomach, several glasses of hot water with two teaspoons of common salt, and follow this with a glass of cold water.

If one will change over from a constipating program to the laxative one, his constipation will usually disappear like the dew before the sun. The Automatic Menu Planner offers normal meals which are laxative, and if followed, will correct most cases of constipation. For those who need a very laxative program, the following menu for one day is provided as an example:

(Let it be noted that you are more sure of success in conquering constipation if you follow the higher of the two levels of diet and abandon the use of all foods coming from animals.)

One Day's Program Which Is Very Laxative

Morning:

At least a half hour before breakfast, a glass of juice—grape, prune, or fresh apple.

Breakfast

Whole wheat zwieback with vegetable butter and one cup of ripe olives.

A liberal serving of either prunes, figs, or apricots.

A few nuts, other than roasted peanuts.

Any other fruits desired, some raw, until satisfied.

No drink.

Dinner (not closer than five hours to the breakfast)   1

Baked potato, eat the skin. Make palatable with vegetable butter, cream and salt, or such additions as are agreeable.

A liberal serving of cooked spinach or other greens or of well-cooked onions.

One serving of a root like beets, carrots, parsnips, or turnips.

A large serving of a raw vegetable. Mayonnaise, if it has no vinegar or mustard, is all right.

A protein dish—beans, peas, lentils, cottage cheese, soy cheese, or nuts, or some meat substitute.

No dessert; no drink.

Supper (not closer than five hours to dinner)

Large serving of a laxative fruit such as prunes, figs, pears, or apricots.

A liberal supply of other fruit, both raw and cooked.

If not specially hungry, no bread. If hungry, one or two pieces of whole wheat bread and a few ripe olives.

No dessert; no drink.

At Bed-Time

A glass of fruit juice from the list offered for breakfast.

If you awaken in the night too hungry to sleep, take a glass of water or half a glass of some sort of fruit juice.

NOTE: It is recognized that some people have sinned against their bodies so long that their stomachs and colons will not tolerate at first the full amount of cellulose contained in the above. They will have to "baby" themselves for a time and come back to a normal diet by degrees. If every constipating practice listed in previous paragraphs is discontinued, possibly normal conditions may be restored.

ECONOMY

If any reader feels that any of the items in the laxative program are too expensive, let him look at the Constipating Program and note the items he does not now have to buy, and he will find one pays for the other. Also remember that mineral oil costs a dollar a bottle. The Journal of the American Medical Association, October 18, page 1335, 1941, published a list of eleven harmful effects of mineral oil purgatives. It never corrects constipation but helps one to tolerate it.

The Cost of Constipation

Americans spend millions of dollars every year for cathartic drugs. It is cheaper to buy healthful foods. But there are other costs accruing from constipation—sickness, lost time, lost earnings, sickness expense, physical and mental agony. It is always cheaper to be well.

Note 1

"Indigestion and constipation," says Dr. Lane of London, "are the starting causes of the diseases of civilization."

"If you wish to produce cancer with a fair degree of certainty, supply a constipated subject with plenty of meat, and endeavor to deal with his constipation by means of irritating purgative drugs." (7)

It is not necessary to use yeast, mineral oil or laxative drugs. There are serious objections to all of them. None of them correct the condition, but merely help you to tolerate it. So long as one has to use any of them he is constipated.

Note 2

"When properly prepared, olives, like nuts, supply the place of butter and flesh meats. The oil as eaten in the olive is far preferable to animal oil or fat. It serves as a laxative. Its use will be found beneficial to consumptives, and it is healing to an inflamed irritated stomach." (8)

"Olives may be so prepared as to be eaten with good results at every meal. The advantages sought by the use of butter may be obtained by the eating of properly prepared olives. The oil in the olives relieves constipation, and for consumptives, and for those who have inflamed irritated stomachs, it is better than any drug. As a food it is better than any oil coming second-hand from animals." (9)

BIBLIOGRAPHY

(1) J. H. Kellogg, M.D., in "The Itinerary of a Breakfast," pages 13, 14, 87, 88.

(2) C. Ward Crampton, M.D., Chairman National Committee on Education, National Congress of Parents and Teachers; and Director Health Service Clinic, Post Graduate Medical School, New York City.

(3) Dr. Rose of New York, in "International Journal of Medicine and Surgery," quoted in "Good Health," October, 1935, page 317.

(4) I. H. Moore, foremost medical authority, in "Northwest Medicine," Volume 25, 1926.

(5) Dr. Leonard Williams, physician to the French Hospital, London.

(6) Dr. Jamieson, New York.

(7) "Modern Living," May, 1935.

(8) "Ministry of Healing," page 298.

(9) Mrs. E. G. White, Volume 7, page 134.

Degenerative Diseases

The widespread prevalence and rapid increase of degenerative diseases such as those which affect the heart, arteries, kidneys, liver, pancreas, glands, and nerves are utterly baffling to the workers for public health. All present efforts are unavailing in lessening their incidence. Mental diseases and cancer may well be added to the list.

It is claimed that one person in six over forty years of age will die of heart disease, one in six of kidney trouble, and one in five and a half of cancer.

Great advance has been made in the control of contagious and infectious diseases since scientists have discovered micro-organisms and have learned how to control them. Great strides have been made in lessening deaths at maternity, and in bringing more babies and children safely past their early hazards, so that a much larger per cent of persons born grow to maturity; but after age forty, degeneracy of vital organs appears so that with the passing of each decade fewer people reach vigorous old age.

Degeneracy is usually caused by human habits, while contagious diseases are caused by germs. Germs are more easily controlled than habits because it is easy for a man to impose his will on a germ, but for a man to yield his will to the Author of his life and obey the rules of life, is more than he is usually willing to do.

The Book says: "The curse causeless shall not come." But too many scientists today refuse to acknowledge their Creator. They have put so many millions of years of the operation of the theory of evolution between Him and them that He is now so remote from them that He has no more jurisdiction over their lives, and they no longer recognize any fundamental obligation to Him. Therefore each person is a law unto himself, and if he wishes to live to unnaturally indulge his physical senses and take the consequences thereof, he feels that no one is concerned but himself, and that no one will call him to an account.

This chapter will seek to strike at the root causes of the degenerative diseases.

THE HUMAN BODY

The human body is the most marvelous thing in the world. It consists of myriads of cells which are assembled into tissue, muscle, nerves, glands, organs, bones, teeth, skin, and hair.

Every cell has to be fed with oxygen, water and food. These supplies must be of the right kinds, in balance, and unfailing. If there be failure, the cells must suffer and then the organs suffer.

As each cell carries on its work, the foods are used, and their use produces by-products which must be carried away from the cells without delay or they will suffer or die from these wastes, which are poison.

Each cell is continually wearing out and being rebuilt. These cell wastes are toxic and must be carried away as well as the by-products.

Two Systems

To supply all of these necessities there are two systems in the body. One system takes in oxygen, water, and food, and prepares them for use and delivers them to the cells. The other begins at the cells and takes their wastes and by-products by the lymph and blood to the elimination outlets—lungs, pores, and kidneys. If these toxic wastes are not efficiently removed, the cells suffer and then the organs must suffer.

As the blood passes through the liver one of its functions is to convert certain toxic elements into non-toxic ones and to discharge some of these elements into the bile for elimination through the colon.

A very fine balance has to be maintained between the operation of these two systems.

They both are operated by the heart which is the principal means of causing the blood and lymph to circulate, carrying the supplies in and wastes out.

This circulatory system which keeps the body clean within, is very efficient. It is said that if the cells were bathed in two hundred thousand quarts of water, the water would have to be changed every few days to avoid the cells being poisoned by their own wastes; but the blood does this work with about seven quarts of fluid in conjunction with co-ordinated facilities.

Suppose an automobile could earn and secure its own supplies, feed itself with gas, oil, water, and oxygen, and drive itself; and suppose the supplies it gives to itself would preplace all of its losses so that no part would wear out in less than one hundred years; and if a fender were broken or tire injured, these supplies would mend the injuries; and that it could gradually renew its coat of paint as it goes over the highways so it always looks new—what a wonder it would be! That is a crude illustration of the human body.

Degenerative diseases are caused by putting in wrong "fuel" and a failure to keep the cells and blood stream of the body clean.

There Is No Argument

In order to go deeper into our subject we must understand the effects of poisons on cells and consequently on organs. There is no argument over the fact that cells must be nourished. Likewise there is no argument over the fact that poisons injure them. Let us see what happens.

The Kidneys

These magic filters handle nearly a quart of blood every minute, and in seven minutes handle an amount equal to all of that in the body; at least 600 quarts of blood pass through the normal kidneys every twenty-four hours for certain wastes to be removed; all the blood of the body passes through the kidneys many times each day.

The wastes are removed by the action of the selective cells in the circular-shaped glomeruli and in the tubules which together constitute one unit of filter mechanism of which there are said to be two million in each kidney (some say four million), each composed of cells, many of which have the power of selection akin to intelligence. The glomeruli drain into the tubules, which are so small each one can handle a fourth of an ounce in sixty years. The glomeruli extract about sixty quarts of fluid from the blood in twenty-four hours, and pour it into the tubules which put back into the blood, all except about two quarts, which are eliminated as urine, and in which are the wastes that have been extracted. The kidneys thus use one quart of water to extract forty-five grams of waste. If there is a deficiency of water in the body, the urine is too concentrated and the kidneys are handicapped in the elimination of wastes. They remove the waste products of metabolism. The glomeruli remove glucose, sodium chlorine, and water which are put back by the tubules to certain levels which must be maintained, which level is called the "threshold," and all amounts above that level are allowed to escape into the urine. Acids and bases both filter through the glomeruli, but the tubules reabsorb bases so as to preserve the right acid-base balance of the blood. There is no mechanism more marvelous than this known to man outside of himself.

The kidney mechanism and functions bear witness to an infinite Mind which designed their structure, and an infinite being Who continues to maintain their existence and Who supervises their functions. To suggest that such an organ could originate of itself without a Designer and Creator is so foolish that no scientist or school boy would even consider applying the same argument to an automobile. Why not be consistent?

But, remember, that the kidney is only one of many parts of the human body, each as wonderful as it, and all of which work together in unison and with as much delicacy as do the various parts of the kidney with each other.

Furthermore, He who created and still maintains this organ will someday call all men to account for their misuse of this marvelous mechanism. To believe that, is inescapable. Therefore, the acceptance of the duty of man, to obey his Maker's will in the use of the organs of his body must be a most vital part of religion when a genuine and complete religion is found and accepted. Little wonder is it that such a religion would have to have within it, as a cardinal feature, a memorial of creation to ever remind man of all of his obligations to do his Maker's will in the use of the organs of his body as well as in the observance of the Ten Commandments. That memorial of creation, and the acceptance of the laws of physiology whose origin it memorializes, must be a most vital part of religion. Such a memorial is found in the fourth commandment.

Poisoning the Kidneys

But men do not reverence God or have regard for their own organs. They overwork their kidney cells to the point of the destruction of many of them. They fail to provide sufficient water for elimination. They live so as to allow poisons to develop within the body which ought never to be there. And worst of all, they daily, knowingly, deliberately put into the body substances which are defined as poisons in every pharmocopeia on earth. These extra poisons destroy the cells of the organ and so lessen its efficiency or perhaps terminate its usefulness.

The kidney cells were designated to handle only the wastes of the cells, and with only that work to do they would last throughout life. They work in "shifts"—part of them rest while others work, and change about so that no portion of the kidney ever need be even "tired."

These extra poisons lessen the vitality of cells and even destroy some of them, and then their places are taken by scar cells which have no powers of selection and cannot help in the work. When a cell is gone, its work is left for others, which increases their work, so they are in greater danger than before. Thus each step in destruction brings successive destructive steps in ever-increasing rapidity until "Bright's disease" is the diagnosis. Now the injury is irreparable. Each year a hundred thousand Americans die of diseased kidneys, many of them in the prime of life.

The kidneys have so great an excess of capacity that two-thirds of one kidney can take care of the wastes of metabolism which is all the wastes the kidneys should be asked to handle. Because of this excess capacity, a great portion of the kidney cells can be destroyed before the owner or his doctor detects any warning sign; there is no pain. You may tell a man he is daily destroying his kidney cells and he will laugh in your face because he feels perfectly well. Too late will he discover the truth. "A normal kidney has been estimated to contain about 1,250,000 glomeruli. When more than 400,000 have been destroyed, signs of chronic nephritis appears." (35)

There are also several types of infection which injure the kidney cells, but their presence in the blood stream whence they may enter the kidney, is a matter of general "immunity" of the body, which is to be discussed in another chapter. There are other kidney conditions but this chapter is concerned specially with the effects of poisons on the kidneys.

Poisoning the Arteries

The blood containing these poisons is flowing through the arterial system—nearly a thousand miles of arteries and veins, besides many more thousand miles of capillaries. Wherever blood vessels are it goes with its poisons—into organs, glands, tissue, brain, etc. The walls of the arteries consist of cells which are subject to the same injury from poisons as the cells in the kidneys. Therefore the arteries degenerate at the same time as do the kidneys and from the same causes. There are various types of degeneracy, but that does not matter so far as our objective in this lesson is concerned.

The inner, middle, and outer layers of cells in the artery walls may develop differing pathology, but the point is they are being injured and their ability to function is decreasing.

As the cells degenerate, the walls thicken and harden. Now it is called "hardening of the arteries," or "arteriosclerosis." As they harden they become more brittle—easier to burst under pressure.

As the walls thicken, the passageway through them diminishes in size so that more pressure from the heart is required to maintain the proper circulation. Now it is called "high blood pressure." It is true that an increase in blood pressure can be caused by an accelerated heart-beat, or by anxiety, or by "nerves," but that is not the dangerous type of blood pressure under consideration just now.

As the hole through the arteries grows smaller and the pressure increases and the walls become more brittle, a little extra pressure at some time from any cause may result in the rupture of a blood vessel. The most delicate ones are in the brain, and consequently such an accident often happens there. That is called a hemorrhage. A blood clot forms. If it is fatal, it is called apoplexy; if not fatal, a stroke of paralysis. Ninety thousand Americans die that way each year.

Poisoning the Heart

The blood which carries the poisons which injure the cells of the kidneys and the arteries is surging through the cavities of the heart which push it on its never-ending journey throughout the body as long as life lasts. But more; the heart has its own circulatory system by which its own muscle and nerve cells are fed, so that the injury to the arteries of the body extends throughout the heart as a part of the body. Sometimes this injury to the arteries becomes pronounced in the heart first; but in either case, the heart is now degenerating.

At the same time it is being weakened it is required to work harder than normal to maintain normal circulation through a thousand miles of arteries with thick walls and a small opening. This extra work plus the weakened condition of the heart handicap the owner and sooner or later bring disaster—heart failure.

The death rate from heart disease in Philadelphia doubled in 20 years from 1922 to 1942, and the increase was entirely in the age group past forty. (38)

A great flood of light has been shed upon this subject by a notable experiment made in the Rockefeller Institute under the direction of Dr. Alexis Carrel who placed a living section of a chicken's heart in a bottle in 1912. He fed its cell scientifically and removed the wastes, and the cells lived and continued to grow for 34 years although a chicken does not live over twelve years as a rule. Dr. Carrel said that so far as he can see the cells are "immortal" so long as they receive proper nourishment and have their wastes removed. The experiment was abandoned in 1946.

If a man would take as good care of his heart from youth up as Dr. Carrel and his associates did with the chicken heart, it would never degenerate; and if the same man would take as good care of his other organs, they would never degenerate, and the heart would not wear out, he would some day quietly die of old age all at once, like the Deacon's One-Hoss Shay.

Poisoning the Liver

The liver is, perhaps, the most versatile organ-gland in the body. One of its duties is to work over poisons so they will be nontoxic. It goes without saying that an extra load of poisons in the blood will greatly add to its work, entail a hardship upon it, and without a doubt tend to the same injury and destruction of cells as occurs in the organs already discussed. And then how can it perform efficiently its dozen different kinds of work upon which normal health depends in more ways than can be told in this book. (5) "Liver complaint" is the liver complaining of its over load of poisons.

Poisoning the Glands

Very brief explanations have been made in other chapters of the work of the glands which are styled the "life activators" of the body. Each gland picks out of the blood the elements it requires to elaborate its own type of secretion. Each gland is a mystery; no scientist fully understands any one of them. However, it is easy to see that if the blood is continually laden with poisons, the glands will be handicapped in elaborating pure secretions out of a poisoned blood stream. The body as a whole exists and functions because of the work of these glands, and so when their source of supply is poisoned, the life of the body is poisoned at its source, and all life processes are diminished.

Poisoning the Nerves

It is impossible in the confines of this book to adequately explain the work of the nervous system. Suffice it to say that it carries all conscious stimuli from the brain outward, giving orders for motion, from the exterior inward, bringing sensations to the brain, and an unnumbered host of automatic, sympathetic, reflex messages of which we are not always conscious. This is the way by which all parts of the body are combined into a coordinate unit so that all can work together—so that two fingers can be placed on the same spot and the eyes look at that spot at the same time. Manifestly when the nerves are out of order, nothing can go right in the body.

The nerves can degenerate from want of proper nourishment and from extra and foreign toxins just the same as other organs do. Now we have seen how to develop many nervous diseases which we will not even take time to name.

Poisoning the Brain

The brain is a living organ whose cells are as dependent upon nutrition and the removal of wastes as any other part of the body. It is the most delicate and intricately constructed of any part. It has power to think, reason, choose, love, hate, etc. It is the head of the kingdom over which it rules. All orders go from it.

Suppose it is not properly nourished! Or, suppose it is poisoned! Can it be undernourished? Can it be poisoned? Why not? How can it help it if the blood is laden with poisons of various kinds every hour of the day?

And when it is poisoned, what will happen to its functions? How might it be affected? How different would it act from normal? How might a man with a sick brain act? Any way except normal. Could he not become "mental"?

Enough of this! How do people poison themselves?

LOADS OF POISONS

Indigestion

One very common way of adding to the body's load of poisons is to practice some of the twenty-seven habits which cause indigestion. This has already been covered and nothing more need be said here.

Constipation

The poisons from constipation are more deadly than from indigestion. It is said that constipation can treble the load of the kidneys. The physiology of this has already been explained.

Salt

The body uses salt; a little is necessary, but too much is not good. Many people use too much. Be conservative. If you find yourself wanting more than other people do, cut it down. People who perspire much will need more salt than those who do not. In my opinion it matters little what kind of salt is used. Although iodized may be needed in goiter sections.

Sugar

Sugar (exclusive of honey) is an irritant. The body can tolerate a limited amount, but doubtless would be better off without the use of any artificial concentrated sugar. The least that can be said is that most people use far too much. The ways in which it is eaten are innumerable. The world would be infinitely better off if candy, ice cream, and many other concoctions were unknown. The advice may be unwelcome, but it is that you cut your consumption of sugar to a very, very low minimum if you want the best of health. One of the results of the free use of sugar is an exhausted pancreas —diabetes.

"Nutritionists agree that of all food, sugar unquestionably is the worst." (36)

Eggs

It is easy to eat eggs to excess and so get an excess of protein. Eggs are quick to putrefy in the digestive tract. They have a large amount of cholesterol, which, when in excess in the body, is said to be one cause of degeneration of the arteries. There are other counts against eggs which do not belong in this chapter.

Excess of Acid-Forming Foods

This matter has been so fully explained in previous chapters that it is not necessary to do more here than mention it. It is important that persons suffering from any of these degenerative diseases increase their akaline foods to 90 per cent and decrease the acid-forming ones to 10 per cent.

Excess of Vegetable Proteins

The work of Nuzam and Sansum (1) showed that an excess of vegetable proteins, even when the diet was highly alkaline, could raise the blood pressure and injure the kidneys in rabbits.

Excess of Proteins, Especially Animal

The same work of Nuzam and Sansum on rabbits showed that an excess of animal protein caused more injury then the same excess of vegetable protein.

Other workers have confirmed this. *Good Health,* of December, 1937, cites the work of Newburgh of the University of Michigan as follows:

"Newburgh and other investigators have shown that meat proteins are far more harmful to the kidneys than milk and vegetable proteins. Rats fed on meat proteins showed symptoms of nephritis within two weeks, or even in less time."

Following is a summary of the report:

Dr. L. H. Newburgh, a professor in the Medical Department of the University of Michigan, reported May, 1922, at a meeting of the American Medical Association in St. Louis his experiment on feeding meat to animals.

Summarizing the results, it appears that of twenty-four animals fed on bread containing about one-half its weight of lean meat, fourteen, or 58.3 per cent, developed in less than eight and a half months, disease of the blood vessels, or arteriosclerosis.

Of the animals fed on bread containing about one-third its weight of lean meat, out of eleven animals that lived more than six months, eight showed typical arteriosclerosis and in seven the changes in the arteries "were advanced and extensive."

Not one of the animals kept in the laboratory under the same conditions as the experimental animals, without meat, showed any evidence of disease of the arteries, although two-thirds of them lived more than six months. (2)

"The result to the person who eats too much meat and other forms of animal food will probably be a liability to gradual development of digestive disorders and thickening of the arteries, with high blood pressure, kidney disease, gout, rheumatism, etc., while the person who takes habitually too much fat and carbohydrate food tends toward increasing stoutness with enfeeblement of the heart's action and possible development of diabetes." (3)

"Dr. Fox, of Philadelphia, has examined all of the animals that have died in the Philadelphia Zoological Garden. His conclusions are of interest in this connection. He pointed out that the carnivora had chronic vascular and renal lesions, and that they were practically the only ones that had such lesions. I wrote to Dr. Fox, asking him whether I was justified in assuming that definite relationship existed between the carnivorous diet and these chronic lesions of the arteries and kidneys. In his reply, he stated that this certainly was true, and that the meat-eating animals showed a high incidence of chronic disease of the arteries and the kidneys as compared with all the other animals on which he had performed necropsies." (4)

Hindhede's notable experiment in Denmark during the World War, which has been retold until it is familiar to all, demonstrated on a nation-wide scale that a low protein diet safeguards from Bright's disease and improves the health remarkably. (5) See Denmark's Food Experiment in this book.

The records of thousands of individuals have shown that the blood pressure of those who eat no meat averages to be lower than in those who do eat it. (6)

It has been shown that a meal heavy in meat protein greatly increases the work of the heart for many hours. One published statement follows:

"After a meal of meat the increase in heart rate regularly amounts to a 25 to 50 per cent rise above the fasting level, and persists, in experimental subjects, from 15 to 20 hours, to reach a total of many thousand extra heart beats. Moore points out that a protein meal thus throws an extra burden of work on the heart which is comparable in extent to the heart's total performance during three or four hours. Obviously, he concludes, a high protein diet is incompatible with cardiac rest." (7)

Some authorities claim that the cholesterol in meats and animal fats is more injurious than the excess protein; that in excess it causes atherosclerosis which makes up 95 per cent of the lesions called arteriosclerosis. Vegetable oils contain no cholesterol, and should take the place of animal fats in the diet. There is much difference of opinion concerning cholesterol which is found in the blood and all body cells and in large amounts in eggs and animal fats. Some say it may be a waste product of metabolism; (Cannon) some hold that it is a necessary part of every cell (Leary) and therefore necessary in the diet. However, those who hold that it is necessary in the cells warn us that an excess of it is dangerous in that it is the chief agent in producing damage to the arteries,— arteriosclerosis. Others contend that it is not a cause of such injury. Yet, an excess of it fed to rabbits is said to produce notable injury to arteries in one month. It is advised that we remove most of the cholesterol from the diet as we grow older. Manifestly it would be to our advantage to exclude from the beginning that derived from animals.

The amount of cholesterol consumed in the ordinary American diet is one third of the amount which produces notable arterial damage in rabbits in one month, given in proportion to their weight. (37) After reading the variety of opinions on the subject the present writer believes that the wise course is to avoid those foods which are high in this substance, and therefore two tables are produced here showing the cholesterol content of various foods. It will be noted that most of those with high content are foods not advocated in this book. In the first seven articles listed, only eggs can be considered necessary, and even they may be discarded by those who follow this book through carefully and secure from other foods the elements found in eggs.

CHOLESTEROL IN FOODS
(mg. per 100 gr. fresh weight)

Cod liver oil	400
Eggs, whole, average	313
Butter	240-340
Oysters	215
Pig's liver	130-140
Lard	110
Chocolate	56
Margarine	43
Cheese	42-62
Beef	38-78
Fish	21-95
Bread	19
Cream, full	11.9

CHOLESTEROL IN FOODS

Foods	Maximum
Brain, cattle	3.7
Liver	3.4
Kidney, mutton	3.4
Pancreas, calf	3.12
Thymus, calf	2.3
Roe, salmon	2.2
Egg, yolk	2.15
Chicken	0.527
Meat, chicken	0.108
Lard, suet	0.35

Butter	0.22
Blood, beef	0.194
Rabbit, whole	0.117
Bacon, fat	0.108
Meat, veal, beef, pork	0.088
Milk, cows	0.03

These are the averages of many estimates, published by American Medical Association, December 9, 1933, page 1845.　(40)

RABBIT EXPERIMENTS BY NUZUM AND SANSUM
BLOOD

Diet No. 1. Liver Diet, High Protein, Acid Ash

Blood Pressure	N.P.N.	Alkalinity	Arteries
Increased in 6 weeks	Increased after 6 weeks	Decreased	Hardened in 7 out of 10

Diet No. 2. Oat Diet, High Protein, Acid Ash

Increased in 6 months	Increased in 6 weeks	Decreased	Hardened in 7 out of 11

Diet No. 3. Soy Bean Diet, High in Protein, Alkaline Ash

Increased in 4 months	Increased in 9 months	Increased	Normal

Diet No. 4. Herbivorous Diet, Low Protein, Alkaline Ash

Normal	Normal	Normal	Normal

URINE

	A. and C.	Reaction	Kidneys
Diet No. 1	In 6 weeks	Acid	Nephritis 8 out of 9
Diet No. 2	In 4 and 5 months	Acid	Nephritis 9 out of 12
Diet No. 3	In 1 year	Alkaline	Nephritis 8 out of 10
Diet No. 4	None	Alkaline	Normal

N.P.N.—Normal waste
A. and C.—Albumin and casts　(8)

To say the least, these animal feeding experiments are very enlightening.

Spices and Condiments

Spices and condiments—pepper, mustard, ginger, cloves, horseradish (especially the things that are "hot" when they are cold), injure the cells of the organs which have to handle them, and they should be excluded from the food. Note the following:

"In this fast age, the less exciting the food, the better. Condiments are injurious in their nature. Mustard, pepper, spices, pickles, and other things of like character, irritate the stomach and make the blood feverish and impure. The inflamed condition of the drunkard's stomach is often pictured as illustrating the effects of alcoholic liquors. A similar condition is produced by the use of irritating condiments. Soon ordinary food does not satisfy the appetite. The system feels a want, a craving for something more stimulating." (9)

"a. Their constant use prevents one from really appreciating good, wholesome food flavors.

"b. The highly seasoned food tends to cause overeating with its troubles.

"c. Their constant contact with the stomach mucosa produces irritation, which eventually results in disease.

"d. The liver, kidneys, and other vital organs are forced to fight constantly against irritant bodies; this eventually causes damage to their structure.

"e. The use of these substances produces a thirst for drink stronger than water.

"f. Those who use condiments find it necessary gradually to increase the amount used to satisfy the unnatural appetite created by them." (10)

Vinegar

This is wholly unfit for food. The acetic acid in it will prevent the action of saliva. One teaspoonful can stop the starch digestion in an ordinary meal. It is an irritant. The "eels" in vinegar often take up their abode in the intestine and become parasites there. It is twice as active in producing "gin liver" as is alcohol. (11) It reduces the alkaline reserve of the blood; is said to aid in destroying red blood corpuscles; and hinders the digestion of protein. (12)

Therefore vinegar should never be used. This, of course, eliminates pickles made with vinegar. Pickles have also been *hardened* by the action of acetic acid and salt until they are almost indigestible. (13)

Coffee

" 'The addition of a strong coffee infusion to a purin (uric acid) free diet causes a marked increase in the excretion of uric acid. The analyses showed that the amount of uric acid after tea drinking was doubled.'—Professor Mendel. There is more uric acid (xanthin purin) in a cup of coffee than in the same quantity of urine."

"The damaging effect of this increase of uric acid will be better appreciated when the recently ascertained fact is recalled that the human liver does not possess the ability to destroy or detoxicate uric acid, which is an important function of the liver in all carnivorous animals."

"Coffee cripples the liver. Tibbles, an eminent English authority on diet, calls attention to the pernicious influence of caffeine on the glycogenic function of the liver which leads him to condemn the use of coffee altogether. This observation suggests that the coffee habit may be one of the causes for the notable increase of diabetes in this country in recent years." (14)

The following are abstracts:

Coffee with children may cause night terrors, insomnia and tremulousness, active delirium, dilated pupils, tremor in the facial muscles and extremities, marked increase in pulse rate, hallucinations.

With adults it invariably leads to persistent functional disturbance of the nervous system, and disturbed digestion, nervous excitement, insomnia, anxiety, apprehension, palpitation of the heart, vertigo, heartburn, dyspepsia, constipation, distressed breathing, weakness of muscles.

Caffeine paralyzes the absorbing power of the convoluted tubules of the kidney.

Causes tetanic contraction of the heart.

Inhibits peptic and salivary digestion.

Accelerates fatigue.

Tea and coffee numb the sense of fatigue which is a warning as a safety measure to protect the body.

Coffee overstimulates the glands of the stomach that secrete hydrochloric acid.

Tannic acid in tea precipitates pepsin.

Tea and coffee cause headaches, nervousness. (15)

"The writer has in many cases seen the blood pressure drop twenty to forty points in cases of high blood pressure after the disuse of coffee, and with a notable improvement in health." (16)

"Dr. W. Faessler of Zurich summarizes (in the *British Journal of Physical Medicine*) the results that well-known investigators have elicited by experiments on men and animals. He quotes Professor Mendelsohn as stating: 'Caffeine is a dangerous substance, and any doctor who frivolously maintains the contrary makes himself responsible for injuries to many of his fellow men.' This view is confirmed by many others. . . .

"Rudolf Bayer says: 'Caffeine as a strong uric acid former has a bad influence on the metabolism, inasmuch as, given in large doses, it disturbs the balance of the glandular functions.' . . .

"Among the effects of caffeine on the heart and circulation of the blood are 'palpitation from irritation of the cardiac nerves, lessened expansibility of the chambers of the heart, due to increased muscle tone, resulting in a weakening of the circulation with rapid and irregular beats.'

"With regard to the nervous system, caffeine may be looked upon as an evil genius. Many authors describe the symptoms of chronic caffeine intoxication as follows:

" 'By irritating the cerebal cortex and spinal and heart centers, pressure and congestion of the head are produced, also general unrest and excitement, sweating, hallucinations, increased tendon reflexes, cold and numbness in hands and feet, rapid fatigue of body and trembling of muscles and hands, shortness of breath, increase of respiration, palpitation, rapidity and reduction of pulse volume, cardiac and pulse irregularity, nausea, diarrhea, constipation, colic, dyspepsia, gastralgia, flatulence, loss of flesh and loss of appetite.'

"Dr. Faessler concludes with the following statement of his own experience: 'In my practice of thirty-eight years I have never seen anything but disadvantage from the frequent enjoyment of coffee, and have therefore felt it my duty to give a warning against that so-called "harmless" poison, caffeine.' " (17)

"With the use of three to six or eight cups of coffee a day, which is not uncommon, serious nerve disorders occur which are even more disturbing than those occasioned by the smoking of two or more packages of cigarettes daily."

"Tea, coffee, and cola drinks are all habit-forming." (18)

"Tea is an intoxicant, a habit-forming drug, and one which leads to the forming of other drug habits. . . . Cases of delirium tremens resulting from the use of tea have been reported." (19)

"Chronic tea poisoning is a frequent affection whose most common symptoms are loss of appetite, dyspepsia, palpitation, headache, vomiting and nausea, combined with nervousness, and hysterical and neuralgic affections, frequently accompanied by constipation and pain in the region of the heart." (20)

"The Texas State Board of Health, after a careful investigation of the causes of nervousness and stupidity among school children, brought in the following report:

" 'Children who drink coffee for breakfast come to school exhilarated. They work strenuously in the morning, and are overflowing with energy and vitality; but they do not last under the school routine. They become fatigued more quickly than the other pupils; and by the close of school in the afternoon, they are exhausted to the point of stupidity. They are nervous and therefore unstable in their deportment.' " (41)

The following table shows the amount of caffeine found in various caffeine-containing preparations:

	Per cent
Cocoa (theobromine)	1.00
Coca-Cola	1.00-1.2
Coffee (roasted)	.75-2.05
Cola	2.00
Mate	1.115
Tea	1.35-1.75

As usually prepared, tea and coffee both contain about the same amount of caffeine. Dry tea contains about one-third as much caffeine as does the same weight of coffee. Cocoa contains about the same amount of caffeine as does coffee. Cocoa nibs also contain caffeine. (21)

MEATS, EXTRACTS, TEA, COFFEE, COCOA COMPARED
Uric Acids and Purines

	Grains per lb.
Lamb (cold roast leg)	3.50
Soup (made from bones)	0.48
Soup (made from meat)	1.40
Hospital beef tea (cooked 8 hours)	7.00
Saddle of mutton	1.40
Mutton (cold roast leg)	1.10

Veal (cutlet)	3.50
Beef (cold sirloin)	1.10
Kidney of sheep	3.50
Liver of sheep	6.50
Fowl (breast)	1.70
Rabbit	1.00
Mackeral	2.00
Herring (Loch Erne, kippered)	6.40
Meat juice	49.70
Meat extract	63.00
Tea	175.00
Coffee	70.00
Cocoa	59.00

(22)

Mate

"Its properties are essentially the same as those of tea and coffee." (23)

Cocoa

The Government has warned farmers not to feed the residue to chickens or cows because they will lay fewer eggs and give less milk; and not to put it on the land because it lessens the fertility of the soil. (24)

"Experiment upon animals has proven that the action of caffeina, theina, and theobromia is identical in kind, though the latter is poisonous and fatal in much smaller doses." (25)

"All cocoa contains theobromin, a nerve poison. . . . Chocolate and cocoa are altogether unwholesome, and if freely indulged in may easily induce conditions which may be attributed to some nerve disorder." (26)

Cocoa is what is left of chocolate after the fat is removed, which was about half of the original content.

Coca-Cola

There are seventy brands of cola drinks listed by U. S. Government. (27)

"Besides flavoring material, the principal constituent of importance is caffeine. Comparing this beverage with others containing caffeine, J. W. Mallet says, that of caffeine, tea, per cup, ordinarily contains 2.02 grains; coffee, per cup, 1.74 grains; coca-cola, as ordinarily dispensed, contains 1.21 grains per glass." (28)

Stimulating Soft Drinks

"It is now the daily custom of many thousands of city workers to prepare themselves for the day's work by drinking at a soda fountain some caffeine-containing soft drink. This practice cannot be too strongly condemned. Many are simple-minded enough to believe the statements of the advertisers that such drinks 'rest you in five minutes.' This is a false statement, and has misled thousands. What such drinks do is to relieve the immediate sensation of fatigue, and enable one to perform with alacrity for a time duties which one would, without the aid of caffeine, do less efficiently. They also relieve the tired feeling with which many who are violating one or more of the fundamental laws of health start each day.

"In purchasing temporary relief from the sensation of fatigue, however, one does not gain something which he would otherwise not have. Fatigue goes on just the same, and continues to do so until additional rest is taken. This is also the case with those who 'brighten up' by drinking coffee or strong tea. The temporary gain in efficiency purchased in this manner leaves one jaded so that after the effects have worn off a period of inefficiency or of extra rest must follow before one returns to the normal state." (29)

Keep Poisons Out

"Among the poisons which must be kept out of the body should be mentioned habit-forming drugs, such as opium, morphine, cocain, heroin, chloral, acetanilid, alcohol, caffeine, and nicotine. The best rule for those who wish to attain the highest physical and mental efficiency is total abstinence from all substances which contain poisons, including spirits, wine, beer, tobacco, many much-advertised patent drinks served at soda-water fountains, most patent medicines, and even coffee and tea." (30)

Alcohol is a narcotic and a strong poison. A summary of its effects on the organs of the body is in a chapter by itself, entitled "Health and Alcohol." That information will not be repeated here.

Its use today is a very grave menace to normal bodies and minds and to posterity.

Tobacco

There is only one other poison known to science which is stronger than nicotine. The only use of nicotine is to kill. One drop put into the blood will kill a man instantly. Why health authorities should tolerate the daily use of such a poison is a mystery. Why doctors and nurses should use it is unexplainable. An entire chapter is devoted to the subject of "Health and Tobacco."

OVERWEIGHT

Overweight is often associated with high blood pressure. It is highly important for many reasons to keep the weight down to the average. It is safer to be underweight than overweight. The mortality rate for people 50 lbs. underweight is 100, while for those who are 10 and 20 lbs. underweight it is 92; at average weight it is 94, and for 50 lbs overweight it is 153. The lowest death rate is found among those who are 10 and 20 lbs. under the average weight. (31)

MEN

Age	5 ft. 0 in.	5 ft. 1 in.	5 ft. 2 in.	5 ft. 3 in.	5 ft. 4 in.	5 ft. 5 in.	5 ft. 6 in.	5 ft. 7 in.	5 ft. 8 in.
15	107	109	112	115	118	122	126	130	134
20	117	119	122	125	128	132	136	140	144
25	122	124	126	129	133	127	141	145	149
30	126	128	130	133	136	140	144	148	152

Age	5 ft. 9 in.	5 ft. 10 in.	5 ft. 11 in.	6 ft. 0 in.	6 ft. 1 in.	6 ft. 2 in.	6 ft. 3 in.	6 ft. 4 in.	6 ft. 5 in.
15	138	142	147	152	157	162	167	172	177
20	148	152	156	161	166	171	176	181	186
25	153	157	162	167	173	179	184	189	194
30	156	161	166	172	178	184	190	196	201

WOMEN

Age	4 ft. 8 in.	4 ft. 9 in.	4 ft. 10 in.	4 ft. 11 in.	5 ft. 0 in.	5 ft. 1 in.	5 ft. 2 in.	5 ft. 3 in.	5 ft. 4 in.
15	101	103	105	106	107	109	112	115	118
20	106	108	110	112	114	116	119	122	125
25	109	111	113	115	117	119	121	124	128
30	112	114	116	118	120	122	124	127	131

Age	5 ft. 5 in.	5 ft. 6 in.	5 ft. 7 in.	5 ft. 8 in.	5 ft. 9 in.	5 ft. 10 in.	5 ft. 11 in.	6 ft. 0 in.
15	122	126	130	134	138	142	147	152
20	128	132	136	140	143	147	151	156
25	131	135	139	143	147	151	154	158
30	134	138	142	146	150	154	157	161

(Normal weight according to height for persons of medium framework)

These tables are based upon the weight taken at a life insurance examination with indoor clothing. The height is taken with shoes on. If the weight is taken without shoes or clothing, the proper deduction should be made for the height of the heels of the shoes and for weight of the clothing. (32)

Instruction for reducing the weight will be found in a chapter on "Overweight."

BLOOD PRESSURE

The figures for normal blood pressure as given today are:

B. P. Ages	Normal Millimeters	B. P. Ages	Normal Millimeters
15-20	120	41-45	129
21-25	123	46-50	131
26-30	124	51-55	132
31-35	124	56-60	135
36-40	127		(33)

As a safety measure one should have his blood pressure checked at least once each year.

A CORRECTIVE REJUVENATING PROGRAM

Much of the matter on the last few pages is negative in character, but it seems necessary to give the information therein contained.

Now it is appropriate to recall that the injurious foods and drinks are not included in a balanced ration—they are outside of it and unnecessary. Every hurtful indulgence should be abandoned.

If one could start at the beginning of life and live according to the rules laid down in the preceding pages of this book, these degenerative diseases would rarely occur, if ever.

If one is now suffering with these conditions, he should make some modifications from the diet of a normal person. He must more severely cut down his sugar and salt, must be extra careful to live above constipation, should remove all animal fats from the diet, and for a short time bring his protein consumption down to about twenty-five grams a day (see the next chapter for this instruction). and should bring up his alkaline foods to constitute 90 per cent of his daily ration. He should partake very freely of fruits and of vegetables; the coarse, leafy vegetables, both raw and cooked, are especially beneficial. The Automatic Menu Planner should be followed as a guide to planning the meals, but with the modifications named above.

CONCLUSION

Danger Without Warning

The heart, arteries, kidneys, liver, pancreas and glands give no warning cry when they are hurt by poisons. Even "well defined symptoms do not appear until disease is far advanced. The earliest symptoms observable indicate, in fact, that the vital reserve has been consumed." (34) The first warning may mean that they are ready to fail, that they are about destroyed, that the end of their usefulness has come, that the end of their life and yours is at hand.

Each organ has a large excess capacity as a safety margin, but it is impossible for one to know when the safety margins have disappeared or when the remainder has been so far destroyed that calamity is near.

It Is Not a Mystery

The prevalence and rapid increase of degenerative diseases is no mystery. In view of the manifold self-destroying habits daily practiced by mankind, the wonder is that the race still exists. The diseases are common because their causes are popular. But though a hundred million people daily practice life-destroying habits, they are *still* life-destroying habits. ·

A Change of Attitude Needed

The great need is for an entire change of attitude. The common attitude is, "A little won't hurt me." While it is true that a little won't do very much harm, it is also true that the continuous accumulation of small injuries sooner or later bring great disaster. A skyscraper is built of little stones.

Rather than to plead for small indulgences, and whine because our best interest calls us from them, why not change our attitude and take the opposite view and ask, What can I do to add the merest trifle to my mental and physical fitness, to my usefulness, to my length of days and the joys of living?

The Great Conquest

Many people know that they ought not to indulge their appetites with these hurtful things, but they are too weak to withstand the examples without and the cravings within. Man can save himself from bacteria by the aid of science, but when it comes to saving himself *from himself*, that is a different task; man needs to surrender to someone stronger than himself—to a Divine Being. For this reason, the teacher of religion must take on the duty of teaching physiology from the sacred standpoint and hold mankind amenable to the laws the Creator established within the body. But too many religionists have gone modernistic, and having made the theory of evolution their god, repudiated all accountability to a Creator, and so put out of their lives all connection with a power strong enough to give them victory over themselves. A reverse in this attitude is the great need of the hour, even for the sake of health, but even more for the sake of a high type of character, and the acceptance of genuine Christianity.

BIBLIOGRAPHY

(1) "High Blood Pressure," by G. K. Abbott, M. D., page 110.

(2) Condensed from "New Dietetics," by John Harvey Kellogg, M.D., pages, 409, 410.

(3) Quoted from "British Journal of Physical Medicine," in "Good Health," September, 1935, page 275.

(4) "New Dietetics," by J. H. Kellogg, M.D., page 411.

(5) "High Blood Pressure," by G. K. Abbott, M.D., pages 85, 86.

(6) "High Blood Pressure," by G. K. Abbott, M.D., page 58.

(7) "Journal American Medical Association," quoted by J. H. Kellogg, M.D., in "Good Health," January, 1933.

(8) "High Blood Pressure," by G. K. Abbott, M.D., page 110, 2nd edition.

(9) "Ministry of Healing," page 325.

(10) "Foods, Nutrition, and Clinical Dietetics," by Risley and Walton, pages 90, 91.

(11) J. H. Kellogg, M.D., in "Question Box," pages 276, 282, 286, 312.

(12) "Health," October, 1935, page 29.

(13) J. H. Kellogg, M.D., in "Question Box," page 276.

(14) J. H. Kellogg, M.D., "New Dietetics," pages 494, 495.

(15) Abstracted from "New Dietetics," by J. H. Kellogg, M.D., pages 495-500.

(16) J. H. Kellogg, M.D., in "Good Health," August, 1938, page 231.

(17) "Good Health," November, 1934, page 25.

(18) G. K. Abbott, M.D., in "Health," April, 1934, page 7.

(19) "Good Health," October, 1935, page 308.

(20) Information given by Dr. Bullard in a paper read before the Massachusetts Medical Society, cited by J. H. Kellogg, M.D., in "New Dietetics," page 493.

(21) "New Dietetics," by J. H. Kellogg, M.D., page 491.

(22) "High Blood Pressure," by G. K. Abbott, M.D., page 48, 2nd edition.

(23) "New Dietetics," by J. H. Kellogg, M.D., page 501.

(24) Department Bulletin No. 1413, cited in "Good Health," May, 1939, page 153.

(25) "Digest of Materia Medica and Pharmacy," by Dr. Albert Merrell, cited by J. H. Kellogg, M.D., in "New Dietetics," page 503.

(26) "Health Question Box," by J. H. Kellogg, M.D., page 360.

(27) "High Blood Pressure," by G. K. Abbott, M.D., page 46.

(28) Bailey, in "Food Products, Their Source, Chemistry and Use," 1921, page 497. Quoted by Risley and Walton in "Foods, Nutrition and Clinical Dietetics," page 89.

(29) "Foods, Nutrition and Health," McCollum and Becker, pages 80, 81.

(30) "How to Live," Fisher and Fisk, page 76, 18th edition.

(31) From "Treatment of Diabetes Mellitus," by Joslin, reprinted in "Foods, Nutrition, and Clinical Dietetics," by Risley and Walton, page 187.

(32) "Common Sense in Diet," by Life Extension Institute, Inc., New York.

(33) G. K. Abbott, M.D., in "High Blood Pressure," page 20.

(34) J. H. Kellogg, M.D., in "Good Health," July, 1931, page 207.

(35) Harold C. Lueth, M.D., Ph.D., in "Journal of the American Dietetic Association" December, 1940, page 988.

(36) "Annals of Internal Medicine," June, 1941.

(37) "High Blood Pressure" by G. K. Abbott, M.D., page 104.

(38) "Philadelphia Enquirer," May 31, 1942.

(39) R. P. Cook, "Cholesterol Metabolism," in "Nutrition Abstracts and Reviews," December 1, 1942.

(40) G. K. Abbott, M.D., in "High Blood Pressure" page 104.

(41) D. H. Kress, M.D., in "Southern Tidings," February 2, 1944.

Eating for Strength

There can be no life in the body without protein.

Protein is a constituent of many of the enzymes. It enters into the formation of hemoglobin in the red corpuscle. (1)

Protein is the substance which builds and repairs tissue, including muscle, but it does not cause the muscle to move—the energy foods do that. These foods were named in the Classification of Foods. This chapter is concerned with protein, the muscle-builder.

Proteins contain carbon, hydrogen, and oxygen as do fats and carbohydrates; but to construct proteins nitrogen is added, and a small amount of sulphur; the protein in brain and nerve tissue also contains phosphorus.

Proteins are complex substance built up of amino acids, of which there are about twenty-four. (Deming 399, Weiner 56). By mysterious forces they are put together into an unlimited number of different arrangements to form the many kinds of living organisms something the same as the 28 letters of the alphabet are used to build up all of the words in the dictionary. Therefore the amino acids are sometimes called "building stones." They are absorbed from the intestines into the blood as individual "stones" and then put together to form any kind of tissue or organ as is needed.

To accomplish all of their manifold tasks all of the amino acids must be available in the body or some cell or function will suffer. Several of these amino acids are elaborated within the body so that only ten of them must be taken in foods. If a single food contains all ten, its protein is said to be "complete" or adequate. Some foods which contain all ten of them have too small a quantity of certain ones; such a deficiency needs to be made up from other foods which have an excess. Wheat is an example, as its lysine content is low, while in the soybean it is high. When 25 parts of

151

soy flour are mixed with 75 parts of wheat flour it becomes adequate for normal growth because of the extra lysine it borrowed from the soy flour, so that its protein now compares favorably with that of meat, milk, and eggs. Such estimates are usually based on patent white flour which has already lost about half of the lysine which was in the whole grain of the wheat.

Therefore when foods are properly combined, adequate protein can be secured without using any one food containing all ten amino acids. However, for the sake of safety it is well to include in the daily ration some of those foods in which all ten are found. There is good evidence that each of the following foods contains all ten of the amino acids:

Meat	Almonds	Rice, whole
Eggs	Brazil nuts	Potatoes
Milk	Wheat, when bran and	Peanuts
Soybeans	germs are included	Sweet potatoes
Garbanzas	Corn, whole	Leafy vegetable
	' Oats, whole	

Certain of these foods do not contain sufficient amounts of some of the amino acids, but they do contain all ten of them.

The proteins of grains have long been held in question by research workers who have given first place to meat, milk, and eggs. It is possible that feeding experiments were conducted with refined grains. However, during recent years when there has been a world shortage of protein foods very careful study has been given to the *germs* of the grains and they have been found to contain the essential amino acids and are now placed alongside of the animal proteins. Thus does science come one step nearer to accepting Mother Nature and revelation. The following brief clipping refers to one of the latest conclusions.

"Grade A Protein Foods"

"In an article entitled 'The Nutritive Value of Wheat Germ, Corn Germ, and Oat Proteins' Doctors Stare and Hegsted, of Harvard University, state: 'Data on the amino acid content of protein content of wheat and corn germ have recently been presented by Block and Bolling. The content of the essential amino acids compares favorably with excellent proteins such as milk and meat. It appears evident from the available studies that the proteins of these germs must be considered as essentially the equivalent of first class animal proteins, both when used as the sole protein or as protein supplements in the diet." (66)

Wheat Proteins

"That the proteins of wheat are of much higher nutritive value than those of white flour has been conclusively shown by independent experiments. . . ."

"Osborne and Mendel found that the proteins of whole wheat are in themselves sufficient for all the protein requirements of normal growth. . . ."

"Several of the legumes, including soybeans, peanuts, and our ordinary garden or field peas, contain proteins very similar chemically and nutritionally to those of meat and are well qualified for the position of main dish at dinner. Ordinary baked beans when eaten as sole protein food are not quite as efficient in protein, but become so when supplemented with the proteins of wheat as in the familiar Boston baked beans and brown bread." (67)

There exists in many minds an erroneous idea as to the best sources of protein. Many people think it is necessary to eat meat to get an adequate supply. Let it here be remembered that the proteins are not an animal product, but are elaborated by plants, and therefore the plant kingdom is the true and original source. Furthermore, it is a plentiful source.

For instance, U. S. Department of Agriculture Bulletin No. 975 on "How Foods Meet Body Needs" contains diagrams comparing the quantity of proteins in various foods, as follows:

One pound of	Contains per cent of one day's ration	One pound of	Contains per cent of one day's ration
Beef	67	Cornmeal	42
Shelled peanuts	117	Rice	36
Dried beans	102	Milk	15
Cottage cheese	95	Spinach	10
Walnuts	84	Raisins	10
Oatmeal	73	Potatoes	8
Macaroni	61	Bananas	4
Wheat	60	Honey	2
Eggs	54		

Soy bean flour contains twice as much protein as meat, and its protein is complete, and it is the cheapest source of protein. These beans have been almost the sole source of protein for the Chinese race for a hundred generations. Note in the above table those foods which contain more protein than does meat.

Proteins are much more plentiful in common foods than most people understand. Herewith is a list of foods which will be very enlightening. No meats are in this list.

Grams of Protein Contained
in Foods

Almonds, salted, 10 to 12 nuts	3.0
Almonds, chopped, 1 cup	18.00
Apple, baked, 1 large, 2 tablespoons sugar	0.5
Apple, fresh 1 large A P	0.75
Applesauce, ⅝ cup	0.25
Apricots, canned, 2 large halves with 2 T. juice	1.25
Apricots, dried, 9 halves	1.75
Apricots, dried, stewed, sweetened, ¼ cup	1.0
Apricots, fresh, A P 5 apricots	2.0
Asparagus, canned, 5 large stalks	2.0
Asparagus, fresh, 20 large stalks 8 in.	8.0
Asparagus, cream soup ½ cup	4.0
Avocado pear, 1 medium	2.5
Bananas, A P 1 medium	1.2
Beans, dried lima, one sixth cup	5.2
Beans, dried soy, 1¾ T	8.0
Beans, string, 2⅓ cups	5.5
Beets, ⅔ cup	2.0
Beet greens, cooked, 2¼ cups	4.0
Blackberries, fresh, ½ cup	2.2
Bread, Boston brown, 1 slice, 3 in. x 3 in. x ¾ in.	2.5
Bread, white, 2 slices, 3 in. x 3½ in. x ½ in.	2.2
Bran porridge, ⅝ cup	4.5
Bran, unwashed, 1 cup	4.5
Brazil nuts, shelled, 2 nuts	2.5
Bread, whole wheat with raisins, 1 slice, 3¾ in. x 3⅛ in. x ½ in.	2.7
Butter, 1 T	0.0
Buttermilk, 1 cup	7.2
Cantaloupe, A P 4½ in. diameter	1.5
Carrots, chopped, 1⅔ cup	2.5
Carrots, fresh, grated, 1 T	0.25
Cauliflower, 1 small head	5.7
Celery, chopped, 4 cups	6.0
Celery, cream soup, ½ cup	2.5
Cottage cheese, 5 T	10.0
Corn, ½ cup	3.0
Corn, cream soup, ½ cup	3.0
Corn meal, uncooked, 1 cup	13.0
Cranberries, 2 cups	0.75
Cream, thick, 40% fat, 1 T	0.25
Cream, 40% fat, 1 cup	4.0
Cup custard, ⅓ cup	4.0
Currants, dried, 1 cup	4.0
Dates, stoned, 1 cup	4.0
Eggs in shell, 1	6.0
Eggs, scrambled, ¼ cup	5.0
Egg white, 1	3.2

Egg yolk, 1	2.75
Figs, dried, 1½ large	1.25
Flour, white, sifted, 1 cup	12.5
Grapefruit, A P ½ large	1.75
Grapes, Malaga, 20 to 25	1.2
Hickory nuts, A P 12 to 15	2.2
Honey, 1 T	0.25
Ice Cream, Commercial, ¼ cup	1.0
Lemons, A P 3 large	2.2
Lentils, dried, 2½ T	7.2
Lettuce, 2 large heads	6.2
Macaroni, cooked, ¾ cup	4.0
Milk, malted, 3 T	3.5
Milk, whole, 1 cup	8.5
Milk, skimmed, 1 cup	8.0
Milk, Soy bean	8.5
Muffins, corn meal, 1, 2¾ in. diameter	4.2
Oatmeal cookies with raisins, 1, 3 in. diameter	3.0
Oats, rolled, cooked, ½ cup	4.0
Okra, 5 to 6 pods, small	0.75
Olives, ripe, 5	0.4
Onions, 3 to 4 medium	3.0
Peanut butter, 1 T	4.75
Peas, ½ cup	7.0
Peas, split dried, 1 cup	47.0
Pecans, 8	1.5
Potatoes, baked, Irish, 1 medium	2.7
Prunes, A P 4 medium	0.75
Radishes, 1 dozen red	1.5
Raisins, seeded, ¼ cup	0.75
Rice, steamed, ¾ cup	2.2
Spinach, cooked, 1 cup	1.2
Spinach, cream soup, ⅔ cup	4.0
Squash, Hubbard, cooked, ½ cup	1.5
Strawberries, fresh, 1⅓ cups	2.5
Tapioca, cream, ½ cup	3.0
Tomatoes, canned, 1 cup	3.0
Tomato, cream soup, ⅝ cup	2.7
Turnip greens, cooked, 2½ cups	9.0
Waldorf salad, ½ cup	2.0
Walnuts, 3	2.6
Watercress, 5 small bunches	3.0
Walnuts, chopped, 1 cup	15.7
Wheat, shredded, 1 biscuit	3.0
Yeast, 1 cake	1.5
Zwieback, 3 pieces, 3¼ in. x 1¼ in. x ½ in.	2.2
Flour, whole wheat, sifted 1 cup	15.0

T means "tablespoon" A P means "as purchased"

GRAMS OF PROTEIN CONTAINED IN FOODS (*Continued*)

SPECIAL FOODS

Soy cheese, slice 3" diameter, ¾" thick ......26.7 grams protein
Stakelets, slice 3" diameter, ¾" thick ....15.1 grams protein
Vigorost, slice 3" diameter, ¾" thick ....18.4 grams protein

Used by permission from "Food for Life" and other sources.

The average percentages of protein contained in dried fruits and vegetables are given as follows:

Alfalfa, with water	18.00
Apples	2.60
Apricots	8.70
Artichokes	9.00
Asparagus	28.80
Barley	12.70
Beets	12.80
Blackberries	8.80
Brussels Sprouts	23.80
Cherries	5.00
Carrots	7.70
Cauliflower	27.70
Celery	20.00
Corn	11.20
Cucumbers	27.30
Dandelions	20.00
Eggplant	17.00
Figs	7.40
Garlic	19.00
Grapes	6.00
Green Corn	12.60
Huckleberries	3.70
Kohlrabi	35.00
Leeks	22.60
Lettuce	24.50
Mushrooms	23.80
Olives	7.50
Oranges	6.10
Oats	11.90
Onions	12.90
Okra	15.80
Pears	4.00
Prunes	4.40
Plums	4.70
Pineapples	4.80
Peaches	6.60
Potatoes	8.00
Pumpkins	11.00

Parsnips	9.00
Raspberries	7.00
Raspberries, black	10.00
Rice	9.00
Rutabagas	12.00
Radishes	14.70
Rye	13.50
St. John's Bread	6.80
Savoy cabbage	26.00
Spinach	30.00
Salsify	29.40
Swiss Chard	20.40
Tomatoes	15.80
Turnips	35.00
Wheat, whole	15.70

These foods present the primary sources of proteins. (65)

From this list it becomes perfectly apparent that there is no need for eating the flesh of animals in order to secure an adequate protein ration. This will be still clearer as we proceed in this chapter.

A Day's Supply of Protein

What is a day's supply of protein and how may one know that he secures enough and no more?

It should be understood that muscular activity results in very little wearing away of the tissue so that only small amounts are needed for repair. An excess is injurious.

The long-accepted Chittenden standard of Calories called for the 2½ ounces mentioned on previous pages, which is about seventy grams. Authorities do not all agree on this point but the trend is downward, as the following statement shows:

"One of the lessons derived from the war was demonstration of the fact that throughout the whole civilized world there was an excessive consumption of meat, especially in Great Britain. Studies of Taylor, Benedict, Roth, Lusk, Sherman, and others—especially those of Sherman, since the war—have shown that the protein requirement is far lower than even Chittenden maintained many years ago." (3)

"At a meeting of the interallied Council of Physiologists during the war it was decided that meat was not a physiological necessity. The following statement was made: 'It is not thought desirable to fix a minimum meat ration, in view of the fact that no absolute physiological need exists for meat, since the proteins of meat can be replaced by other proteins of animal origin—such as contained in milk, cheese, and eggs—as well as by proteins of vegetable origin.' " (4)

"There is no danger of protein deficiency except in poverty or famine, and in diseases preventing eating, or absorption of food from the digestive tract." (5)

"Surely we need no longer worry lest a few days' shortage of nitrogen (protein elements) in the intake will lead to a prompt nutritive debacle, so long as the supply of the other essentials is not threatened." (6)

"Reliable human experiments have shown a necessity of not over forty grams of protein a day for a man of 154 pounds weight, even though 60 grams may be taken without harm, and be a safer rule. Kon and Klein, of Warsaw, kept two adults (man and woman) in protein equilibrium and in good health for a period of 167 days on a diet the protein of which was derived solely from the potato. The protein intake for the man was 35.6 grams daily, and for the woman 23.7 grams daily."

"Hindhede, of Copenhagen, kept a man in a perfect state of nutrition and in full working capacity for many months on a diet the protein of which was derived solely from the potato, averaging 23 grams daily. One man has been seventeen years on various diets low in protein, and is in perfect health and is doing hard work." (7)

"Demonstration of ability to maintain health and to do vigorous physical work on a very low protein ration, is given by a German, Dr. C. Rose. He lived for fifteen years on an average daily protein intake of thirty-eight to forty grams (one to one and one-third ounces). During an experimental period lasting for several years, he took only twenty-six grams, at times dropping to twenty. When he was almost seventy, he climbed several mountains, over four thousand meters (13,000 feet) in height. A friend, Dr. Schmidt, a Swiss, also ate only thirty to forty grams of vegetable protein daily for twenty-five months. In this period he made twenty-two mountain ascents, some of them very difficult, without signs of great fatigue. He, however, was only thirty-five years old." (8)

A man weighing 154 pounds needs only 44.4 grams of protein daily. Americans average 106, more than double the amount needed. (9)

Sherman states that many hundreds of diets have been examined without finding one of them deficient in protein if the caloric values were sufficient. (10)

When considering the amount of protein needed one should know that when the total diet contains the right proportion of alkaline foods he does not need as much protein as formerly because the abundance of alkalies causes a saving of protein so that a smaller amount of protein will accomplish as much work now as the larger amount formerly did when the ration was too strongly acid-forming. For this reason the vegetarian needs less protein than those who eat animal foods. This is a very important point. Following is a scientific report on this point:

"A big excess of bases in the organism as well as in the food is a necessary precondition for an optional utilization of protein.

"Therefore, a real minimum for protein requirement can be found only when there exists an excess of bases in the organism as well as in the food.

"With the increase of the excess of acids in the food as well as in the organism itself the nitrogen requirement mounts uninterruptedly until finally the physiological impossibility of an immediate excretion of the by-products through the kidneys prevents a further rise and produces the illusion of a storage." (11)

The present author is an untiring observer of the trends of nutritionists, and has been deeply impressed by the fact that in several matters scientists are slowly coming to conclusions which are in accord with instruction given long ago in writings which have been his guide throughout his lifetime in studying and teaching the principles of nutrition and healthful living. The instructions referred to have never yet been proven to be wrong in any matter. Following are a few statements taken from them, with the dates when they were first given, which indicate clearly that a ration relatively low in protein is correct.

(1870) "Some fall into the error that because they discard meat, they do not need to supply its place with the best fruits and vegetables, prepared in their most natural state, free from grease and spices." (55)

(1883) "Meat is not essential for health or strength, else the Lord made a mistake when He provided food for Adam and Eve before their fall. All the elements of nutrition are contained in the fruits, vegetables, and grains." (56)

(1890) "Where plenty of good milk and fruit can be obtained, there is rarely any excuse for eating animal food." (57)

(1902) "Parents can secure small homes in the country, with land for cultivation, where they can have orchards and where they can raise vegetables and small fruits to take the place of flesh meat; which is so corrupting to the life-blood coursing through the veins." (58)

(1905) "When flesh is discarded, its place should be supplied with a variety of grains, nuts, vegetables, and fruits." (59)

(1905) "It is a mistake to suppose that muscular strength depends on the use of animal food. . . . The grains, with fruits, nuts, and vegetables contain all the nutritive properties necessary to make good blood." (60)

(1901) "There must be other ingredients combined with the nuts, which will harmonize with them, and not use such a large proportion of nuts. One-tenth to one-sixth part of nuts would be sufficient, varied according to combinations." (61)

(1905) "With nuts may be combined grains, fruits, and some roots, to make foods that are healthful and nourishing. Care should be taken, however, not to use too large a proportion of nuts. Those who realize ill effects from the use of nut foods may find the difficulty removed by attending to this precaution." (62)

None of these statements indicate that a large amount of protein is needed. The high protein foods mentioned are the nuts which we are instructed to mix with other foods so that the nut content will be small. They also indicate that the protein supply may be obtained wholly from the vegetable kingdom.

Therefore, the vegetarian diet, high in alkaline foods as directed in this book and in the Automatic Menu Planner, calls for a minimum amount of protein, 40 to 60 grams, and constitutes the ideal diet.

The Ministry of Health of Great Britain and the nutrition committee of the British Medical Association have agreed "that accumulated evidence indicates that the total daily need for protein per man unit probably lies between 80 and 100 grams. (50) It is understood that a large part of this protein would come from meat, an acid-forming food. Thirty-six per cent of the protein in American diets comes from grains, also acid-forming. Therefore the high alkaline balance secured by our Menu Planner is not anticipated by these authorities. Their high acid-forming diet requires more protein, as already explained. Our plan of getting no protein from meat or eggs, less from grains, and more from alkaline sources particularly the soybean and other legumes, makes practical the lower protein ration suggested by our Automatic Menu Planner.

Between the standard in our Menu Planner and the British standard the readers of this book will be able to adjust their protein requirement to the individual needs. They are asked to remember that excess protein cannot be stored, and is not as readily converted into heat and energy as are other foods and consequently must be excreted by the kidneys, and is counted as one cause of injury to those organs. It has been shown that an excess of vegetable protein is not as injurious as the same excess of animal protein, and therefore the vegetarian might safely consume protein up to the higher standards.

The following tables, by G. K. Abbott, M. D., show how easy it is to eat unwittingly a dangerous excess of protein. If one wishes to secure his entire protein ration without using either milk or eggs, the chapter "The Ideal Vegetarian Regimen" explains how this can be done.

Suggestion No. 1	Grams
Milk, 1 cup	8.1
Cottage cheese, 2 tbsp.	6.0
Cereal, 1 serving	2.0
Bread, 6 slices	19.2
Almonds, 10 small	2.1
Potatoes, 1 serving	4.4
Total Protein	41.8

Suggestion No. 2	Grams
Milk, 2 cups	16.2
Bread, 3 slices	9.6
Potatoes, 1 serving	4.4
Spinach, 1 serving	2.4
Oatmeal, 1 serving	2.0
Green peas, 1 serving	5.7
Tapioca pudding, 1 ser.	3.3
Total Protein	43.6

Suggestion No. 3	Grams
Milk, 2 cups	16.2
Bread, 3 slices	9.6
Egg, 1	6.7
Baked beans ½ cup	8.0
Oatmeal, 1 serving	2.0
Potatoes, 1 serving	4.4
Total Protein	46.9

Example of meals with average protein ration for the day of from 40 to 60 grams:

Breakfast

3 tablespoons oatmeal
2 tablespoons cream
9 dates
1 dozen ripe olives
2 tablespoons apricots

3 tablespoons fresh strawberries
1 slice 100% entire-wheat bread toasted
1 tablespoon vegetable butter

Dinner

2½ tablespoons squash, or
  1 baked potato
  1 large onion, boiled
  7 stalks creamed aspara-
    gus
  3 tablespoons carrots

Raw tomato and lettuce
  salad
Half cantaloupe
2 tablespoons stewed pea-
  nuts
1 tablespoon cottage cheese

Supper

1 baked apple
6 tablespoons cherries

1 slice 100% entire-wheat
  bread

The above provides about 2100 calories of food, and contains about fifty grams of protein. If more calories are eaten there will of course be more protein eaten.

Example of low protein ration of about 25 grams (to lower blood pressure) :

Breakfast

1 shredded wheat biscuit
  with 1 tablespoon of cream
1 orange or 1 slice pineapple

1 dozen ripe olives
4 figs
1 small banana

Dinner

1 small baked potato with
  vegetable butter
3 tablespoons carrots
1 heart of lettuce

3 tablespoons string beans
1 small tomato
3 tablespoons spinach

Supper

1 orange
2 heaping tablespoons apple-
  sauce

1 slice 100% entire-wheat
  bread, toasted, with vegetable butter

The above provides a total of 1,100 calories, which is intended to reduce body weight, as many people with high blood pressure are overweight. If the person is not overweight, more fruit may be added to the breakfast and supper and more low protein vegetables may be added to the dinner.

Meat Not Necessary

Further opinion is here given that meat is not a necessary article of diet. Literature on this point is so voluminous in the various nations that an entire book would be required to reprint them. Only a few are given here.

"Even the most ardent advocates of a meat diet can not produce any scientific evidence to show that intestinal putrefaction to high degree is in any way beneficial to the organism; hence, in seeking the best form of diet, meat as a source of protein may well be excluded and the requisite protein secured from milk, nuts, cereals, and vegetables. If in the average diet a pint of milk daily is substituted for whatever meat portions have theretofore been taken, there would be no danger of protein lack." (12)

"I have not the slightest hesitation in saying that a vegetarian diet, supplemented with fairly liberal amounts of milk, is the most satisfactory type of diet that man can take. . . . I feel that you would be doing much better by your patients than is now being done in many of the best hospitals in the land, where patients are attempting to recover from wasting diseases or from surgical operations on diets of the cereal, tuber, muscle meat type. Palatable and attractive as they may be, I feel confident that they are not very satisfactory as human foods when adhered to over appreciable periods." (13)

"I am convinced that anyone who eats the average amount of meat consumed in this country will improve, rather than suffer, by cutting it all out of his diet. Meats greatly increase intestinal putrefaction. There is no other class of foods which so greatly tends to promote intestinal putrefaction and unwholesome decomposition products." (14)

"The first element of treatment (for cancer) is an absolutely correct vegetarian diet, with the avoidance of coffee and alcohol in every form. A vegetarian diet needs no defense, for millions of human beings naturally live thus and escape cancer, and those in civilized lands are adopting it for health." (15)

"That it is easily possible to sustain life on the products of the vegetable kingdom, needs no demonstration for physiologists, even if a majority of the human race were not constantly engaged in demonstrating it; and my researches show, not only that it is possible, but that it is infinitely preferable in every way, and produces superior powers of both mind and body." (16)

The long disputed question of the value of wheat protein compared with protein from animal sources seems at last to be coming to a settlement in favor of wheat.

E. V. McCollum states that the growth value of the protein of whole wheat is a little higher than that of milk or eggs. (63)

A report of the rat feeding tests made in the Pillsbury Research Laboratory gives the comparative biological value of wheat as follows:

Wheat germ 2.12 Skim milk 1.83 Egg white 2.02 Casein 1% cystine 1.88 and then comments,—

"From these results it can be concluded that wheat-germ protein is at least as good in quality as are the animal proteins." (64)

A notable health magazine editor in commenting on this report said,—"Thus, one ounce of wheat germ contains as much protein as two-thirds of an ounce of average meat and four ounces of milk and protein that is equal to that of milk and meat. . . . An ounce or two daily will be sufficient to insure a plentiful supply of excellent protein and without meat, milk, eggs, or other protein of animal origin." (65)

"Soy beans and soy bean products constitute the chief source of protein food of hundreds of millions of people—Chinese, Japanese, Koreans, and Manchus. Soy beans play a much greater role in the nutrition of these people than does wheat in this country, or rye in Germany, Scandinavia, and the U.S.S.R., for, unlike the cereals, which are chiefly used in the preparation of baked products (mostly bread), soy beans are converted into numerous products which can be substituted, in a general way for such foods as cow's milk, cheese, eggs, and meat. For nearly fifty centuries the people of the Orient have subsisted on the products of the soy bean, and hundreds of millions of these people have never even known the taste of cow's milk. While these people are essentially vegetarians, the protein fraction of their diet, supplied or supplemented largely from soy bean products, is adequate and, according to Horvath, their diet is well-balanced. It is well known, furthermore, that the soy bean eaters of Northern China have greater stamina than the inhabitants of Southern China who subsist largely on rice. The soy bean is a highly nutritional and adequate food." (17)

"Cuthbertson, writing in *"Nutrition Abstracts and Reviews"* in 1940 stated 'there is no need to include protein of an animal origin in the diet of man whatever the needs to be satisfied, provided that the choice of plant foods is not too restricted.' " (51)

"All the evidence from both animal experimentation and human experience supports in a manner that can never be broken down the viewpoint that meat is not necessary in the human diet." (18)

"I have not the slightest hesitation in saying that a vegetarian diet, supplemented with fairly liberal amounts of milk, is the most satisfactory type of diet that man can take." (19)

DENMARK'S FOOD EXPERIMENT

"It seemed desperate, but the solution was nevertheless extremely simple. The fact merely was that both people and pigs could not live. In Germany the pigs were allowed to live, and therefore the people died. In Denmark we killed our pigs, and lived directly on pigs' food—their barley and potatoes. We took all the wheat bran from the cows, and put it in our whole-rye bread. The half of our bread consisted of bran."

"Moreover, we took the grains from the distillers, which left us without brandy and whiskey, while the English deprived us of coffee. Some doctors were angry, and wrote that Hindhede put the people on pig food, and hen food. Yes, I did. It was my intention to put my people on pig food, a natural diet, to show how foolish we humans have lived!"

"The whole country was placed on a low protein diet. Believers in high protein suggested that the resistance against disease would decrease. My expectations were to the contrary. Who won? Well, the result was a great victory for the low protein diet. The state of health improved as never before. The doctors lost their business. The death rate went down during this period of rationing, October 1, 1917, to October 1, 1918, to 10.4 per one thousand, the lowest known death rate of any European country at any time." (20)

Thus does science today confirm as correct the counsel given many years ago for the guidance of a group of workers entrusted with the responsibility of operating the largest chain of sanitariums in the world, beginning with Battle Creek in 1866 and circling the globe.

Note this example written in 1906:

"In grains, vegetables, fruits, and nuts are to be found all the food elements that we need." (54)

SIXTEEN REASONS FOR VEGETARIANISM

(1) *Avoid Excess Protein*

Those who eat meat are almost surely getting too much protein, as has already been made plain. Americans eat much more protein than is needed. Therefore a "meat substitute" is no more necessary than is meat. The need is for a balanced ration. The meat "substitutes" are useful in satisfying the appetite and in preparing attractive and tasty foods when meat is discarded, but when used, other heavy protein foods should be omitted so as to avoid excess.

(2) *Animal Tissue Wastes*

Meats all contain the poisonous wastes of the cells, which are on the way to the lungs, skin, and kidneys for elimination. A major problem in the human body is to eliminate its own wastes, and when the wastes of animals are added, they become a menace. Meat extracts and broths contain practically no food value and are heavily loaded with wastes similar to uric acid.

"Dogs fed with extracts of meat die more rapidly than dogs which receive nothing at all. A person in health may use extracts of meat in small quantities, but it is necessary to prohibit meat extract for invalids." (21)

"Says Gautier with further reference to these extractives: 'We must not forget that these bases are poisonous.' ...

"According to the analyses of Gautier, a quart of beef tea contains enough creatin to kill nine guinea pigs, besides potash salts, purin bodies and other substances even more toxic than creatin."

"Meat extracts of all sorts are concentrated preparations of the toxins of meat." (22)

(3) *Meat Stimulants*

The toxic substances in meat are stimulating. A half pound of meat contains one and a half times the nerve stimulant found in one ounce of dry tea. The reason the meat-eater misses his meat and feels weak when he does not get it is not because it gave him strength but because he did not get his accustomed stimulant—the same reason the coffee drinker misses his coffee. (23)

(4) *Meat Is Acid-forming*

Meat is highly acid-forming. The harm resulting from acidosis has been explained in a previous chapter. A balanced ration does not call for meat and has no room for it.

(5) *Lacks Minerals and Vitamins*

Meat is lacking in minerals and vitamins and so contributes to deficiency diseases.

(6) *Hyperacidity*

Meat contributes to hyperacidity of the stomach. This was explained in a previous chapter.

(7) *Meat Is Constipating*

Oysters, fish, fowl, and meats of all kinds putrefy rapidly and contribute to constipation.

(8) *Degenerates Vital Organs*

This has been explained in the previous chapter. The opinion of one additional writer is offered here:

A meat diet acidifies the blood and diminishes the oxidation. It charges the humours of the system with a superabundance of nitrogenous wastes, uric acid in particular; it increases the urinary alkaloids; it congests the liver; it brings on obstinate constipation and causes dyspepsia, gastric difficulties and enteritis; it leads to psoriasis, eczema, etc.; it develops rheumatic, arthritic, gouty and nervous tendencies. An alimentation not even exclusive, but only too rich in meat, could not be endured for long. It produces arterial hypertension and heart fatigue, and becomes one of the most active predisposing causes of arteriosclerosis (Buchard). M. Houssaye has shown that in the case of birds, a carnivorous diet produces sterility, arrest of development and an excessive proportion of males (C. Rend. 1903). (24)

Furthermore, meat extractives are a favorite ingredient of media used for the growth of bacteria in the laboratory. They likewise assist in the growth of bacteria in man.

(9) *Loads of Bacteria*

Microscopic count has been made of the bacteria to be found in meats of various kinds so that people may know what they are getting when they eat meat.

	Bacteria per Gram	
Beefsteak	1,500,000	
Corned beef	31,000,000	
Hamburger steak	75,000,000	
Pork Liver	95,000,000	
Limburger cheese	18,000,000	(25)

It is interesting to compare the above figures with the number of bacteria found in manure.

	Bacteria per Gram	
Oyster juice	3,400,000	
Fresh droppings of calf	15,000,000	
Fresh droppings of goat	20,000,000	
Fresh droppings of horse	25,000,000	(26)

Perhaps a deeper impression can be made by looking at a table giving the number of putrefactive bacteria in each ounce of food.

	When Purchased	Putrefactive Bacteria per Ounce After 20 Hours at room Temperature
Small sausage	19,800,000,000	19,200,000,000
Roast beef	16,800,000,000	22,500,000,000
Round steak	16,800,000,000	25,200,000,000
Large sausage	12,600,000,000	14,700,000,000
Sirloin steak	11,340,000,000	—————
Tenderloin (rare)	5,040,000,000	—————
Hamburger steak	3,870,000,000	21,000,000,000
Pork	3,781,000,000	31,000,000,000
Smoked ham	1,293,600,000	22,500,000,000
Porterhouse steak	900,000,000	21,000,000,000
Tenderloin (well-done)	756,000,000	(27)

If we multiply these figures by sixteen we get these foods by the pound, the way most people buy them. The farther we proceed in this study the less interesting it becomes.

Oysters seem to be a very good source of bacteria, as this report shows:

"A few years ago a paper by Hindman and Goodrich, of the University of Washington, published the results of an extended study of bacteria of oysters and oyster juice, which showed from 100,000,000 to 200,000,000 bacteria to the teaspoonful of juice. These bacteria were not of the innocent kind such as those which produce sour milk, but were gas-producing organisms of the sort which cause putrefaction. These pernicious organisms were found in great abundance, in one series in twenty-three out of twenty-four specimens. In another series the gas-producing organisms were found in all but one of twenty-two specimens." (28)

If two colon germs are found in a glass of water, it is condemned as unsanitary because they can multiply to be millions tomorrow.

The standard for certified milk is 1,000,000 to the glassful.

If the law concerning water were applied to milk it would require all milk to be thoroughly sterilized; and if it were applied to meat, it would utterly destroy the meat business. (29)

(10) *Disease from Animals*

Eating the flesh of animals is the most prolific source of human disease. Not only does it contribute to the degenerative diseases discussed in a previous chapter, and fill the body with putrefactive bacteria, but often the animals themselves are afflicted with diseases which may be passed on to the consumer.

The prevalence of disease among domestic animals, and the increasing frequency at which these occur among human beings, are of so great importance that it seems best to devote a section of this book to authoritative statements setting forth the existing conditions and the dangers confronting us from this source. See the chapter on "Animal Kingdom A Reservoir of Disease."

CANCER

It would hardly be fair to the reader if we did not include the opinions of several eminent medical authors concerning the relation of the use of meat to the incidence of cancer.

"The best dietetic method of combating a cancerous hereditary tendency is to give up flesh foods entirely, to reduce the quantity of starchy foods and cereals, and to increase to a larger extent the use of salads, fresh vegetables, fruits, and oils." (30)

"What we should do then, if we would avoid cancer, is to eat whole-wheat bread and raw fruits and vegetables, shunning all meat; first, that we may be better nourished; second, that we may more easily eliminate waste products, and thus adequately drain the house in which our cells live."

"Whoever will correct his diet to a reasonable extent, take reasonable exercise, and keep his digestive tract absolutely clean, need have no fear of cancer." (31)

"Indigestion and constipation are the starting causes of the diseases of civilization."

"If you wish to produce cancer with a fair degree of certainty, supply a constipated subject with plenty of meat, and endeavor to deal with his constipation by means of irritating purgative drugs." (32)

(11) *Not a "Strength" Food as Supposed to Be*

A few records of tests are given here. A mass of material could be exhibited because such tests have been numerous. These few will suffice:

(a) Running Test

Race of 125 miles:

Entrants—thirty-two persons, of whom twelve were meat-eaters and twenty were vegetarians.

The race was won by a vegetarian eight hours ahead of the foremost meat-eater. He had been a vegetarian for nine years, and ate two meals daily.

Only three meat-eaters finished in forty-five hours.

Ten vegetarians finished in forty-five hours.

(b) Holding the arms extended

Meat-eaters averaged .... 10 min.
Vegetarians averaged .... 49 min.
Longest time held by a meat-eater was .... 20 min.
Longest time held by a vegetarian was .... 200 min.

(c) Deep knee bending

Meat-eaters averaged .... 383 times
Vegetarians averaged .... 833 times

(d) Arm holding

"The first comparison (for arm holding) shows a great superiority on the side of the flesh-abstainers. Even the maximum record of the flesh-eaters was barely more than half the average for the flesh-abstainers. Only two of the fifteen flesh-eaters succeeded in holding their arms over a quarter of an hour; whereas twenty-two of the thirty-two abstainers surpassed that limit. None of the flesh-eaters reached half an hour, but fifteen of the thirty-two abstainers exceeded that limit. Of these, nine exceeded an hour, four exceeded two fours, and one exceeded three hours." (36)

"A group of eleven soldiers and another of eight college athletes were chosen upon which to experiment. Both were accustomed to a mixed diet, that is, a high-protein diet including flesh foods, eggs, cheese, and beans. Such a diet contains from 100 to 120 grams (30 grams to the ounce—about three or four ounces) of albuminous or protein material. They were carefully examined, and placed upon a diet containing 48 grams of protein in the daily ration. No attempt was made to make the diet exclusively vegetarian, but, of course, very little flesh foods could be given with this reduction in protein content. The tables below give the strength tests at the beginning and the close of five months on such a diet. Both groups were kept in good physical condition by systematic exercise.

(e) Soldier Group		
	October	April
Broyles	2560	5530
Coffman	2835	6269
Cohn	2210	4002
Fritz	2504	5178
Henderson	2970	4598
Loewenthal	2463	5277
Morris	2543	4869
Oakman	3445	5055
Sliney	3245	5307
Steltz	2838	4581
Zooman	3070	5757

(f) Athletic Group		
	January	June
W. W. Anderson	4913	5722
W. L. Anderson	6016	9472
Bellis	5993	8165
Callahan	2154	3983
Donahue	4584	5917
Jacobus	4548	5667
Schenker	5728	7135
Stapleton	5351	6833
		(37)

(g) *Fifty-three per cent higher*

"Ioteyko, in determining the endurance of individuals by means of the ergograph, found vegetarians to exceed the meat-eaters by fifty-three per cent in mechanical work done." (38)

Flesh-eating animals do not have the endurance of those which eat no flesh. (39)

(12) *Filled with Fatigue*

A further explanation of why meat-eaters tire more quickly than vegetarians should be made.

"The chemical changes which occur in muscle tissue during work afford a clear explanation of the diminished endurance of meat-eaters, either animals or men, when compared with vegetable feeders.

"During contraction, lactic acid is produced in the muscle tissue. While the muscle is relaxing, the acid is neutralized by the alkalies present in the tissue fluids. This enables the muscle to contract again. Later, after relaxation, the lactic acid is burned up by the oxygen of the blood stream. Fatigue begins as soon as the lactic acid begins to accumulate in the muscle.

"It is evident that if the tissue fluids are only slightly alkaline, fatigue will occur sooner than if they are more strongly alkaline. The tissue fluids of flesh-eaters are much less alkaline than those of vegetable feeders, as shown by the fact that the urine of flesh-eaters is always highly acid. This is one of the reasons why mixed feeders invariably show themselves inferior to flesh-abstainers in tests of endurance." (40)

But that is not all. Not only does the meat hinder the disposal of the lactic acid, but it carries within it the fatigue wastes of the animal so that the meat-eater adds the weariness of the animal to his own. All animal tissue is wearing out and being rebuilt. These wastes are acid, and will add to the fatigue of the eater. The vegetarian rests five times faster than the meat-eater. (41)

(13) *A Second-Hand Food*

The animal gets the first benefit of the food which came from the earth, and the eater of the animal gets the second—what is left.

(14) *Not a Natural Food; Is Cruel*

It is not natural that life be taken for human food. If the meat-eater had to kill and dress his own meat, very few would eat it. I will not ask another man to follow the conscience-hardening occupation of constantly taking life that I may have food, even if it were a good food.

"Some animals that are brought to the slaughter seem to realize by instinct what is to take place, and they become furious and literally mad. They are killed while in that state, and their flesh is prepared for market. Their meat is poison, and has produced, in those who have eaten it, cramps, convulsions, apoplexy, and sudden death. Yet the cause of all this suffering is not attributed to the meat. Some animals are inhumanely treated while being brought to the slaughter. They are literally tortured, and after they have endured many hours of extreme suffering, are butchered." (52)

"The moral evils of a flesh diet are not less marked than are the physical ills. . . . Think of the cruelty to animals that meat-eating involves, and its effect on those who behold it. How it destroys the tenderness with which we should regard these creatures of God!

"The intelligence displayed by many dumb animals approaches so closely to human intelligence that it is a mystery. The animals see and hear and love and fear and suffer. They use their organs far more faithfully than many human beings use theirs. They manifest sympathy and tenderness toward their companions in suffering. Many animals show an affection for those who have charge of them far superior to the affection shown by some of the human race. They form attachments for man which are not broken without great suffering to them.

"What man with a human heart, who has ever cared for domestic animals, could look into their eyes, so full of confidence and affection, and willingly give them over to the butcher's knife? How could he devour their flesh as a sweet morsel." (53)

A GUILTLESS FEAST

No flocks that roam the valley free
To slaughter I condemn;
Taught by the power that pities me,
I learn to pity them.

> But from the mountain's grassy side
> A guiltless feast I bring;
> A script with herbs and fruits supplied,
> And water from the spring.
>
> *—Goldsmith*

(15) *Expensive*

The reason for the high cost of animal-derived foods is that much land, labor and expense are required to produce feed for stock, 80 to 90 per cent of which is lost in producing the animals, so that the eater of the animals gets only a small per cent of the value of the land and feed used to grow the animals. For instance, it is claimed that 100 acres of potatoes will feed 420 persons for one year, while 100 acres of grass fed to cattle will grow enough beeves to feed only 15 people for a year. A fat ox has eaten 64 pounds of dry grain for every pound his carcass weighs. Therefore if people would live directly from the products of the soil, many more people could live from a hundred acres than by getting their living from the animals which lived off the same hundred acres. In the United States the livestock consume enough food to supply five hundred million people. (42)

(16) *Character*

The eating of flesh more or less affects the disposition, the morals, and the character. A great deal might be said on this point, but we will let the opinions of a few writers express it all.

In one of his masterly works, Materlinck wrote as follows in regard to a fleshless diet:

"It was only yesterday that man learned that he had probably erred hitherto in the choice of his nourishment, . . . that a little fruit or milk, a few vegetables, farinaceous substances—now the mere accessories of the too plentiful repast he works so hard to provide—. . . are amply sufficient to maintain the ardor of the finest and mightiest life. It must be admitted that of the objections urged against vegetarianism, not one can withstand a loyal and scrupulous inquiry. I for my part can affirm that those whom I have known to submit themselves to this regimen have found its result to be improved or restored health, marked addition to strength and the acquisition by the mind of a clearness, brightness, well-being, such as might follow the release from some secular, loathsome, detestable dungeon. Were the belief one day to become general that man could well dispense with flesh food, there would ensue not only a great economic revolution, but a moral improvement as well. . . ."

For we find that a man who will give up meat will give up alcohol also, and to do this is to renounce most of the coarser and more degraded pleasures of life." (43)

Gautier Observes:

"Carnivorous animals are generally fierce and dangerous, whilst the herbivora, on the contrary, are easy to live with and to domesticate. More or less exclusive carnivorous alimentation is, to a greater extent even than race, one of the factors of the gentle or violent character of an individual. It is known that the white rats of our laboratories, as long as they are fed on bread or grain, are very manageable and easy to tame, whilst they become snappy and given to biting from the time they are fed on flesh. The same observations have been made in the case of a horse and even of a dog, although the latter is omnivourous. Liebig relates that a bear kept at the museum at Giessen was gentle and quiet when it was fed exclusively on bread and vegetables, but a few days of animal diet caused it to become fierce and dangerous to its keeper. They used to amuse themselves by thus periodically altering the animal's character. It is known, adds Liebig, that the irascibility of pigs may be increased by a meat diet to such an extent as to cause them to attack men (*Nouvelles tellres sur la chimie; 35th letter*)."

"Its (vegetarianism) advantages are those which result from temperance: by this method of alimentation the tendency to arthritic, gouty or rheumatic diathesis, to neurasthenia, etc., disappears or is weakened; the character becomes supple and the mind seems to enjoy more rest and perhaps acuteness."

"I have shown what the influence of meat food is on the character of animals. As to the action of a vegetarian diet on the intelligence, here is the opinion of two celebrated men who were keen observers of themselves."

"Writing to his friend Firmus, who gave up the Pythagorean doctrine to eat meat, the philosopher Porphyre says:—

" 'It is not amongst the eaters of simple and vegetable foods, but amongst the eaters of flesh that assassins, tyrants and thieves are met with. . . . I cannot believe that your change of diet is due to reasons of health, for you yourself have constantly affirmed that a vegetable diet is much more suitable than any other, not only to give perfect health but even a philosophic and balanced judgment, as a long experience had taught you.' "

"And Seneca, who, preoccupied with the same considerations had slowly adopted vegetarianism, writes (Epistol., 108) : 'Struck by such arguments, I also have given up the use of the flesh of animals, and at the end of a year my new habits have become not only easy to me, but delicious; and it even seems to me that my intellectual aptitudes have been more developed.'" (45)

"If the main objective point of progress among mankind were peacefulness and quiet, and the life in common—as in Paradise—of wild and tame animals, without mutual annihilation, an exclusively vegetarian diet would be the best way to attain this result. A quieting influence is exerted upon the mind by such a diet, and violent criminals may be subdued by means of it." (46)

"Flesh food has a tendency to animalize the nature, to rob men and women of that love and sympathy which they should feel for everyone, and to give the lower passions control over the higher powers of the being." (47)

Meat "excites the animal propensities to increased activity, and strengthens the animal passions. When the animal propensities are increased, the intellectual and moral powers are decreased. The use of the flesh of animals tends to cause a grossness of body, and benumbs the fine sensibilities of the mind." (48)

"Meat should not be placed before our children. Its influence is to excite and strengthen the lower passions, and has a tendency to deaden the moral powers." (49)

Nobility of character is of far higher value than strength of muscle, and if there were to be a choice between the two, the former should be preferred, but in the case under consideration the right food increases both. The conquest of the appetite is fundamental to the development of character. To conquer oneself is greater than to conquer a city. Confucius, the Chinese sage, said, "Eat not for the pleasure thou mayest find therein; eat to increase thy strength; eat to preserve the life thou hast received from Heaven."

BIBLIOGRAPHY

(1) "Neighborhood Health," Vol. VII, 1941, page 10.
(2) Wheat, see McCollum, "Newer Knowledge of Nutrition," 1925, page 129; Sherman in "Chemistry of Food and Nutrition," 1924, page 56; Sherman in "Food and Health," page 163; L. B. Mendel and T. B. Osborne, in "Journal Biol. Chemistry," Vol. 41, pages 275-295; McCollum, Simonds and Pits in "Journal Biol. Chemistry," Vol. 25, pages 105-131; F. A. Csonke in "Journal Biol. Chemistry," Vol. 118, pages 147-153.
(3) "How to Live," 18th edition, page 263.
(4) "How to Live," 18th edition, page 47.
(5) "High Blood Pressure," by G. K. Abbott, M.D., page 164.

(6) "Journal American Medical Association," May 26, 1928.

(7) "High Blood Pressure," by G. K. Abbott, M.D., page 167.

(8) "Good Health," March, 1938, page 85.

(9) "Food and Health," by H. C. Sherman, pages 74, 75; "The Normal Diet and Healthful Living," by Sansum and Hare, page 6.

(10) "Food and Health," by H. C. Sherman, page 76.

(11) A. A. Horvath, "The Nutritional Value of Soy Beans," in "The American Journal of Digestive Diseases," Vol. V, No. 3.

(12) "How to Live," Fisher and Fisk, page 250.

(13) Prof. E. V. McCollum, in answer to a questionnaire sent out by a committee appointed by Board of Trustees of Beth Israel Hospital concerning a meatless diet in their hospital. In "How to Live," Fisher and Fisk, page 266.

(14) "Health," September, 1934, in article, "Why I Am a Vegetarian," page 32. Quoted from Prof. E. V. McCollum of Johns Hopkins University, eminent scientist and America's leading authority on diet.

(15) Dr. L. Duncan Bulkley, for years senior physician of New York Skin and Cancer Hospital. From "Why I Am a Vegetarian," by Charles H. Wolohon, M.D., published in "Life and Health," June, 1935, page 26.

(16) Dr. Alexander Haig, in "Uric Acid in the Causation of Disease," page 864.

(17) "Cereal Chemistry," September, 1935, page 487; L. H. Bailey, R. G. Capen, and J. A. LeClerc, Food Research Division, Bureau of Chemistry and Soils, U. S. Department of Agriculture, Washington, D. C.

(18) E. V. McCollum, Johns Hopkins, quoted in "Good Health," January, 1941.

(19) E. V. McCollum, Ph.D., Sc.D., Johns Hopkins University.

(20) "High Blood Pressure," by G. K. Abbott, M.D., page 75.

(21) J. H. Kellogg quotes this from Roger, the successor of Bouchard, "New Dietetics," page 398.

(22) J. H. Kellogg, "New Dietetics," pages 398-400.

(23) "Foods, Nutrition and Clinical Dietetics," by Risley and Walton, pages 80, 81.

(24) "Diet and Dietetics," by Armand Gautier, page 417, 1906.

(25) "The New Dietetics," by J. H. Kellogg, page 407.

(26) "The New Dietetics," by J. H. Kellogg, M.D., page 408.

(27) A. W. Nelson, Bacteriologist, Battle Creek Sanitarium, from paper by Dr. J. H. Kellogg, read at National Nut Growers' Convention, Jacksonville, Florida, 1930, and printed in "Annual Proceedings."

(28) "The New Dietetics," by J. H. Kellogg, M.D., page 397.

(29) J. H. Kellogg, M.D., in "Good Health," February, 1937, page 46.

(30) Dr. Josiah Oldfield, prominent English physician and author, in the "London Daily Chronicle."

(31) Sir Arbuthnot Lane, one of England's eminent surgeons.

(32) Sir Arbuthnot Lane, diet authority on cancer and cathartics.

(36) "A Fleshless Diet," by Buttner, page 139, and "High Blood Pressure," by Abbott, page 52.

(37) "High Blood Pressure," by G. K. Abbott, pages 40-43.

(38) Buttner's "A Fleshless Diet," page 121; "Food, Nutrition and Clinical Dietetics," by Risley and Walton, pages 103, 104.

(39) "New Dietetics," by J. H. Kellogg, M.D., page 824.

(40) "New Dietetics," by J. H. Kellogg, M.D., page 418.

(41) "High Blood Pressure," by G. K. Abbott, M.D., page 51.

(42) J. H. Kellogg, M.D., in "Good Health," February, 1935, page 48.

(43) "Good Health," February, 1935, page 61, and June, 1937, page 188.

(44) "Diet and Dietetics," by A. Gautier, translated by A. J. Rice-Oxley, page 376 (second edition). Published by Archibald Constable and Co., 16 James Street, Haymarket, London.

(45) "Diet and Dietetics," by A. Gautier, translated by A. J. Rice-Oxley, pages 408, 409 (second edition). Published by Archibald Constable and Co., 16 James Street, Haymarket, London.

(46) Arnold Lorand, M.D., Carlsbad, in "Health Through Rational Diet," page 23.

(47) Mrs. E. G. White, Vol. 9, page 159.

(48) Mrs. E. G. White, Vol. 2, page 63.

(49) Mrs. E. G. White, Vol. 2, page 352.

(50) "Food and Life" in the U. S. Dept. Year Book 1939, page 183.

(51) "Nutrition" Vol. 6, No. 4.

(52) "Counsels On Diet and Foods," page 386.

(53) "Ministry of Healing," pages 315, 316.

(54) "Counsels On Diet and Foods," page 310.

(55) Id., page 399.

(56) Id., page 395.

(57) Id., page 394.

(58) Id., page 400.

(59) Id., page 397.

(60) Id., page 396.

(61) Id., page 365.

(62) Id., page 363.

(63) "Newer Knowledge of Nutrition," page 129.

(64) "Cereal Chemistry," March, 1942.

(65) "Good Health," June, 1942, page 84.

(66) "Life and Health," May, 1949, page 32.

(67) "Principles of Nutritive Value of Foods," by Henry C. Sherman in U. S. Department of Agriculture, Miscellaneous publication, No. 546, June, 1944.

(68) Otto Carque.

The Animal Kingdom A Reservoir of Disease

The general public is not aware of the wide-spread prevalence and rapid increase of disease among domestic and wild animals, and the serious nature of many of these diseases; therefore they are not awake to the possible dangers involved in the use of animal flesh and other animal products, for human food.

The compiler has gathered data concerning this matter from sources which will be acceptable to all classes of people because they are above question. This information is classified in this treatise.

That the reader may get the full force and importance of the statements of authorities consulted, their original statements are used almost entirely even though portions of them are somewhat technical. Considerable pathology caused by these diseases is explained.

The reports of these authorities also deal, in certain instances with methods for eradicating these diseases, and some of these methods are of unusual concern to those considering using animal flesh and animal products as human food.

It is hoped that the reader will take a deep interest in every fact presented.

Very few comments have been made by the compiler because the significance of each statement is clear without doing so.

The above title was used by Karl F. Meyer, M.D., Director of the Medical Center, The George Williams Hooper Foundation, University of California, San Francisco, as the title of a treatise on animal diseases published in the "Proceedings of the Institute of Medicine of Chicago," May-June 1931, pp. 234-261. It is used here with his consent.

The following statements taken from that treatise are typical ones.

"Diseased animals play an important role in the realm of human pathology." "The Biological laws which govern the general principle of human and animal pathology are essentially the same." "Contemporaneous treatises and reviews detail the role of the domesticated and the most important wild game animals as *spreaders of disease*. In fact, this aspect of communicable diseases is stressed." "The problems involved in the continuous flow of parasites from the wild animals to domesticated ones, from the latter to man and from man to domesticated animals, are, however, only a small fraction of the multitude of other unsolved questions which are met by the student of the animal kingdom as a reservoir of parasites." "The end of this cursory trip through the animal kingdom has been reached. The main lesson to be gathered from the incomplete data is that there are within the environment of man reservoirs of disease which cannot be ignored." (1)

Dr. Meyer did not write his treatise in the interest of vegetarianism, but the facts he records concerning the diseases prevalent in the animal kingdom are of intense interest to vegetarians.

THE TESTIMONY OF AUTHORITIES

This chapter will consist almost exclusively of quotations from and citations to the writings of workers who are specializing in the field of animal diseases of whom there are no better authorities in the United States. The facts presented are so astounding that some readers might be tempted to doubt them unless thus documented. The purpose is to awaken those who read this book to universal sources of human disease that they may become interested in the way of living which offers greater freedom from disease as presented in this book.

NEARLY HALF OUR DISEASES

"Nearly half of the diseases that attack human beings are also diseases of animals." (279)

ANIMAL AND HUMAN DISEASES

"Although disease processes have affected men and animals since prehistoric times, certain circumstances of civilization have definitely permitted many of the diseases due to bacteria to become more prevalent as civilization advanced. Crowded conditions of living, artificial housing, unnatural food, pampering of the physically unfit, and the opportunity for pathogenic bacteria to be transported great distances within a comparatively short time, all contribute to the difficulty of controlling infectious diseases among animals and human beings. The fact that many of the most important bacterial diseases of animals may occasion serious sickness or even death in human beings makes it imperative that knowledge of the transmissibility of animal diseases be better understood by both the physician and the veterinarian. . . .

"When it is realized that animals are susceptible to a list of diseases almost as large and as varied as those which affect human beings, the general public will better appreciate that there are other than economic reasons for the control and eradication of animal diseases. . . .

"In this discussion no attempt will be made to deal specifically with all of the diseases of animals which are transmissible to man."

He then gives the following partial list of animal diseases communicable to man.

(A) *Diseases of domestic animals and birds*

Tuberculosis	Swine erysipelas
Anthrax	Cow-pox
Foot and mouth disease	Glanders
Malta fever and abortion	Rabies
disease	Psittacosis
Milk sickness	Certain parasite diseases

(B) *Diseases affecting rabbits and small rodents*

Plague	Rat-bite fever
Tularemia	Rocky Mountain spotted fever
Infectious jaundice	

(280)

BACTERIAL INFECTIONS COMMON TO
ANIMALS AND MAN

"Man is indebted to the animals for food, furs, clothing, leather, fertilizer, and medicines, besides work and companionship, but on the other side of the ledger, many human diseases are traceable directly or remotely to contact with diseased animals or their by-products.

"The publicity given in recent years to research on brucellosis, psittacosis, rabies, tularemia, encephalomyelitis, and other animal maladies transmissible to man has called attention to the fact that diseased animals are potential hazards to human health. The intimate associations between man and his household pets and his direct contact with other domestic animals create a public health problem of universal importance, and the necessity for a closer bond between physicians and veterinarians is becoming apparent. Many physicians are now making use of the scientific facts established by veterinary research workers in the field of animal diseases.

"Lower animals may harbor four general types of diseases common to man: (1) infections caused by animal parasites, of which trichinosis, acquired from eating raw pork, is an example; (2) virus diseases, such as encephalomyelitis, or sleeping sickness, in equines and man; (3) mycotic, or fungus diseases, illustrated by actinomycosis, or lumpy jaw; (4) infections of bacterial origin. The fourth group will be considered first, and a discussion of the parasitic diseases will follow. Virus and fungus diseases are not included in this article. . . ." Then follows a discussion of several diseases. (216)

PARASITES COMMON TO ANIMALS AND MAN

"Man probably owes most if not all of the parasites that he may harbor to his long and intimate association with animals. Comparatively few intestinal worms or other parasites live exclusively as adults in or on human beings. Among the worm parasites (helminths), only seven that are more or less widespread and important are said to be confined to human beings. Two of these are acquired by man from the flesh of domestic animals used for food. The other five are transmitted from one human being to another directly or through the agency of invertebrate animals acting as carriers (vectors) for the worms in their infective stages.

"Included in the group of adult helminths common to animals and man are a small number of species that are frequently found in human beings. It is believed, however, that some of them are rarely or never transmitted from animals to man and that despite the identical appearance of worms of these species from human and animal hosts, those found in man are distinct biological strains or varieties. Man is merely an occasional host of adult worms of many species usually found in dogs, cats, swine, sheep, cattle, and other animals; and he may become parasitized by the larval stages of certain worms that occur as adults in some of these animals. Such infestations are traceable to direct or indirect association and contact with the normal hosts or the invertebrate carriers of the parasites.

"Some of the parasites transmissible from domestic and wild animals to man act as carriers for virus and bacterial diseases, and others directly and seriously affect his health, sometimes causing death. Many kinds of parasites do not produce well-defined, acute symptoms following a more or less regular course, as do bacterial and virus infections, and the injury caused by parasites usually depends on the number present.

"By no means all the parasites transmissible from animals to man, or even from domestic animals to man, are included in this article, but most of the important ones and most of those reported as having been found in human beings in the United States are mentioned or briefly discussed." (He then discusses several groups of parasites) (217)

PROTOZOA

"So far as is known, man does not acquire any protozoan parasites by eating the flesh of meat animals. Some of the protozoans that live in domestic animals are apparently transmissible to human beings, infection following ingestion of the infectious stages passed with the feces of animals. Thus *Balantidium coli*, a ciliate (having hairlike organs for locomotion) occuring in the intestines of man and sometimes causing a type of dysentery, is also found in pigs, and these animals are thought to serve as reservoirs of infection. Though some authorities deny the probability, others have considered it likely that cats and rodents serve as reservoirs and disseminators of infections with *Giardia*, a flagellate (having whiplike organs for locomotion) that occurs in man's intestines and sometimes causes a recurrent diarrhea and other disturbances.

"Some investigators believe it probable that pigs, rats, and especially monkeys act as reservoir hosts for *Entamoeba histolytica*, which causes amoebic dysentery and is one of man's most important intestinal protozoans. Wild and domestic animals are suspected of being reservoir hosts for certain of the trypanosomes that cause disease in man. The type of sleeping sickness caused by trypanosomes, which is widespread in Africa, is transmitted by insects and ranks as one of the most important diseases of man. . . .

"Perhaps the most important protozoan disease of man in this country is malaria." (218)

WORM PARASITES

"The roundworm, or nematode, *Trichinella spiralis*, is undoubtedly the most important worm parasite transmissible from domestic animals to man. This worm causes trichinosis.

"Two other worm parasites that man acquires by eating infected meat, either raw or imperfectly cooked, or improperly processed meat products are the beef tapeworm and the pork tapeworm. The adults live in the small intestine of man, and the eggs or segments containing eggs pass out with the feces. Cattle or swine that swallow the eggs of the respective tapeworms become infested with the larval stages, known as bladder worms, which become localized in the muscles of these intermediate hosts. When a human being swallows the live bladder worms in meat, he becomes infected with the adult worms. Man can also serve as an intermediate host of both tapeworms, and if a person swallows their eggs as a result of unsanitary conditions he becomes infected with the bladder worm stages. The pork tapeworm is the more dangerous to man in this respect, since the bladder worms may lodge in the heart, brain, or eye and cause serious consequences." (219)

BACTERIAL INFECTIONS AND PARASITES
COMMON TO MAN AND ANIMALS

"Livestock diseases are a public health problem because many of them affect human beings as well as animals. This article considers only those caused by bacteria and parasites. Fungus diseases common to animals and man may be illustrated by lumpy jaw and virus diseases by sleeping sickness (encephalomyelitis of horses, encephalitis of human beings.)

"Stiles briefly discusses the bacterial infections. In the case of diseases covered elsewhere in this book, further details will be found in the separate articles.

"Brucellosis affects cattle, swine, goats, and according to recent evidence, horses. It causes undulant fever in human beings, who can acquire the infection from unpasteurized milk or by careless handling of diseased animals and their products. Bovine tuberculosis can be passed on to human beings, children being the most susceptible. Usually it is acquired by drinking raw milk. Hence both Bang's disease (brucellosis) and the tuberculosis eradication campaigns are important public health measures as well as being of benefit to farmers.

"Septic sore throat in human beings is often traceable to the consumption of raw milk from cows harboring *Streptococcus epidemicus*. The common mastitis organisms in cows (*Streptococcus agalactiae*) have not been shown to be capable of setting up a disease process in man. Milk, of course, can easily be contaminated after it leaves the cow.

"Tularemia affects many wild animals, including rabbits, and is passed on to human beings by contact with diseased animals, by the eating of undercooked infected meats, and by the bites of ticks, deer flies, and other arthropods. The wearing of heavy rubber gloves will protect persons who dress rabbits and other game.

"Anthrax affects many species of animals, including domestic livestock, and is readily passed on to human beings. Efficient methods of sterilizing hides, wool and hair should prevent infection from these sources. Persons who handle carcasses of animals that have died of anthrax must use the utmost precautions.

"Swine erysipelas can affect turkeys, ducks, pigeons, and sheep; possibly it is now becoming more widespread among domestic animals. It causes erysipeloid in human beings, the organism usually entering through broken skin. True human erysipelas is an entirely different disease, not caused by the swine organism.

"Glanders, a disease of equines that can affect human beings, has been practically wiped out in the United States.

"Bubonic plague (black death), a disease of wild rodents, is carried to human beings through the bites of fleas that infest rats, three species of which harbor the plague organism. Small areas of infection among rodents have been found in 11 Western States. Serious epidemics have occurred elsewhere in the world within recent years.

"Food poisoning of various types may result from eating products contaminated with *Salmonella* bacteria and staphylococci, which infect animals. Botulism is caused by three types of botulinus organisms which produce deadly toxins in perishable foods. The poison of each type can be neutralized by its own antitoxin. Botulinus spores are extremely resistant to destruction even by boiling, and they can infect many kinds of food products.

"The parasitic infections are discussed by Lucker, who comments that man probably acquired most, if not all, of his parasites from his long association with animals.

"Among the external parasites, the fleas of dogs and cats infest man as does the sticktight flea of chickens, which can carry endemic typhus fever virus. A rat flea transmits bubonic plague to human beings. The red mite of poultry can parasitize man. Several kinds of ticks are transmissible from animals to man, and some carry the organisms of such diseases as Rocky Mountain spotted fever, tularemia, and sporadic relapsing fever.

"It is suspected that wild and domestic animals act as reservoirs for certain protozoan diseases of human beings, notably African sleeping sickness.

"Perhaps the most important worm parasite transmissible from animals to man is the nematode that causes trichinosis. It usually is acquired from infected pork that has not been thoroughly cooked. The beef tapeworm and the pork tapeworm are also acquired by **human beings from raw or undercooked meat.** If eggs of the pork tapeworm are swallowed, bladder worms may lodge in the heart, brain, or eye. Several species of worm parasites that normally infest animals can develop to maturity in the human body.

"The common liver fluke of sheep and cattle has been reported as an accidental parasite of human beings in this country, and a liver fluke of dogs and cats not uncommonly infests human beings in Europe. In the Phillipines certain flukes of dogs and cats are associated with a form of heart disease in man. Two tapeworms of dogs and cats are transmissible to man. A number of species of hairworms of sheep and goats, certain eye worms of dogs and sheep, the threadworm of swine, the giant kidney worm of dogs and mink, and the common thornheaded worm of pigs have been reported occasionally in human beings.

"The larvae of the hydatid tapeworm of dogs and other carnivores can produce huge hydatid cysts in the liver, lungs, or brain of human beings, and the larvae of several other worm parasites of animals are capable of developing in the human body. The larvae of blood flukes of birds sometimes invade the skin of bathers in the lakes of Michigan, Wisconsin, Minnesota, and elsewhere, producing a temporary inflammation called swimmer's itch. A skin disease reported in the South and called creeping eruption is caused by the larvae of hookworm of dogs and cats." (220)

Viruses and Bacteria

"Viruses are too small to be seen under a microscope, and they pass through a filter fine enough to hold back bacteria. Only in recent years has it been possible to propagate some viruses artifically, by the use of living tissues; and these studies have revealed many facts and led to the development of certain immunization methods. More than 35 virus diseases of animals are now known. Some viruses attack nerve tissue primarily, as in rabies and encephalomyelitis; others skin and membrane tissues, as in foot-and-mouth disease; and still others, several or all kinds of tissue. After a virus has weakened the body's defenses, bacteria that may not ordinarily be very harmful will often become secondary invaders, with serious results, as in hog cholera complications.

"Bacteria and viruses invade the body in various ways, mainly through the respiratory, digestive, and genital tracts and the skin. They are transmitted from animal to animal by biting insects, by the blood, excretions, and secretions of infected animals which contaminate the surroundings, and by carriers—that is, animals that harbor an infective agent without apparently getting the disease themselves or continue to harbor the agent after recovering as in foot-and-mouth disease." (221)

VETERINARIANS AND PHYSICIANS COOPERATE

"Recently public health authorities have become cognizant of animal diseases being a greater source of human disease than was formerly thought. Tuberculosis, trichinosis, undulant fever, septic sore throat and encephalitis have received much attention as diseases of animal origin. But the enteric infections are now moving up into this group of diseases. In a recent Army medical bulletin attention was called to the fact that physicians may often be able to predict the occurrences of disease by finding out what diseases are occurring in animals. The medical literature has called attention to this editorially by saying that physicians should have close professional relationship to veterinarians in the community so that they may know what epizootics or enzootics are occurring. In Ohio we are developing this relationship in pointing out to local health officers to contact veterinarians for information about animal diseases. By having local veterinarians participate in health programs we may even develop to the point where the health authorities can predict enteric disease outbreaks. For example, hog cholera occurs in the community and the health officer is notified. He may know from experience that some ill hogs will be slaughtered and offered for sale with ensuing enteritis. The possibilities of improved public health procedures by closer relations between the veterinary profession and health authorities are immense." (222)

VETERINARY AND HUMAN MEDICINE

"The close relationship that exists between veterinary and human medicine is manifest when one considers the list of animal diseases to which man is susceptible, and this list is rapidly growing as our progress in research develops.

"Among the virus infections alone which may be transmitted

from animal to man are rabies, enquine encephalomyelitis, lymphocytic chorio meningitis, cowpox, foot and mouth disease, and psittacosis. We know that these may be communicated to man by various modes of transmission, as by direct contact, by inhalation of infective particles and by direct insect vectors.

"However, a vast number of problems still await solution in relation to the virus diseases which are acquired by man from animals." (223)

"Veterinary medicine has had a notable history, and it is more closely associated with human medicine than most persons realize. Many of the discoveries of human medicine are applied by the veterinarian, but the reverse is as often the case; some of the discoveries made in animal-disease research have been of inestimable value in human medicine. The lines cross at many points. To take a single example, the virus that causes sleeping sickness of horses also causes sleeping sickness of human beings, and in its action it is not unlike other viruses that produce a group of dreaded diseases of the brain and spinal cord." (224)

WILDLIFE DISEASES AND PARASITES AND FARM-RAISED GAME BIRDS

Shillinger deals with the following diseases and parasites:

"Pullorum disease is only occasionally observed in pheasants and quail.

"Tuberculosis is often transmitted from domestic to game birds.

"Ulcerative enteritis is the most destructive disease of quail and grouse on game farms. Unchecked outbreaks may kill 70 to 100 per cent of the birds.

"*Salmonella* infection produces a disease of obscure character among quail.

"Blackhead is especially destructive to wild turkeys but also affects quail and ruffed grouse.

"Coccidiosis is as destructive to young game birds as to young chickens.

"Trichomoniasis causes severe losses among quail and wild turkeys.

"Aspergillosis is a fungus disease that may cause losses as high as 90 per cent in affected broods of quail.

"Thrush is another fungus disease that affects quail and wild turkeys.

"Worm parasites of several kinds attack various internal organs, as in the case of domestic fowl.

"Nutritional diseases—especially vitamin A and vitamin D deficiencies—are responsible for disease among farm-raised game birds; and cannibalism (corrected by feeding extra salt) also occurs.

DISEASES OF FUR ANIMALS

"Shillinger covers some of the more important diseases of silver foxes and minks; the latter, as he notes, are particularly subject to infection because they are so often kept in crowded quarters. For further information on some of these diseases the reader should refer to the articles on dogs and cats in this book.

"Paratyphoid, which occurs fairly frequently in severe outbreaks among silver foxes, can be checked by the use of a vaccine, preferably prepared from material on the farm where the disease occurs.

"Infectious enteritis, caused by a *Salmonella* organism, produces severe inflammation of the intestinal tract. Careful hygiene is necessary to prevent the spread of infection. A specially prepared buttermilk is sometimes given to sick animals.

"Distemper is so easily spread that the utmost hygienic precautions must be taken when a case occurs. The antiserum used for dogs gives temporary protection to foxes. Experiments are being made to develop a vaccine that will produce more lasting immunity.

"Anthrax among minks has been traced to the feeding of meat from infected domestic animals. Since it entails heavy losses and is very dangerous to human beings, extreme care should be taken to prevent its introduction from this source.

"The internal parasites that infest fur animals include hookworms, ascarids, and lungworms. The use of wire-mesh flooring to reduce infection from droppings is a wise precaution. Anthelmintics, discussed by the author, are used for hookworms and ascarids.

"Fleas, which may damage pelts, can be controlled by the use of sulfur, pyrethrum, or derris, preferably used as a dust rather than a dip. Body mange seldom affects fur animals; when a few are affected, it may be better to destroy rather than treat them. Ear mange, which is common among silver foxes, can be treated with various preparations suggested by the author.

"Food poisoning, chiefly botulism, sometimes occurs on fur farms, especially among minks. It is due to inadequate refrigeration or unsanitary handling of feed.

"Chastek paralysis, a disease of silver foxes fed liberally on certain kinds of fresh fish, is apparently due to a factor that destroys vitamin B-1. This factor itself can be destroyed by adequate cooking of the fish. Administration of vitamin B-1 cures the disease.

Diseases of Wildlife and Their Relationship To Domestic Livestock

"The fact that many diseases and parasites affect both domestic animals and wildlife poses a threefold problem—how to prevent their spread from domestic to wild animals, and also in the reverse direction; and how to control them in wild animals. Shillinger's discussion of these maladies is brief, to avoid repetition of details given in the articles on livestock; but some of the important facts he brings out will be new to readers not intimately acquainted with wild life problems. The diseases and parasites included are the following:

"Brucellosis is rather common among big-game ruminants. Brucellosis-free herds of buffalo and elk are being built up by vaccination.

"Hemorrhagic septicemia is responsible for extensive losses among deer and buffaloes. An effective bacterin has been produced for the latter.

"Tuberculosis has frequently been diagnosed in deer, foxes, wild ducks, and wild pheasants.

"Necrobacillosis is a rather common cause of losses, especially among the larger wild ruminants fed in concentrated herds by attendants.

"Malignant edema is a fatal disease of deer.

"Tularemia affects not only rabbits but many other animals and has been responsible for heavy losses among dense populations in the wild.

"Foot-and-mouth disease, in one outbreak in this country, affected deer as well as cattle.

"The virus of encephalomyelitis, a disease of equines (and human beings), has been found in wild pheasants and semiwild pigeons.

"Virus tumors, of both fatal and nonfatal types, occur in rabbits.

"Leucocytozoan disease is caused by a protozoan organism that infects wild as well as domestic ducks and is especially dangerous to young ducklings.

"A malarial organism has recently been found in the blood of sharptailed grouse, and its possible relationship to losses in other wild and domestic birds is now being studied.

"Anaplasmosis has been found to be infectious for Columbian blacktailed deer, which may serve as reservoirs of the blood parasite.

"Whether mange mites are transmissible from wild to domestic animals and vice versa is not definitely known.

"Screwworms have caused rather heavy losses among deer.

"Worm parasites of several kinds are parasitic in wild animals, causing damage similar to that in livestock.

"Pollution of water by sewage, oil, and industrial waste has caused considerable destruction of aquatic mammals and birds.

"Botulism has been responsible for many deaths among waterfowl and shore birds around stagnant pools." (225)

DISEASES OF ANIMALS AND MAN

Cattle

DISEASES	CAUSE OF DISEASE	HUMANS Susceptible
Actinomycosis	Fungus, Scattered by animals	Humans susceptible, can contract through milk, meat or scattered fungus
Anaplasmosis (anemia)	Parasites	
Anthrax	Bacillus—fleas carry	Human susceptible
Black leg	Very deadly infection	
Brucellosis	Germ	Human form is undulant fever
Coccidiosis	Parasite	
Cow pox	From human small pox	Vaccinia—mild Smallpox
Diptheria	Germ	Humans susceptible
Foot-and-mouth diease	Virus—rare	Rare in man
Genital Trichomoniasis	Germ	
Johne's disease	Bacillus	
Listerellosis	Bacteria	Humans susceptible
Liver flukes	Parasite	Humans susceptible
Mastitis	Germ	To man as Septic sore throat
Milk sickness	Eating poison plants	Affects man through milk
Pneumonia	Germ	
Q Fever	Virus	To man by barn yard dust
Scarlet fever	Germ—contracted from man	Passed to man through milk

Sleeping sickness	Virus—carried by mosquitoes	Passed to man through mosquitoes
Tape worm	From infected pastures	Passed to man through meat
Tuberculosis	Bacillus	Passed to man through milk and meat

Swine

Actinomycosis	Fungus	Humans susceptible Contact or scattered fungus
Anthrax	Ingestion or biting of fleas	Humans susceptible
Brucellosis	Germ	Humans susceptible By contact or handling carcass
Cholera	Infection—fleas	Enteritis
Coccidiosis	Parasite	
Erysipelas	Bacillus	Erysipoloid in humans through abrasions
Foot-and-mouth disease	Virus	Humans via milk
Glanders	Bacillus	In man by contact and skin abrasions
Influenza	Virus	
Listerellosis	Bacteria	Humans susceptible
Mange	Parasite	Humans susceptible
Mastitis	Bacteria	
Pigpox	Virus	
Sleeping sickness	Mosquitoes carry	Humans susceptible
Tapeworm	Parasite	Humans susceptible
Trichinosis	Parasite	Humans susceptible
Tuberculosis	Bacillus—often acquired from poultry	Humans susceptible

Sheep

Actinomycosis	Fungus	Humans susceptible
Anaplasmosis (anemia)	Parasite	
Anthrax	Bacillus	Contact with animals and their by-products. Humans susceptible
Coccidiosis	Parasite	
Foot rot	Infection	
Foot-and-mouth disease	Virus	
Glanders	Bacillus	Contact with diseased animals. Humans susceptible
Johne's disease	Bacillus	
Listerellosis	Bacteria	Humans susceptible
Liver flukes	Parasite	Humans susceptible
Mastitis	Germ	
Rocky Mountain spotted fever	Spread by ticks	Acquired by humans
Swine erysipelas	Bacillus	Conveyed to man through skin abrasions
Tuberculosis	Bacillus	

Chickens

Blackhead	Parasite	
Bluecomb disease	Source unknown	
Cholera	Infection	
Coccidosis	Parasite	

Epidemic tremor	Infection	
Laryngotracheitis	Virus	
Leukosis	A mystery disease	Seems to belong to a group of diseases affecting certain animals and man
Mycosis of the skin	Fungus growths	Humans susceptible
Pox (Diptheria)	Virus—mosquitoes carry	Humans susceptible
Psittacosis	Virus	Humans susceptible
Pullorum	Germ—through egg and excreta	Eggs may produce colitis in man
Sleeping sickness	Virus	Humans susceptible

Horses

Mules are subject to many diseases of horses

Actinomycosis	Fungus	Humans susceptible
Anthrax	Bacillus	Humans susceptible
Brucellosis	Germ	Humans susceptible
Equine encephalomylitis (sleeping sickness)	Virus—mosquitoes carry	Humans susceptible
Equine infectious anemia	Parasite	
Glanders	Bacillus	Humans susceptible
Horsepox	Virus	Humans susceptible
Johne's disease	Bacillus	
Tuberculosis	Bacillus	Humans susceptible

Goats

Actinomycosis	Fungus	Humans susceptible
Anthrax	Ingestion or biting fleas	Humans susceptible
Brucellosis	Germ	Humans susceptible
Coccidiosis	Parasite	
Glanders	Bacillus	Humans susceptible
Johne's disease	Bacillus	
Sleeping sickness	Virus	Humans susceptible
Tuberculosis	Bacillus	To man by meat

Dogs*

Actinomycosis	Fungus	Humans acquire from contact
Anthrax	Ingestion or biting fleas	Humans acquire from contact
Coccidiosis	Parasite	
Liver flukes	Parasites, acquired by eating fish	Humans susceptible
Rocky Mountain fever	Parasite, carried by insects	Humans susceptible
Sleeping sickness	Virus, mosquitoes carry from horses	Humans susceptible
Tapeworm	Parasites	
Tuberculosis	Bacillus, from meat and milk	Humans susceptible

Turkeys*

Blackhead	Parasites	
Coccidiosis	Parasites	
Sleeping sickness	Virus	Humans susceptible
Pullorum disease	Germ, through eggs and excreta	
Swine erysipelas	Germ	
Trichomoniasis	Infection catarrhal enteritis	

Cats*

Liver flukes	Parasites	Transferable to man
Sleeping sickness	Virus, carried by insects	Man susceptible
Tuberculosis	Bacillus	Acquired from contact

Pigeons*

Sleeping sickness	Virus, contact from horses	Man is susceptible
Psittacosis	Virus	Through contact or dust from excreta (widespread
Tuberculosis	Bacillus, from poultry and sparrow	Man susceptible

Sparrows*

Psittacosis	Virus	Through contact or dust from excreta
Sleeping sickness	Virus	Man is susceptible
Tuberculosis	Bacillus	May be taken by man but not readily

Parrots*

Psittacosis	Virus	Humans highly susceptible

*This list of conditions is not complete but these are considered to be the important ones.

Rodents

Rodents commonly thought of as mice and rats are a serious menace to man. The mouse is a kin to the rat, but is not as seriously indicted, principally because it is not considered to be as prolific a carrier of disease as the rat.

The rat originated in Asia and has been a source of dissemination of disease and destruction throughout all its years of history. Directly traceable to the rat has been the spread of:

Bubonic plague	Tularemia
Endemic typhus fever	Rat-bite fever
Rocky Mountain spotted fever	Leptospirosis
Trichinosis	Numerous food poisoning epidemics

The total number of deaths since the beginning of history, due to plague and diseases, carried by rats, would run into hundreds of millions. Among the animals, the rat may safely be said to rate as man's public enemy number one.

Wild game may also be said to be responsible for spreading several diseases which are communicable to man. Squirrels, woodchucks, chipmunks, opposum and rabbits carry such diseases as Rocky Mountain spotted fever, sleeping sickness, Tularemia. Hull, in *Diseases Transmitted from Animals to Man,* pages 386-389, gives a more complete list of diseases traceable to and spread by these small wild animals.

Too Numerous to Mention

There are many animals and their diseases which it seems unimportant to tabulate here as most of them have been mentioned in some of the general statements preceeding this table. Among them are guinea pigs, rats, mice, ducks, beaver, foxes, geese, pheasants, and other birds, rodents, and wild life.

Not Communicable To Man

Certain diseases and conditions of animals which are *not* communicable to man are included in this table because many of the readers of this book do not wish to be associated with animals which are diseased, or eat their flesh, or use their products,—they do not like the idea even though disease may not be directly incurred.

Diseases Increasing

"Every farmer realizes that diseases both in his crops and herds are more numerous than a generation ago." (2)

INDIVIDUAL DISEASES CONSIDERED

TUBERCULOSIS FROM CATTLE TO MAN

"For centuries it was strongly suspected that scrofula or consumption of cattle was transmissible to man. After Villemin, Chauveau and Gerlach proved that tuberculosis is transmissible from animal to animal, Koch discovered the tubercle bacillus, Theobald Smith described the bovine type and Ravenel proved conclusively that this type causes tuberculosis in man, there were few unbelievers and doubters. . . . From this came the greatest victory ever won over tuberculosis. It included the solution of one of man's greatest economic problems and also one of the most serious public health problems. . . .

"There is no doubt that large numbers of human beings of all ages formerly developed primary tuberculosis from the bovine type of tubercle bacillus and this markedly increased the incidence of tuberculin reactors wherever human beings associated with tuberculous cattle or consumed the products of these animals.

"Thus, the rapid decline in the incidence of tuberculin reactors among children of this country in the past ten or fifteen years is probably due more to the protection you have afforded them against the bovine type of tubercle bacillus than any other single factor. . . .

"There can be no doubt that in the past much of the tuberculosis that caused illness and death of human beings in this country was due to the bovine type of tubercle bacillus. In fact, in 1910 Park estimated that in about 10 per cent of all infants dying from tuberculosis, the bovine bacillus was responsible. He later reported that from bacteriologic examinations 66 per cent of fatal generalized tuberculosis in children was found to be due to the bovine bacillus. In 1914 Mitchell studied cervical lymph nodes of 72 children and 8 adults who were treated surgically for tuberculosis and found the bovine bacillus was responsible for the disease in 65 of the children and 6 of the adults.

"Since accurate typing of tubercle bacilli has been possible, the seriousness of the bovine type of tuberculosis in man has been better appreciated. For example, in 1937 Dr. A. Stanley Griffith of Cambridge University pointed out that in England 50 per cent of the cases of cervical lymph-node tuberculosis and 50 per cent of the cases of tuberculosis of the skin were caused by the bovine type of tubercle bacillus. Moreover, approximately 25 per cent of the cases of tuberculosis meningitis and 20 per cent of the cases of tuberculosis of the bones and joints and genito-urinary tract, respectively, were due to this type of organism. . . .

"For a long time it was thought that chronic, pulmonary tuberculosis in man was almost never caused by the bovine type of tubercle bacillus. . . . Hedvall of Lund, Sweden stated that there is reliable evidence that bovine tuberculosis can be transmitted from cattle to man, from man to man, and from man back to cattle. He found that the bovine type of tubercle bacillus causes just as serious disease in man as the human type.

"The control of tuberculosis in cattle, therefore, has markedly reduced the incidence of tuberculosis infection, the morbidity, and the mortality from tuberculosis." (226)

"We should ever be mindful of the fact that tuberculosis of animals, and particularly of cattle, may be transmitted to human beings." (227)

TUBERCULOSIS FROM OTHER ANIMALS

"As you well know, in addition to man, tuberculosis affects many of the lower animals, including practically all of the domestic species, many of the captive wild animals, as well as fish and reptiles. . . .

"Tuberculosis in cattle is usually due to the bovine form of the organism, whereas chickens, pigeons, turkeys, geese, ducks, and pheasants are affected with the avian type. Each of the three varieties of the bacillus mentioned may cause tuberculosis in swine. The human being seems to be extremely resistant to the avian form of the organism and infection from this source is rare.

"Other possible sources of danger to man from tuberculous animals are dogs and cats. Dogs are susceptible to both the human and bovine forms of the tubercle bacillus, but tuberculosis in the cat from the human type of the tubercle bacillus seems unlikely since in none of the reported cases has the bovine type been found to be responsible for the disease. Parrots are usually infected with the human or bovine type of the organism, and, when infected, these birds must be considered a menace to human beings.

"Without question tuberculosis still remains one of the most important diseases with which man has to cope, and an understanding of all possible factors pertaining to the dissemination of the agents responsible for the infection is not only desirable but necessary. . . .

TUBERCULOSIS

"Although the consumption of raw milk from diseased cows is held largely responsible for the bovine infection tuberculosis in man, other modes of transmission are possible. The hands are subject to dangerous contamination, and through carelessness this and other deadly diseases may be contracted or spread. K. A. Hermanson says: 'After examining the carcasses of tuberculous cattle, the meat inspectors washed their hands in sterile water. This was centrifuged and the sediment injected into guinea pigs. Eleven of the fifteen inoculations produced tuberculosis in the guinea pigs. The wash water from the hands of the meat cutters was shown to contain tubercle bacilli. The rinse water from the towels used by the meat inspectors was injected into guinea pigs, producing tuberculosis in every instance.' (228)

Danger in Both Milk and Flesh

The last paragraph above is most revealing concerning the transmission of tuberculosis not only through milk but by the hand towels and wash water from the hands of the cutters of tuberculous meat.

Tuberculosis Is Tuberculosis

"Tuberculosis is tuberculosis, so I should remind you of swine and fowl potentialities, and it might be profitable to consider the danger to cattle of human tuberculosis. In the past from control standpoint too much attention was paid to types. My late respected chief, Dr. C. H. Mayo, always insisted that different types of tubercle bacilli are more a matter of soil than of seed." (229)

TUBERCULOUS CONDITIONS OF CATTLE

TUBERCULOSIS OF UDDER IN COWS

"Tuberculosis of the udder usually commences well up in one or both quarters, and may involve the lymph glands situated above and back of the two rear quarters of the udder. The organ itself becomes progressively hard and swollen, sometimes acquiring enormous size. Milk secretion appears normal until the infection has progressed considerably, when the milk becomes thin, watery, and scanty, and contains flaky and stringy material, and possibly blood and pus.

"This disease, however, may go on unrecognized for years; meanwhile the animal continues to yield milk containing tubercle bacilli, thus endangering the health of other livestock as well as human lives. . . . There is no known cure for the disease." (13)

Forced Lactation Prepares for Tuberculosis

"Animals which are fed on non-nutritious foods as well as those that have too little feed, become weakened constitutionally and lose the power to resist the invasion of the organisms. Stabling animals in dark, poorly ventilated, and dirty barns helps to spread tuberculosis. . . . Any condition that produces constant strain upon the systems of animals, such as continued forced lactation periods of dairy cows, renders them fit subjects for the development of tuberculosis." (11)

No Outward Symptoms

"In most cases the outward appearance of the animal bears no relation to the degree of infection. The disease frequently develops so slowly that in some cases it may be months or even longer before any symptoms are shown." (4)

Danger Undetected

"The tuberculous cow is the greatest source of danger in healthy cattle. Inasmuch as it cannot be determined just when that animal becomes a 'spreader' of the germs unless daily microscopic tests are made of the milk and of the discharges from the body, it is unsafe to keep her with healthy cattle." (5)

Gives No Indication

"It must be understood that tuberculosis is a disease which often gives no indication of its presence by external symptoms." (6)

"Animals that are extensively diseased are often in apparently perfect physical condition." (7)

Milk a Carrier

"Milk is a good medium for the distribution of the tubercle bacilli." (14)

From Milk to Calves

Tuberculosis is spread "by feeding calves with raw milk or other dairy products from tuberculous cows. This frequently occurs where the owner purchases mixed skim milk from the creamery and feeds it to his calves without first making it safe by pasteurization." (15)

From Milk to Hogs

"When hogs were fed on tuberculous milk for only three days the post-mortem examination held 107 days later showed that 83.3 per cent of the animals had become tuberculous. When hogs received tuberculous milk for thirty days and were allowed to live 50 days longer, 100 per cent of the animals had developed generalized tuberculosis." (16)

"In one instance a shipment of 74 hogs showed tuberculosis in 61, and investigation brought out the fact that the swine had been fed on skim milk of a creamery of a nearby town. The separator slime from two of the creameries in this town was obtained for experimental purposes, and the inoculation test showed that one of the samples produced tuberculosis in all of the guinea pigs inoculated." (17)

"A lot of hogs which contained 36 per cent of tuberculous animals was traced to the farms of the raiser, and the authorities were notified. They made a tuberculin test of the cattle that produced the milk; about 22 per cent of them reacted. This infected milk had been separated on the farm with a hand separator and the skim milk fed to the hogs." (18)

From Milk to Children

"Many cases of tuberculosis among children are traceable to the use of milk from tuberculous cows. If milk is properly pasteurized the living organisms of tuberculosis are destroyed, but raw milk and milk improperly pasteurized may be sources of danger." (19)

Viability

"The germs of the disease may live for months in manure or litter." (12)

Only One Cow in Two Hundred Now Has Tuberculosis

"Practically all animals are subject to tuberculosis, particularly cattle, hogs, and poultry. Human beings, especially children, can get it from cow's milk. . . . The relentless campaign of eradication between 1917 and 1942 has reduced the number of tuberculous cattle in the United States from 1 animal in 20 to less than 1 in 200." (230)

"All states are now in the modified accredited status, that is, there is infection in less than 0.5 per cent of the cattle in any state." (231)

This marked reduction of tuberculosis in cattle is a notable achievement. If the same gains can be made with other animals it will help much in the fight against tuberculosis in human beings.

Tuberculosis Remains One of the Greatest Killers

"The tubercule bacillus is a microbial gangster that makes its own rules and gives no quarter. . . .

"When considering the control and eradication of tuberculosis in cattle one must not be unmindful of the fact that tuberculosis remains one of the greatest killers of mankind. . . . This disease kills 160 every day in the United States. This represents one death every nine minutes. . . . It kills more people between the ages of fifteen and forty-five than any other disease." (232) These are the years of greatest endurance.

Tuberculosis

"Of all the infections, tuberculosis continues to be the most general and damaging. Though it now is seventh on the mortality table, having occupied first position less than 20 years ago, a significant fact is that in increase in non-infectious conditions largely due to the deteriorating process of middle and old age it has had some influence in this result. As an infection, tuberculosis is still preminent. Even when considering the top-flight killers such as heart conditions and other circulatory ailments, cancer, diabetes, and nephritis, the tuberculosis germ still represents the most devastating factor in the age group from fifteen to forty-five years." (233)

BOVINE TUBERCULOSIS IN HUMANS

"The large majority of cases of bovine tuberculosis in humans are not found in mortality lists—they do not result in death. They result in suffering, incapacitation, and crippling to which death might be preferable." (234)

TUBERCULOSIS IN MAN

"Institutions for the tuberculous cost $75,000,000.00 annually to maintain." (235)

TUBERCULOSIS IN SWINE

The Incidence

In a given year 46,688,860 hogs were slaughtered in the United States. Only 65 per cent of them were inspected for tuberculosis. Of these 5,321,352 were found to have the disease; 42,381 of these were condemned, and the remaining 5,278,971 were sold to and eaten by the unsuspecting public. It is claimed that the incidence of tuberculosis is still greater in the 35 per cent which are not inspected. (21)

The Sources

"Tuberculous fowls are the main source of tuberculosis in hogs." (22)

Also from manure dropped by infected cows and from using the milk from tuberculous cows. (23)

Prevention

"Prevention lies in the eradication of tuberculosis in poultry flocks and keeping poultry from feeding with hogs or roosting where their droppings may contaminate the hogpen." (24) (25)

If poultry is so dangerous to hogs is it safe for humans?

Sold Unawares

"It is very probable that many farmers have sold tuberculous hogs without suspecting that they were unsound, for few of these diseased hogs ever show the presence of tuberculosis by outward symptoms. In fact, the hogs that disclose the affection after slaughter are frequently the finest-appearing animals in the drove." (26)

Plan for Eradication

To eradicate tuberculosis from hogs "there can be no doubt that the best and surest method of procedure, in nearly every case, is to slaughter the entire drove as soon as the animals can be put in a marketable condition." (27)

To eradicate tuberculosis from swine "it is not necessary to apply the tuberculin test to all the swine herds because it is more economical to send the entire herd, with the exception of valuable breeding animals, to market when fat than to undertake to exterminate the disease in any other way." (28)

TUBERCULOSIS IN FOWLS, CATTLE, AND MAN

"Tuberculosis infections in man, cattle, and fowls are each traceable in the majority of cases to their specific type or organism; the human type is generally found in man, the avian type in fowls, and the bovine type in cattle. The bovine type, however, may occur in swine and is also recognized as an important factor in tuberculosis in children. The avian type has been repeatedly found in swine and occasionally in calves and sheep but is rarely communicated to man. Nevertheless tuberculous fowl carcasses should be regarded as unwholesome and unfit for food even though thorough cooking destroys their infectious character." (29)

Intermediate Types

"Intermediate types of the avian, human, and bovine organisms occur which do not completely conform with the characters of these three main groups. More information regarding these less common aberrant types is necessary before the complete history of the spread of tuberculosis from one species to another can be described. The intermediate, or aberrant, types are less frequently encountered and fortunately constitute a smaller, though still a significant, part of the tuberculosis problem." (30)

This statement reveals that there is yet more to be learned about how the disease spreads from one animal to another and to man.

Widespread in Illinois

"The disease exists in practically every locality of the state. . . .

"In tuberculin-testing 1253 farm flocks in 10 counties in 1933, about half the flocks proved to be infected. These flocks included more than 157,904 fowls. An average of 5.1 per cent of all the fowls in these infected flocks reacted to the test. Approximately 66 per cent of the reacting fowls suffered from mild lesions of the disease and were passed for food. Subsequent reports of tuberculin tests in Illinois flocks confirm in a general way the figures gathered in this preliminary survey. . . ." (31)

Note that 66 per cent of the fowls found infected with tuberculosis were sold for food.

In Wyoming

"In one county where a large number of flocks were examined, one third were found to be infected, and in those infected flocks sixty-six per cent of the birds were diseased." (32)

Throughout the United States

"The disease exists on 80 per cent of the farms in some counties and is a serious menace to the poultry industry in at least 600 counties in the Middle West." (A map accompanying this statement shows in which states the incidence of tuberculosis varies from less than 1 per cent of the flocks to over 7 per cent.) (33)

FIFTY TO SEVENTY-FIVE PER CENT

"In some sections of the Central and North Central States from 50 per cent to 75 per cent of the poultry flocks are affected with this disease." (34)

"A survey was made which involved the inspection of about 115,700 flocks of poultry in 40 states. The number of flocks found apparently free was slightly more than 109,010 leaving 6,690 infected." (35)

"The greater prevalence of avian tuberculosis occurs in the states of the North Central section, an area which forms a large part of the region commonly referred to as the 'Corn Belt.' In some of this territory the number of poultry flocks found infected has represented as high as 85 per cent of the flocks within a certain area, and, over comparatively wide sections in some of the states, tests of the poultry population have revealed a flock morbidity rate of from 40 to 50 per cent.

"A significant fact of some economic concern is the high avian tuberculosis incidence in the greater portion of the area which provides the greatest egg and poultry meat production for this country." (236)

Chickens Most Susceptible

"Of all domestic birds, chickens are by far the most susceptible to tuberculosis. . . . Turkeys, geese, ducks, and guinea fowls have been found to have the disease. . . . Sparrows and pigeons also have been proven to be susceptible." (36)

Conditions Produced

"A very characteristic thing about tuberculosis is the production of nodules. These nodules or tubercules vary in size. . . . In fowls tuberculosis is a disease of the abdominal organs, and any one or a number of these organs may be affected. The most common location for the tubercules or nodules is the liver. The spleen is next in order for frequency of organs affected. . . . The intestines are very frequently the seat of tuberculous growth. . . . Other organs and places where lesions of the disease have been reported with considerable less frequency, are peritoneum, lungs, joints, kidneys, ovaries, testicles, gizzard, skin, inside lining of eyelids, and lymph nodes." (37)

"In some birds that die of tuberculosis there are no lesions that can be seen by the unaided eye, although these birds show symptoms of tuberculosis after the disease has become well-established in the system. Smears made from the liver of such birds, stained by a special method, and examined with the microscope, will show the organisms that cause the disease. For such cases of tuberculosis, because nodules, loss of weight, and lameness, may be found in other diseased conditions, it may be necessary to have a laboratory examination in order to establish a positive diagnosis." (38)

"By far the greatest number of tubercular fowls show no symptoms. But in most diseased flocks there are some birds showing outward signs of the disease. The authors have found in very badly diseased flocks as high as one-third of the birds showing symptoms of tuberculosis, but in general the proportion is much smaller." (39)

"After the disease has been found to exist in the flock it is much more difficult to ascertain which birds are diseased and which are not, since so many diseased ones will show no symptoms. The only way which always finds all birds showing lesions of the disease is to kill and examine every bird over one year old. The young birds then in time may develop lesions of tuberculosis." (40)

"Tuberculosis may be present in the flock for weeks or even months before any symptoms are noticed. . . . The gradual development of symptoms is often overlooked and the flock may be badly infected before the nature of the malady is suspected." (41)

Tuberculosis in Dressed Poultry
"About 3 per cent of the dressed poultry offered for sale in American markets is infected with tuberculosis. In order to test for the possible presence of tubercle bacilli in dressed poultry, W. H. Feldman of the Mayo Foundation removed spleens asceptically from 125 fowls at the time of evisceration by a local dealer."

(Then follows a description of his procedure in making the tests.) "Since virulent tercule bacilli are thus present in about 3 per cent of apparently normal fowls, and since no practical method of postmortem inspection will disclose their presence, Feldman concludes that the rearing of fowls for food markets should be prohibited in environments known to be infected with avian tuberculosis." (42)

How, then, can one be sure the fowls he eats are healthy?

The Egg Question

"There may be some possibility of bringing tuberculosis into a flock with eggs purchased for hatching, but such chances are very slight." (43)

"It is best to restock from eggs or from chicks a few days old. It is possible that eggs may contain tubercle bacilli, but such possibility is rare, and even if a few did, such eggs often do not hatch, or the chicks do not live long enough to become diseased to such an extent that they will be the cause of infection of other chickens." (44)

The author quoted is concerned about his flock and his business, but the eater of eggs might be concerned about his health.

Examination showed that of "876 eggs from tubercular hens less than one per cent of the eggs contain living tubercle bacilli. They also state that indications are that 30 per cent of the tuberculous hens in all stages of the disease do not lay." (45)

But who wants to eat that 1 per cent which is infected? Note also that 70 per cent of the affected hens may lay eggs.

Danger in the Egg

Hull, probably the outstanding authority in this field says that man's chief danger of contracting tuberculosis from chickens does not lie in eating the flesh because it is usually cooked, but rather in eating the eggs. Common methods of cooking the eggs will not destroy the bacillus and so they are eaten in living virulent state. (237)

PARATUBERCULOSIS IN CATTLE
(Johne's Disease; Chronic Bacterial Dysentery)
Spreads Unawares

"The disease affects cattle and, in rare instances, sheep and goats. ... Like tuberculosis, it progresses very slowly in the animal, which therefore, may show no evident symptoms for many months after the disease is established in the tissues. The transfer of such an apparently healthy, but really diseased, animal from one herd to another is very likely to produce another center of infection from which the disease may spread to other herds. The rapidity of distribution of the disease increases as the centers of infection increase." (51)

"In several States, indemnities can be paid for the slaughter of cattle with Johne's disease on the same basis as for the slaughter of tuberculous cattle. Since human beings are not subject to the disease, and it does not damage edible parts of the carcass, the meat is suitable for human consumption, subject of course to inspection." (238)

BRUCELLOSIS

"*Synonyms.* Undulant fever, Mediterranean fever, gastric fever, Malta fever, rock fever, Gibraltar fever, melitococcie, goat fever, Texas fever, Rio Grande fever, Brucella fever, Bang's fever.

"*Definition.* Brucellosis in man is a systemic or focal infection caused by Brucella melitensis, Brucella abortus, or Brucella suis. The disease is characterized by weakness, fever with morning remissions, occipital or frontal headache, muscular pains, profuse sweats, chills, constipation, secondary anemia, nervous disturbances, and metastatic involvement of the joints, the eyes, and the reproductive organs. The course is of indefinite duration, but may be marked by repeated relapses and may become chronic. The mortality is low." (52)

Localized Brucella Infections

"Localization has long been recognized as characteristic of Brucella infections in animals. In guinea pigs, especially those inoculated with Br. suis, we have repeatedly observed suppurative lesions, notably arthritis, osteomyelitis, spondylitis, meningitis, orchitis, and abscesses of the spleen, liver, lymph nodes, and other soft tissues. In cattle brucellosis is typically a localized infection, involving the udder, the pregnant uterus, the lymph nodes, and occasionally the joints. In hogs, according to the observations of Thomsen (344) in Denmark, and Feldman and Olson (96) in this country, focal lesions are not unusual. The pregnant uterus may be affected. Suppurative or non-suppurative epididymitis is relatively frequent. Occasionally the testis or seminal vesicles are involved. Destructive bone and joint lesions, meningitis, soft tissue abscesses, and tenosynovitis are also encountered. In horses, according to Fitch (103, 104), certain rather common suppurative lesions (poll evil and fistulous withers) may be due to Brucella." (74)

World-wide Distribution

"Since Keefer's report, cases of brucellosis in human beings due to either Br. abortus or Br. suis have been found in all parts of the United States, as well as in Rhodesia, Germany, Denmark, France, Great Britain, Sweden, Argentina, and Brazil. Wherever Br. abortus or Br. suis is found in animals, there will also be found infection in humans. The world-wide distribution of brucellosis in both animals and man has recently been summarized and reported by Thomsen (345)." (53)

Annual Loss In the United States $100,000,000

The annual loss to the livestock industry in the United States is estimated conservatively at—

Loss of milk production	$ 50,000,000
Loss of calves	5,000,000
Loss of infected cows	32,000,000
Loss caused in other stock	13,000,000

Total annual loss, not including human sickness $100,000,000

(281)

Costs $5,000,000.00 Annually in Illinois

"No infectious disease of cattle appears to be more widely distributed in Illinois than Bang's disease. . . . Apparently about 12 per cent of the cattle in Illinois react to the agglutination test. . . .

"Conservative estimates place the total loss to cattle owners in Illinois as a result of this disease at a minimum of $5,000,000.00 annually." (59)

Costs $5,000,000.00 Annually in Michigan

"The disease causes a probable annual loss to Michigan dairy farmers of more than $5,000,000.00." (60)

Causes More Losses Than All Other Diseases Combined

Brucellosis causes more loss to cattlemen than all other diseases combined. (61)

Ten to Twelve Per Cent of Animals Tested Are Affected

"Bang's disease, or infectious abortion, exists in nearly all countries where cattle are raised. It appears to be world-wide. The disease has spread in the United States to the extent that many herds, either purebred or grade, show evidence of the disease. The testing campaign so far conducted in Minnesota has shown that 30 to 40 per cent of the herds are infected. In other words, about one herd out of every three has the disease. From 10 to 12 per cent of the animals so far tested in this state show the infection. This is a little more than twice the amount of tuberculosis present in Minnesota." (54)

Wyoming

Two hundred seventy-four herds from sixty-five counties were tested which included every county but one in the state of Wyoming. Only three counties showed no reactors. And only a few in each herd were tested. (62)

One hundred seventy-nine herds showed reactors.

Ninety-five herds showed none.

There were 1086 reactors among 4501 cattle tested, or 24 per cent of those tested. (63)

Three Times as Prevalent as Was Tuberculosis

"Brucellosis is receiving increased attention as a disease of world-wide importance. With reference to its incidence in animals in this country, Dr. Giltner states: 'Brucellosis is perhaps three times as prevalent as was tuberculosis at the time its eradication was begun.' Its prevalence in man in the United States is not known definitely because of differences in the accuracy of diagnosis. It is hoped that this volume will promote more effective diagnosis and treatment of brucellosis." (64)

Will Not Soon Be Eradicated—The Opinion of an Expert

"Bang's disease may some day be fully eradicated from the cattle, but I do not anticipate that the present generation will witness that accomplishment." (65)

Clean Herds Are Impossible

If the elimination of all of the infected cows were required "many a dairy herd would lose from a quarter to a half of its otherwise healthy cows at the first test; and it would require repeated tests at fairly short intervals, with the elimination of still more cows from time to time, over a period of years, before we would be reasonably sure that the milk no longer contained undulant fever germs. The expense of such a program would be prohibitive." (282)

Well-advanced Before Discovered

"Bang's disease strikes slowly and quietly, it gains a well fortified position in a herd before its presence is discovered." (75)

Many Unsuspected Cattle Are Spreaders for Years

"Two degrees of resistance are found among cattle that remain infected. Some of them will become normal breeders and to all appearances will be normal cows. These animals are, however, still spreaders of Bang's disease. Many cattle belong in this group." (76)

Wherever There Are Hogs There is Brucellosis

"Brucellosis, or Traum's disease, in swine, accompanied by premature birth of young, has been reported from nearly every hog-raising section in the United States." (56)

More Hogs, More Brucellosis in Man

"Though the prevalence of contagious abortion in hogs is not accurately defined, it is still evident that in the United States the incidence of recognized brucellosis in man tends to vary directly with the extent of the hog-raising industry." (72)

From Swine to Man

"Brucellosis of swine is communicable to man. The disease in man is known as undulant fever. Persons handling infected animals or aborted materials from infected animals should use every possible precaution to avoid acquiring the infection." (71)

Cattle Infected from Swine

"It has not been established that swine can contract brucellosis from infected cattle, but it is known that cattle can be infected with Brucella suis. Every possible safeguard should therefore be employed to prevent the disease from being passed from swine to cattle." (57)

Brucellosis in Goats

"In the United States Brucellosis in goats is confined principally to southwestern states." (283)

Viability of Brucella Germs

Lives—
        43 days in soil which dries slowly
        60 days in soil which dries quickly
        21 days in damp soil
        42 days in sterilized tap water
        28 days in dry building dust
        15 days in sterilized sea water
Direct sun rays kill it in a few hours
Not destroyed—
        by artificial gastric juice
        by meat-curing brine
        at 10 below zero
        by 7 months in ice chest
        in ice cream for 30 days
        in butter 142 days

Temperature of—
            140 degrees F. kills in 20 minutes
            142 degrees F. kills in 15 minutes
            145 degrees F. kills in 10 minutes   (87)

Brucellosis in Animals Causes Undulant Fever in Man

Methods of Spread From Animals to Man

"Brucellosis, caused by bovine, porcine or caprine strains of brucella, is transmissible from animals to man. Cows and hogs are the usual source of undulant fever in Iowa, apparently also in many other states. Although goats were found to be the source of undulant (Malta) fever in the Mediterranean region, in Texas and other southwestern states, these animals have not thus far been incriminated as the source of endemic human infection in Iowa.

"People usually acquire the disease (1) as the result of direct contact with infected animals or (2) following the use of raw dairy products from infected cows. When the disease is due to contact with infected animals or their tissues, the germ gains entrance to the human body through the skin.

"Persons who live on farms are more subject to undulant fever than those who live in cities. On farms, the disease affects more male workers than females, due to the fact that men on the farm come in contact with hogs and cows to a much greater extent than do women.

"Urban residents, with the notable exception of packing house workers, have little or no occasion for direct contact with infected animals. Undulant fever acquired in city or town is due, as a rule, to the use of raw milk, cream and butter, from dairy cows infected with Bang's disease." (240)

Undulant Fever

"It will be noted that the hazard of exposure to brucella infection is greatest in the group of packing house employees, second greatest among male farm workers, with a far smaller relative hazard among children, housewives and merchant professional groups.

"Among 118 packing house workers who acquired undulant fever during the 6 year period 1936-1941 (see table 3), 98 per cent gave the history of direct contact with live stock; only 20 per cent of this group used raw dairy products during the period preceding onset of illness." (241)

Undulant Fever Average Duration is Four Months

"The victims are often sick for a long time, the average being four months. . . . There are doubtless numbers of low grade ailing cases who never get into the hands of a physician or who are never diagnosed as undulant fever. . . . It is claimed that the more malignant goat and hog strains weave back through cattle to the *human* being. While it is possible that some of this takes place, competent technicians in America have also found the bovine strain in human cases. As far as *milk* is concerned, the cow is responsible for the transmission of the disease whatever strain of organism is present." (242)

Not Always Recognized

"The present or past prevalence of brucellosis cannot be determined reliably. There is reason to believe that this clinical entity occurred in the United States and other countries for many years before it was finally commonly diagnosed. Undoubtedly the present completeness of its recognition and reporting varies markedly. However, it is known to be a widely distributed disease. No broad areas have been conclusively shown to be free of Brucella infection in animals and in man."

"About 10 per cent of the population has become infected with the germ. The chronic form is far more common than the acute." (70)

UNDULANT FEVER

A Public Health Hazard

"From a public health standpoint, human infection with the swine type of Brucella is unquestionably more important than human infection with the bovine type. It is a recognized fact that Brucella melitenis, the goat type, induces the most severe type of undulant fever, the disease in human beings. Next in order is the swine type, and last, the bovine type. This fact has been established by isolating the various types of organisms from infected human beings and observing the severity of the disease, caused by each of the three species. It has been estimated by Public Health Service officials that about 50 per cent of human infection is due to Brucella suis and is the result of contact with infected swine on farms or in abattoirs. The frequent occurrence of the disease in human beings in swine-raising localities is indicative of the danger, and the disease often occurs among workers in packing houses as a result of handling carcasses of infected swine. Studies have shown that in the Corn Belt more than half the cases of undulant fever are caused by the swine type, and that in regions where the infection in hogs is not common this type of infection in man is less frequent." (243)

"It may be . . . that ten years from now (by 1956) brucellosis (undulant fever) will rank first among the infectious diseases." (284)

"Undulant fever continues to be a major health problem." (285)

Rarely Transmitted from Human to Human

"Brucellosis in man rarely if ever spreads to other human beings although it is conceivable that it is contagious from man to man under certain conditions; certainly it is the part of wisdom to take suitable precautions against such a possibility." (73)

The First Case

The first recognized case of undulant fever in man was in the state of Iowa in the year 1926, in December. Now it is a national animal and human health problem.

Milk Glands Chief Seat; Milk Unsafe

"Since the mammary gland or the udder is regarded as the chief permanent residence of the Bang germ, milk from diseased herds usually contains the germs, and, therefore, serves as a medium for spreading the disease." (82)

"Infected cows may give off Brucella abortus through milk for many years." (83)

Milk and Cream Are Carriers

"Does pasteurization destroy Brucella abortus in milk? Yes, provided pasteurization is carefully done. Thirty minutes at 145 degrees F. (63.9 degrees C.) is sufficient.

"Should raw milk from Brucella-infected cows be regarded as dangerous for human food? It is potentially dangerous. Virulent strains might infect man following ingestion. A disease known as undulant fever in man is sometimes caused by Brucella abortus. Compared with the number of persons that consume raw milk, however, there are but few known cases of undulant fever traceable to this organism. Relatively few persons seem susceptible, or it may be that undulant fever is not yet generally recognized. The danger to man from virulent Brucella organisms in milk can be eliminated by efficient pasteurization.

"In what part of the milk is Brucella abortus found in largest numbers? When milk is infected, cream contains relatively larger numbers of the organisms than skim milk." (84)

Seventeen Per Cent of a Group of Children Infected

"Mohler and Traum as early as 1911, on examining the tonsils of children consuming raw milk, isolated Br. abortus in one instance. A few years later Larson and Sedgwick examined the blood of 425 children that had received raw milk in their diet. Of these, seventy-three, or seventeen per cent, gave a positive test. The clinical diagnosis in these cases was tuberculosis or rickets." (85)

"Are We Sure?"

"Are we sure that cases of glandular disease or cases of abortion, or possibly diseases of the respiratory tract, may not sometimes occur among human subjects in this country as a result of drinking raw cow's milk? (86)

Milk Is a Carrier

"The udders of many infected cows, whether they abort or not, contain and eliminate the germs for a widely variable period. . . . The abortion germs may be present in the milk of some infected cows during all the rest of their lives after the malady is contracted." (78)

"In some instances between three and four months was required before a positive diagnosis by the agglutination test was established. . . . A like period may sometimes elapse before the fact is revealed by test." (80)

Who eats the milk during that time?

"The milk of cows that are infected often contains many organisms. It has been found that from sixty to eighty per cent of badly infected cows eliminate the organisms in their milk. The number of abortion organisms in each cubic centimeter, or twenty-four drops, has been found to be from 110 to 4300, and even as high as 50,000 has been reported. The organism may appear in the milk before abortion and remain for from two to four months, and occasionally for life." (81)

Standard Testing Does Not Reveal It
Brucellosis Common in Milk

"Investigators have stated variously that 10 to 40 per cent or even more of market milk contains the organism of Bang's disease. An infected cow is said to shed it in the milk only periodically. In an infected herd only one or only a few cows shed it at one time. Where for instance 40 per cent of the herds are infected with Bang's disease, it can be expected that much market milk will contain the germ and that it will exist in numerical proportion according to the dilution of infected milk with non-infected milk. For the most part it will be thinly distributed in the milk. The use of milk from a single infected cow is likely to lead to a higher intake of Bang's bacilli than from market milk. The germ exists in greater concentration in the cream than in other portions of the milk. When the germ is found in the milk it is because of especial laboratory tests. It takes two or three days to grow a colony on agar media and ordinary bacterial milk counts made in the enforcement of laws and ordinances do not include it. It resists a considerable degree of souring and may be present in the milk for a long time. It is destroyed by proper pasteurization." (244)

There Is No Medicine

"There is no medicine or combination of materials known to be a cure for Bang's disease." (88)

No Cure; Vaccination Disappointing

"Science has not been able to develop a cure for the disease. Vaccination has been disappointing." (89)

For several years experiments were made with vaccination of cattle, but the living Brucellosis germs used were found in the milk and so increased the danger to the public.

Promising Experiments

As this book goes to press there are beginning to appear in research publications, reports of progress being made to prevent and to remedy Brucellosis and undulant fever. These reports seem very promising. One method concerning which very favorable reports are being made is to raise the immunity by balancing the nutrition of animals and humans by restoring to the soil certain minerals which it has lost. The same minerals may be fed direct to animals and humans while the soil is being restored. The same is said to be efficiacious in handling mastitis.

PREVALENCE OF UNDULANT FEVER—PASTEURIZATION OF MILK
VACCINATION OF CATTLE

"Cases have been reported from 68 of the 92 counties in Indiana in 1945. This does not mean the disease is not present in some counties. Persons with mild symptoms often do not seek medical advice. Diagnosis is often very difficult. Furthermore, the State Veterinarian, Dr. J. L. Axby, reveals that he has evidence there is an animal reservoir, especially bovine, in every county of the State. Dr. Axby also calls attention to the possibility that many cases of human brucellosis apparently acquired by ingestion of raw milk from cows may nevertheless have been due to Brucella suis.

"(The highest incidence is among farmers. They use raw milk more than do other classes of people.) Probably the most valuable procedure now available for prevention of the spread of undulant fever in human beings is the use of pasteurized milk. In addition, butter, buttermilk, cream, cottage cheese and other products derived from milk should be produced usually from pasteurized milk. Pasteurization is said not to affect the food value of milk. Milk is such a splendid medium for many types of bacteria and it is inoculated so easily by accident that the use of the raw product is always attended by a certain amount of risk. The risk includes also the danger of infection from several other serious diseases sometimes conveyed by this vehicle.

"Safety is facilitated, but not guaranteed, when the producer is careful to buy only those animals that are negative to laboratory tests. A cow that reacts negatively today may react positively two or three months later. The source of its infection may be determined only with great difficulty or not at all.

"Some dairymen have acquired the false impression that the cow that aborts should be vaccinated. Vaccination performed at this time may prevent abortion, but does not necessarily kill the germs in the animal. Hence the milk of the vaccinated animal may continue to be infectious for susceptible consumers. Apparently these owners do not realize that infections of the cow's udder may be as important from an economical point of view as the loss of the calf. They do not realize that old methods of vaccination with living germs often resulted in spreading the disease to previously healthy animals. However a new technique in vaccination appears to be very helpful. A special strain of the germ is used as the immunizing agent. This strain does not as a rule lead to the permanent infection of the animal with living virulent germs. The vaccination should be done only between the ages of four and eight months. It is believed the proper use of this method may serve a useful purpose in preventing the spread of the disease in infected herds. It may also prevent the occurrence of the disease in clean herds. . . .

"Among humans the disease does not spread from case to case.

It is acquired only by drinking raw milk or by handling infected animals or products from such animals. The disease is believed to be very common. Most cases are mild. Nevertheless they probably constitute an important percentage of undiagnosed physical disability. Brucellosis appears to be a major problem." (245)

The Vaccination Program

Experimentation is still carried on, and the plan now advocated is to vaccinate heifers between six and eight months of age which as yet have no mammary tissue in which the germs can become established. This plan has been widely adopted and is now regarded as an important aid in the control of the disease in connection with the test and slaughter method.

The Ideal Solution

"The ideal solution of the Brucellosis problem would be the eradication of Brucella by destroying all sources or reservoirs of the various species of the organism. These reservoirs are, so far as we know, the infected domesticated animals, especially the goat, cow, pig, and to a lesser degree, the importance of which cannot now be appraised, the sheep, horse, and barnyard fowl." (92)

Eat to Eradicate

"The test-and-slaughter method is similar to the one used so effectively in the eradication of tuberculosis. This method involves the immediate disposal for slaughter of the animals which react to the test. . . . In this plan it is necessary that repeated tests of the herd be made at intervals of from thirty to sixty days, and that the same disposition be made of any subsequent reactors. . . . This method may prove costly in herds where the disease is making rapid headway, as the owners may find it necessary to dispose of many more animals than the original test indicated would be necessary. On the other hand, the test-and-slaughter method is likely to be successful and practical in herds having a low percentage of reactors, those in which the breeding or milk-producing value of the animals is not greatly in excess of their value for beef." (93)

How Eradicate It From Humans?

"In the light of present knowledge the prevention and control of brucellosis in man is directly dependent upon its control and eradication in domestic animals." (286)

A Plan For Perfect Protection

"The one perfect protection against serious injuries from the use of infected milk and infected meat is the return to the original diet of man, which all biologists now recognize as having been derived exclusively from the vegetable kingdom." (287)

The Conclusion

The foregoing information concerning Brucellosis, coming from the authorities indicated, will disturb some of the readers of this book, as it does not add to the zest of eating the flesh of swine, cattle, sheep, goats, or fowl, nor to the use of milk, cream, butter or cheese.

Certain readers may feel that *thorough cooking* of all flesh foods and pasteurization of the milk and its products, will make them appetizing and satisfactory. (The chapter on Pasteurization will be of interest in this connection.)

But there is an increasing number of students of this question who are seeking a way of living which is more appetizing, safer, and more healthful,—a way of nourishing the body direct from the products of the earth. One purpose of this book is to make plain how the body can be scientifically sustained with better foods, more delightful to the eye, and more appealing to the esthetic sense, than is commonly done.

Mastitis (Garget) in Cows

The Incidence

"The development of a high-producing udder has apparently resulted in a gland readily susceptible to injury and infection. This common udder infection called mastitis, 'garget,' or mammitis, is found in almost all countries where dairy cows are kept. This is, economically, one of the most destructive diseases in the dairy industry today. An estimate of fifteen per cent cow replacements annually, because of mastitis, is made for the dairy herds in the United States. In New York state alone, the estimated annual loss from mastitis, due to replacements and reduced production, is seventy-two million dollars." (94)

Forcing a Cause

"Over-feeding and high protein grain mixtures are commonly associated with mastitis and breeding troubles. Avoid forcing production. Rely upon commonly accepted feeding standards and cows bred for production." (95)

Infectious

"In approximately ninety per cent of the cases, mastitis is infectious. The specific cause is usually a type of bacteria technically called streptococci which typically grows in long bead-like chains." (96)

Enter Through the Teat

"These streptococci apparently must enter the udder through the teat canal." (97)

Often Undetected

"Mastitis germs will subsist for a considerable length of time, possibly up to thirty days, outside the cow's udder. These infectious bacteria are kept in constant circulation by the presence of chronically infected cows, some of which may not show physical evidence of the disease." (98)

Progress Unseen

"Usually the disease is not so spectacular. The injury progresses unseen for several months or years, until much of the gland tissue is replaced by useless scar or fibrous tissue. Sometimes such udders develop abscesses or 'lumps' and are called indurated." (99)

HALF OF THE COWS

"It is not unusual to find infectious mastitis in half the cows in many dairy herds. The total annual loss that results from reduced production, poor quality milk, and seriously diseased cows is enormous. There are two forms of mastitis—chronic and acute. The disease usually occurs in the chronic form and is difficult to detect. The acute form, which is a flare-up of the chronic form in most cases, is easily recognized by redness and swelling of the affected quarter, reduced milk flow and marked changes in the appearance of the secretion. In advanced cases of chronic mastitis, the quarter becomes hardened and milk production is greatly reduced. The disease is caused by bacteria, which are spread on the hands of milkers or in the cups of milking machines." (246)

Forty Per Cent Infected

"Once this udder trouble gets into a herd, the dairyman is soon convinced that it will 'spread.' Sometimes it spreads rapidly and causes great injury to the udder. Usually it spreads slowly, requiring several years to establish itself thoroughly throughout the herd. Often this depends on the type or virulence of the mastitis germ, or on the management practices in the herd. An incidence of forty to sixty per cent infection is not uncommon in herds where no mastitis control measures are followed." (100)

Unknown, Undetected

"All tests. . . . *fail to detect* the dangerous occult subclinical case of mastitis. By the term subclinical we refer to the cow that harbors mastitic streptococci or other pathogens in one or more quarters of the udder, without any gross manifestation of the disease, either as regards the physical condition of the udder or the physical or chemical conditions of the milk. Such animals are definite carriers of the infection and potential spreaders of the infective agents of mastitis.

"It is these very subclinical cases, *unknown and undetected* by the ordinary means of diagnosis that are today causing havoc with apparent relapses or reinfections in many herds where the supervising veterinarian thought he had the disease suppressed or eradicated. The incidence of mastitis in a herd can be materially and transitorially reduced by ordinary diagnostic tests in most herds, but it is impossible to entirely eradicate the disease unless the hidden dormant subclinical cases are ferreted out by bacterilogical means and considered and treated accordingly." (247)

No Recovery

"Unfortunately, complete recovery from infectious mastitis rarely occurs. The udder inflammation may subside temporarily and the milk appear normal, thereby giving the appearance of recovery.

"The infection commonly flares up from time to time, however, and the milk will show temporary evidence of garget. These outbreaks may become increasingly severe from one lactation period to another until the injury done produces lumpy, contracted, nonfunctional or lost quarters. Dairymen must appreciate the fact that persistent chronic mastitis constantly may be producing injury to the udder without the cow showing physical evidence of the disease. An animal may fail to react to mastitis tests during these intervals between 'attacks.' Such cases will be detected if the tests are applied at regular intervals throughout the year." (101)

Damages Milk Glands

"Garget is of great economic importance because it damages the tissues upon which milk production depends. The affected quarters may never again come into full production, or they may be entirely lost, and the disease may actually result in the death of the cow. Mastitis also has some public health significance. 'Gargety' milk is frequently seriously impaired in quality for human food because of its obnoxious appearance, its altered flavor and chemical composition, and also because it may contain bacteria such as are occasionally associated with human sore throat and other human infections." (102)

Pus Cells in Milk

"Milk from cows with chronic mastitis may be altered in several ways, some of which can be seen while others are not apparent. The inflammation produced by the streptococci infection commonly causes blood or blood constituents to seep into the milk ducts and hence into the milk. Severely affected udders yield bloody milk. The more severe chronic types of infection yield milk that is watery, discolored, or full of clots or clumps (gargety).

"This well-known clotted or stringy milk, characteristic of garget, is the result of excess leucocytes (white blood cells or pus cells). Abnormal numbers of these cells in milk are the direct effect of udder inflammation." (103)

A Source of Septic Sore Throat

"Streptococcus-infected milk should not be consumed in the raw state because of the possibility of human infection. This may take the form of epidemics of septic sore throat, if a streptococcus of human origin is involved, or isolated cases of human infection when certain bovine as well as some human streptococci are concerned. Only persons free from sore throats and open sores on their hands should milk the cows." (104)

SEPTIC SORE THROAT

"Septic sore throat in human beings is often traceable to the consumption of raw milk from cows harboring the *Streptococcus epidemicus* organism. The onset of symptoms occurs within a few days after exposure. Mastitis (garget, or caked udder) in cows may be caused by a variety of bacteria, including certain types of streptococci and staphylococci. Some scientists state that the bovine mastitis streptococcus is a cause of septic sore throat in man, but others disagree.

"Concerning the relationship of streptococci recovered from man and those isolated from the lower animals, Kelser states that according to some authorities *Streptococcus pyogenes* is common to both man and animals. Others maintain that the organism is primarily a human type." (248)

Gargety Milk Unfit to Eat

"Finally, mastitis milk usually contains streptococci, sometimes in great numbers. These bacteria naturally reduce the quality of the milk. Some of these bacteria have been associated with human infections, and, therefore, such milk must be considered unfit for human use." (105)

No Cure
"No reliable cure for garget is known." (106)
See "Promising Experiments" in section on Brucellosis.

MILK SICKNESS
Milk sickness in man and trembles in animals is caused by cow's eating rayless goldenrod. It is transmitted to man through the cow's milk. (249)

ACTINOMYCOSIS
(In Cattle, Lumpy Jaw)

This is a tumor-like swelling caused by members of the ray fungus group. It affects cattle, man, horses, pigs, and sheep. It less often affects dogs, goats, guinea pigs, rabbits, and geese. Many wild animals have it.

When Such Cattle Are Slaughtered
In most cases only the head is discarded and the remainder of the animal is eaten. (108)
The disease may involve the lungs, liver, spleen, muscles and brain. (109)

The Udder May Be Involved
"When the udder is involved, pus may escape through the abscessed wall or the teat canal." (110)
In 1936 out of 16,000,000 animals 215,870 cases were reported. (111)

SMALL POX; COW POX
Is primarily a disease of man; secondarily it infects cattle and is then called cow pox. From cattle the disease may be passed back again to man but in a modified form called vaccinia which is not fatal. (250)

ANAPLASMOSIS
(A disease similar to Tick Fever)

Affects bovine, antelope, buffalo, camel, deer, sheep, goats. Is spread over the Southern States and into the North. (112) Is transmissible to man.

BLACKLEG

"Blackleg is a rapidly fatal, infectious disease which is confined to certain areas where the soil is infected with the blackleg organism." (113)

"Blackleg is caused by a specific micro-organism (germ) which produces spores (seeds) which are very resistant to destruction and may survive in the soil of a pasture for several years. Animals are infected through small punctures of the skin by thorns, briers, stubble, burs, barbed wire, etc." (114)

ANTHRAX

Universal, Infectious

"Anthrax is an infectious disease of livestock caused by a germ that exists in the soil of certain regions known as 'anthrax districts.' Such districts exist in practically all countries where livestock is raised." (153)

Losses Great; Endangers Public Health

"The disease causes annual losses of many millions of dollars to the livestock industry. It is also infectious to man and is a menace to public health." (154)

Germs Multiply Rapidly

"Once in the body, the germs multiply rapidly; after death every drop of blood contains myriads of the disease-producing organisms." (155)

All Livestock, and Man

"Practically all species of livestock are susceptible to this disease, which is transmissible to man. Cattle, horses, sheep are most commonly affected and develop the disease in an acute form, with a high resulting death rate. Hogs acquire the disease for the most part in a chronic form from which they frequently recover." (156)

Effects on Human

"Anthrax is infectious to man also, being contracted through the handling of anthrax-infected carcasses, hides, wool, or hair, and manifesting itself as a local infection of the skin or as an infection of the respiratory or digestive tracts. In the latter forms, the disease spreads rapidly throughout the entire body and terminates in death." (157)

May be carried by wool, bone meal, fertilizer, or forage. (158)

"It may terminate in fatal septicemia or blood poisoning." (159)

"The inhaled spores may set up a rapidly fatal form of pneumonia." (160)

Infection of animals usually takes place by ingesting the organism. It may be passed from animal to animal, or from animal to man by biting flies. Shaving brushes made with hair from abroad have been a source of infection.

Fields once infected are difficult to cleanse.

Viability

The spores "are very resistant to heat, cold, drying, and exposure to disinfectants. In the soil these spores may live for years, ready to reproduce the disease in susceptible animals that may come in contact with them." (161)

FOOT AND MOUTH DISEASE

Universal Among Cattle

"Foot and mouth disease is one of the most universal diseases of cattle, as well as one of the most difficult to suppress. Although essentially a disease of cattle, most other farm animals are susceptible in varying degrees." (162)

Taken by Man

"Foot and mouth disease is transmissible to man." (163)

Highly Contagious

"Because of the highly contagious character of the disease, strict quarantine regulations are put into effect as soon as foot and mouth disease is suspected." (164)

Mortality High

"The mortality reached from thirty to fifty per cent of the adult animals in some affected areas." (165)

Carried by Other Animals

"It may be carried by dogs, cats, rats, chickens, pigeons and other birds." (166)

Various Media

It may be spread through the medium of "manure, hay, utensils, drinking troughs, railway cars, animal markets, barnyards and pastures." (167)

In Animal Secretions and Excretions

"The contagion may be found in the serum of the vesicles and vesicle coverings on the mouth, feet, and udder; in the saliva, milk, and other secretions and excretions; also in the blood during the rise of temperature." (168)

Cattle Spread It Undetected

"Infected animals even before they show any visible symptoms of the disease may eliminate virus from their bodies in large quantities, thus acting as an unexpected source of spread of the disease." (169)

May Exist Inside and Not Show Outside

"The disease may attack some of the internal organs before it appears on any of the external tissues. These cases are very likely to prove quickly fatal. The animal dies from paralysis of the heart, due to formation of poisonous substances within the system, or it may suffocate by reason of the action of these same positions on tissues of the lungs, or it may choke to death as a result of paralysis of the throat." (170)

Milk "Dangerous"

"In cases of serious affection of the udder the erosions will often be found located within the passages of the teats, resulting in a 'caked' udder, and the same toxic poisoning which is the cause of death in the apoplectiform types just mentioned may arise from this source. In any event, the milk from such cases will be found to be dangerous for use, causing fatal diarrhea in sucking calves or young pigs, and serious illness in human consumers." (171)

"Milk in a raw state may transmit the disease to animals fed with it." (172)

This disease is so infectious and so dangerous that it is watched with extreme care. No outbreak has occured in the United States for several years.

In 1947 an outbreak occurred in Mexico which spread into 32 states of that country and threatened to extend into the United States. Our government officials were alarmed and by Dec. 1947 had spent $35,000,000 fighting the disease. (288)

DISEASE X

In 1948 a new disease of cattle was reported having been found in 26 states. For want of a name it was called "Disease X." It was reported to cause serious losses of meat, milk, and other animal products. (289)

Q FEVER

This disease of cattle was first noticed in Queensland, Australia in 1937. It was reported by the U. S. Public Health Service in May 1948, as already having attacked humans among stock yard workers.

It is a virus disease which cannot be distinguished from virus pneumonia except by blood tests.

It is understood to pass to human being by inhaling barnyard dust carried by the wind.

TRICHINOSIS

There are no figures showing the prevalence of Trichinella spiralis in swine. The reason, in part, is that—

"It is almost impossible to detect infected hog flesh by inspection because the cysts are so very small and because they are of the same general color as the muscular tissue in which they are imbedded ... Government microscopic inspection of pork for trichinae was discontinued in 1907." (173)

"As there is no test for trichinosis meat except by actual destruction of meat fibers and microscopic examination, government authorities cannot combat it. So the protection lies in proper cooking—pork of any kind must be cooked until white. Pink pork is dangerous and should never be eaten." (174)

Pork has well been called a "diet of worms" even when "well done."

In Man

"Its clinical picture may simulate typhoid fever, its abdominal pain, appendicitis, the muscle pain and weakness, neuritis, or arthritis, the dropsical swelling, kidney trouble, and it may have deceptive meningeal, heart, and lung complications to help mislead a diagnosis."

"Usually following the consumption of infected or undercooked food there is a short incubation period in which the larvae taken into the intestine reach maturity and the females penetrate the intestinal mucosa. In about eight days the embryos are discharged fully formed and penetrate into the intestinal lymphatics, are carried to the messenteric lymph nodes and the thoracic duct and thence to the general circulation."

"After reaching the capillaries they may wander into various regions, as lungs, heart, brain, etc. The majority reach the voluntary muscles finally, these being most suitable for encystment."

"The most pronounced symptoms occur when the trichinella embryos are invading the tissues and organs of the body."

"Following a variable incubation period of five days to two or three weeks there is a sudden onset of gastro-intestinal symptoms, the severity of which depends on the number of parasites ingested, and the clinical picture of a febrile disease resembling typhoid fever supervenes." (173)

At a conference of New York and New Jersey health officers these statements were made: "Particularly disturbing is the fact that the medical profession as a whole does not recognize this parasitic infection but writes down a diagnosis of typhoid, intestinal 'flu,' or may even operate for appendicitis. In all, some sixty diseases have been confused with trichinosis." (175)

Cannot Be Diagnosed

From the foregoing it can be seen that there is no other way to accurately diagnose trichinosis except at the autopsy.

Inasmuch as there is "No successful treatment for trichinosis . . . known," (176) there is no alternative for the autopsy.

The following paragraph summarizes the reports of autopsy findings.

Autopsy Findings

The recent evidence from necropsies that thirty-six per cent of the inhabitants of Cleveland have trichinosis must not be interpreted as proof that Cleveland is the most highly infested area in the United States. It suggests rather that the routine diagnostic methods employed by earlier investigators were fallacious. Routine examinations of the diaphragms of adult cadavers by the Baermann digestion method led previous investigators to the conclusion that approximately 13.67 per cent of all persons in or around Washington, D. C., are infested with trichinae, 17.5 per cent in Minneapolis and Rochester, N. Y., 24 per cent in San Francisco and 27.6 per cent in Boston. Hall and Collins (Hall, M. C., and Collins, B. J.: Pub. Health Rep. 54:468, April 16, 1937) however, showed that the routine Baermann technic failed to detect about 29.3 per cent of the positive cases. Evans (Evans, C. H.: J. Infect. Dis. 63:337, Nov.-Dec., 1938) of the Institute of Pathology, Cleveland, therefore supplemented this routine diagnostic method by application of the newer compression microscopic technic. In this technic 1 gm. samples of the diaphragm, intercostal muscle and sterno-mastoid muscle are compressed between two pieces of plate glass and examined microscopically. Parallel digestions were made with one hundred gm. samples of the same muscles. Diaphragmatic digestion alone revealed the presence of twenty cases of trichinosis in one hundred consecutive necropsies. This is about the average of the percentages reported by previous investigators. Many cadavers, however, whose diaphragms were negative showed trichinae in one or both of the skeletal muscles. Combining all positive data, Evans found thirty-six positive cases of trichinosis in the first hundred Cleveland necropsies studied by his double technic. Applying the implied correction coefficient (36-20) to the percentages previously reported from other cities, one would conclude that there are presumably the following percentages of trichina infestation in other American cities: Washington, D. C., 24.6 per cent, Minneapolis and Rochester, N. Y., 31.5 per cent; San Francisco, 43 per cent; and Boston 49.7 per cent (an average of 37 per cent infestation of the urban population of the United States.) There is no way, of course, of estimating the resulting social or economic loss; but the estimated forty-eight million cases of trichinosis in the United States is far from being a national asset. (177)

These figures indicate that there are 48,000,000 "worm-eaten" Americans.

ERYSIPELAS IN SWINE

"The specific cause of swine erysipelas is the erysipelas bacillus (Erysipelothrix rhusiapathiae), a slender, small rod 1.0 to 1.5 microns in length, as it occurs in the organs of actually affected swine. There they tend to form small conglomerations and as such they are frequently found to be contained in leucocytes. On artificial culture media, long thread-like forms of the organism may be seen; such forms have also been found to be occasionally associated with the more chronic lesions in swine. The erysipelas bacillus is non-motile and it does not form spores." (178)

Can Be Passed to Man

"Cases of the human disease in which the initial infection could be attributed to the consumption of meat either are exceedingly rare or have escaped attention. That there may be such a possibility is, however, indicated by a report of an otherwise also unusual case by Fiessingen and Brault (20). In this instance the patient developed the disease after the ingestion of salted pork, in a manner comparable to the acute septicemic form commonly observed in swine. The diagnosis was confirmed by blood cultures. The patient improved rapidly under serum treatment, but in the course of convalescence an acute nephritis and cardiac failure developed which terminated in death." (179)

Swine Erysipelas to Man

"Swine erysipelas can affect turkeys, ducks, pigeons, and sheep; possibly it is now becoming more widespread among domestic animals. It causes erysipeloid in human beings, the organism usually entering through broken skin. True human erysipelas is an entirely different disease, not caused by the swine organism." (251)

"This disease is pathogenic to man, and it seems that we should not lose sight of the public health angle of this problem." (252)

Hog Cholera

"Destroys more hogs in the U. S. than all other diseases combined." (180)

Sometimes exceeds six million hogs in one year. (180)

Is not transmissible to man. (181)

Swine Influenza to Man

"Healthy hogs brought into contact with affected animals develop influenza in three days. McBryde suggested the possibility of man becoming infected with influenza by contact with infected pigs, and emphasized the close relationship between the two diseases." (253)

Equine Encephalomyelitis

(Sleeping Sickness)

This is a disease of horses and mules which is widespread. It is also called brain fever and sleeping sickness. It is a disease of the central nervous system.

The same virus can cause sleeping sickness in man,—"encephalitis."

"Both maladies belong in a group of serious diseases of the central nervous system that includes poliomyelitis. (infantile paralysis) of human beings." (254)

It is spread by mosquitoes.

"Every indication points to the fact that it is spread by bloodsucking insects. Experiments have proved that several species of mosquitoes and the Rocky Mountain spotted fever tick can transmit the virus, and it has been found in the field in one species of mosquito and in the assassin bug. It has also been proved that over 20 species of birds, as well as cattle, swine, sheep, goats, dogs, cats, guinea pigs, rabbits, monkeys, rats, mice, gophers, hedgehogs, and woodchucks can be infected; and since 1938 the virus has been definitely found in cases of brain disease in human beings. In fact, so far as is known, no other virus is capable of infecting so many different species of animals." (255)

It (encephalitis in humans) is spread by fowls, domestic and wild.

"Fowls have been found to be the principle reservoir of the virus"

"While men and horses may suffer severely, the birds show no symptoms. Human encephalitis occurs mainly in rural areas and in the suburbs of large cities where chickens are kept." (291)

GLANDERS

This is primarily a disease of horses; man may become infected by contact with animals. Infection takes place through broken skin, by ingestion or by inhalation.

The most susceptible other animals are guinea pigs, cats, dogs, ferrets, moles, field mice, sheep, goats, hogs, and rabbits.

It can be passed from person to person but this is rare. (256)

Internal Parasites of Horses and Mules

"Horses, mules, and donkeys, 'provide shelter and subsistence'— as Foster puts it—for about 150 different internal parasites, which are of two kinds, the protozoa, or minute one-celled animals, and the worm, or helminths. Practically speaking, it can be said that no horse or mule is ever entirely free of internal parasites of some kind. Some of these parasites are confined to certain geographic regions; others are found everywhere. Many are highly specialized in the parts of the body they attack; some do a good deal of wandering in the body, often following certain regular routes. Thus practically every organ of the body has its parasites. The importance of these enemies is not generally recognized, partly because the damage they do is seldom in the nature of a specific or spectacular disease; rather it is a general sapping of the animal's vitality, and efficiency.

In general, the protozoa are of two types, those that live in the blood and those that live in the intestines, and the former are the ones that cause serious diseases, though fortunately they are limited in distribution." (257)

WORMY FOOD

Following is a list of parasites found in swine:

*Dysentery Protozoa	(182)	Intestinal Thread Worm	(192)
Coccidia	(183)	Large Intestinal Round-	
Liver Fluke	(184)	Worm	(193)
Lung Fluke	(185)	Thorn-headed Worm	(194)
*Tapeworms	(186)	Nodular Worms	(195)
*Pork Bladder Worms	(187)	Whip Worm	(196)
*Thin-neck B. Worms	(188)	Swine Kidney Worm	(197)
*The Hydatid	(189)	Lungworms	(198)
*Round Worms	(190)	*Trichina	(199)
Stomach Worms	(191)	Total 18 kinds	

(*) These parasites may be passed to human beings.

LISTERELLOSIS

"That many bacterial diseases of animals were not known until the last few decades is demonstrated by the recent discovery of another malady affecting both man and lower animals. The English investigators, Murray, Webb, and Swann described in 1926 a disease of animals characterized by a monocytosis (an increase in one of the types of white blood cells), the causative agent of which they named *Bacterium monocytogenes.* This name was later changed to Listerella monocytogenes.

"Merchant states that this organism affects a variety of species, including swine, sheep, cattle, foxes, and man. It is a small, motile rod with round ends. The mode of transmission is unknown. Guinea pigs, rabbits, mice and rats were found experimentally to be susceptible, the animals usually dying within 48 hours after exposure." (258)

TULAREMIA

"The germ that causes tularemia, *Pasteurella tularensis,* has been discovered during the last 25 years by workers in the United States Public Health Service. The disease was first observed in ground squirrels. In different localities it is known as deer fly fever or rabbit fever, and is now recognized in a wide variety of wildlife, including birds. Although discovered in Tulare County, California, the disease has been found in every part of the United States, and in foreign countries. In recent years its prevalence in this country has increased. Parker and others have recovered tularemia organisms from flowing streams in the Rocky Mountain region. A recent Public Health Report, devoted to a discussion of the sources, symptoms, and prevention of tularemia, states that there were 2,088 cases and 139 deaths from this disease in the United States alone in 1938. In 1939, 2,200 cases were reported.

"Human beings acquire infection through the bites of ticks, blood sucking flies, lice, and bedbugs, and by contact with diseased animals, especially wild rabbits. The bacteria from infected material can penetrate even unbroken skin. Eating partly cooked flesh from sick animals occasionally causes illness." (259)

TULAREMIA A HUMAN MENACE

This was once thought to be limited to certain areas but is now found in all parts of the United States.

"The infection is carried by various species of animals which suggests the possibility of its becoming a constantly growing menace to human health, and in this connection a rather widespread epidemic in beaver in Montana during the past year should be noted. . . . The presence of P. tularesis was demonstrated in four of the big streams where beaver had died, the bacteria being found in the water in one case as long as 30 days after any beavers were known to be present in the pond tested.

"The findings indicate that water may be a medium of transmission of tularemia and might be a possible source of human infection." (260)

Dogs and Children

There are several animal parasites which infest most dogs which are a menace to man. Among the most dangerous of these are two tape worms. The larva stage of one of these occurs in lice and fleas which infest dogs. Children can become infected by swallowing such lice and fleas by accident, or by crushing them and then sucking their fingers. (261)

POULTRY DISEASES

"Hardly a year passes without the occurrence of what appears to be a new poultry disease." (115)

Pullorum Disease of Chicks
(White Diarrhea)

"Pullorum disease is a highly fatal and contagious disease of young chicks. A large percentage of losses from disease in chicks under three weeks of age appears to be traceable to this cause. Its ravages have rendered many flocks unprofitable.

"The disease is one of the few affecting adult fowls that may be transmitted directly through the egg to the newly hatched chick. It is rare that mature stock infected with the disease show any symptoms, yet when infected hens are killed and the body cavity opened, abnormal or diseased yolks are found. Infected parent stock and contaminated incubators and brooders are largely responsible for the presence of the disease in young chicks.

"The specific cause of pullorum disease is a microscopic germ known as Salmonella pullorum. This organism gains entrance to the chick through the respiratory or alimentary tract with contaminated air, feed, or water, or, as indicated above, it may have been in the egg from which the chick was hatched. The germ is found in the blood, in the unabsorbed yolk, and in the internal organs of baby chicks, following death from the disease." (116)

"Among baby chicks, in exceptional cases, as high as 90 per cent of a flock may die from the disease during the first three weeks. This is unusual, but losses up to 25 or 50 per cent are common. With a small amount of infection and where good brooding and feeding methods are followed, losses have been known to run less than five per cent." (117)

This disease exists in every part of the United States. (118)

PULLORUM DISEASE

"The poison-forming germ, *Salmonella pullorum,* primarily attacks the ovaries in hens and may produce no visible symptoms or signs except reduced productivity of the hen and hatchability of its eggs. In chicks, however, it produces a devastating disease, formerly called bacillary white diarrhea, which may practically exterminate an entire brood within three weeks after hatching. The germ is transmitted through the egg and also in excreta and on bits of contaminated material, such as fluff, floating in the air. The disease is extremely contagious and infectious. Unfortunately, many of the infected chicks do not die but grow up and in their turn produce infected eggs, perpetuating and spreading the malady. Thus pullorum disease has become exceptionally widespread and has been responsible for enormous losses to poultrymen. It is one of the major problems of the hatchery industry, since a few infected eggs in one of the giant modern incubators are a source of danger to the whole hatch.

"There is no medicinal cure or preventative for pullorum disease and control depends fundamentally on locating and eliminating all carrier hens." (262)

Although Pullorum is a disease of chickens, it is also found in ducks, turkeys, guinea fowls, quail, pheasants, bullfinches, english sparrows, foxes, and rabbits.

"Pullorum disease in turkeys is less prevalent than in chickens. However, it is transmitted from the turkey hen to the poult through the egg and no doubt also in the incubator. Infected chickens may also very likely be a menace to poults." (263)

From Hen to Egg to Chick

"Chicks from eggs laid by infected hens carry infection in their yolk, internal organs and intestines at the time of hatching." (119)

An infected chick may survive, mature, and lay infected eggs. (120)

"The mother hen is the source of infection. Due to the ovarian carrier condition (permanent infection), eggs which are incubated develop apparently normal chicks which carry the specific organism in their yolk and body tissues. The chicks from these hens constitute centers of infection in the broods and thus spread the disease to other chicks, through their droppings. Surviving chicks often continue to harbor the organism, and become permanent carriers, usually ovarian, and thus the cycle is completed." (121)

The progeny of infected hens laid 1012 eggs, of which 24.7 per cent had infected yolks. (122)

One thousand, seven hundred twenty-eight incubator eggs were tested, and infection up to 8.4 per cent was found present. (123)

"Egg-Eating Habit" Unsafe

"Infection spreads among adult birds mainly through unsanitary conditions and the feeding of eggs or as a result of the egg-eating habit. It is very unsafe to feed eggs to chickens at any age because of the danger of spreading pullorum disease." (124)

If it is unsafe for chickens to eat eggs at any age, what about the unwitting public and their children?

Can Be Diagnosed Only in the Laboratory

"An accurate diagnosis of pullorum disease can be made only by laboratory examination." (125)

How is the farmer, the poultryman, or the purchaser to be sure that any individual fowl is free from this disease?

GIZZARD ULCERS IN CHICKS

"If any lot of day-old chicks is selected at random and killed, and the gizzard linings examined, it is probable that at least seventy-five per cent of the chicks will be found to have ulcers or hemorrhages in the gizzard lining. The wide-spread occurrence of this condition has been a matter of concern to many poultrymen."

"The amount of gizzard ulceration present in any lot of chicks at hatching time has no relationship to their early growth and mortality, provided they are given a good ration and kept reasonably free of infection." (129)

Was anything wrong with the eggs?

COCCIDIOSIS OF CHICKENS

"Coccidiosis is one of the most common diseases of chickens in Wyoming. It is a highly infectious disease and causes enormous losses in this state. Turkeys also frequently contract the disease. The mortality runs heavy in chicks from two to six weeks of age. Sometimes as high as sixty to eighty per cent of the flock die with coccidiosis." (130)

LEUCEMIA OF FOWLS

(Synonyms: Range paralysis, Leukemia, Leukosis.)

"One of the most serious diseases affecting poultry flocks. It occurs in both acute and chronic forms and is usually fatal. Chickens and turkeys of all breeds and ages are susceptible." (131)

Wide-spread

"Fowl leukosis is so widely spread and is causing such tremendous losses to the poultry industry that corrective measures must be made available. Otherwise the industry will be faced with economic annihilation." (132)

Mortality High

"The mortality may be very high, in some cases reaching 50 per cent or more." (133)

Increasing

"During the last few years there has been an immense increase." (134)

Conditions Produced

"Two manifestations of the disease are commonly seen, paralysis of the limbs and gray eye. Perhaps the most common and most striking type is that in which the nerves of the legs and wings are affected, with resulting lameness and drooping of wings. . . . The lameness becomes progressively worse so that the bird becomes prostrated in a day or two."

"In advanced cases, the pupils frequently become irregular in outline, very small, or eccentric, and there may be bulging of the eyeballs. In advanced gray eye there is generally partial or complete blindness. Some birds with gray eye appear to be otherwise healthy and may lay fairly well. . . . Other symptoms of disease sometimes associated with paralysis outbreaks are skin tumors and anemia. Skin tumors may be small and almost as numerous as the feather follicles."

"Anemia may be recognized by the extreme pallor of the head or by microscopic examination of the blood. If it is a true leukemia, the leucocytes, or immature blood cells, will be present in the blood in large numbers." (135)

"In the light of recent studies it would appear that a number of tumorous growths of various parts of the body including the internal organs, and particularly an extremely large mottled liver, should be included here. These conditions were at one time considered as being caused by different agents but are now being looked upon as simply different manifestations of fowl paralysis." (136)

"Fowl paralysis very commonly appears in birds which are in excellent flesh, have a good appetite, and red comb and wattles. Even after paralysis of the legs is complete birds may be in fair flesh, have excellent appetite and have a healthy appearance about the head." (137)

Nerves Attacked by Germs

"The changes which occur in the nervous system of affected birds during the course of the disease indicate quite clearly that paralysis is caused by a germ or virus which attacks the nervous tissue. Unfortunately intestinal worms as well as other common intestinal parasites, such as coccidia, have been erroneously considered as causes of paralysis." (138)

"The ovaries may be increased several times in size by tumorous masses. Ovarian leucocytic infiltration is common in leucemia, but other causes of cystic and tumorous masses of ovaries are recognized.

"Leucemic kidneys may show white streaks (urates) or they may be greatly swollen and vary in color from a pale brown to almost white. One or more lobes of the organs may be involved, and the principal kidney tissue appear normal. In some cases noticeable infiltration of lymphoid tissue in the liver, heart muscle, skeletal muscles, kidneys, ovaries, etc., may result in tumorlike growths or masses. Leucemia of the muscle is characterized by yellowish white enlargements or tumefactions which have an altered texture.

"In fowls that show lameness or drooping wings, gross enlargements of the ischiatic and brachial nerves may be present, with resulting atrophy of the muscles. The involved nerve trunks may be enlarged, dull yellowish or glistening and watery, with an absence of normal cross striations.

"A striking anatomical change appearing in connection with leucemia is the grayish-red discoloration of the bone marrow. The marrow in diseased fowls is often firmer than normal and fills the marrow cavity more completely. Sometimes this diseased marrow is almost white, very dry, and contains very little fat. Another manifestation of leucemia occurs in the bones of chicks six weeks old or older. This type of the disease is chronic, seldom fatal, and is characterized by large, irregular swellings of the leg or wing bones. At the distal portion of the bone the marrow cavity is almost obliterated, irregular and is surrounded by dense, greatly thickened bone tissue; the proximal portion of the bone is much enlarged and porous. The periosteum is adherent to the bone and the marrow appears swollen." (139)

"The changes in the spleen of a diseased fowl generally conform to those in the liver. The diseased spleen frequently becomes greatly enlarged, light in color, and may have a mottled appearance. It may be soft and pulpy or a firm, compact mass. Not infrequently it is from two to five times normal size." (140)

"Masses of leucocytes may infiltrate the liver, spleen, kidneys, skin, or muscles; in fact, practically all the visceral organs may show varying degrees of small round-cell invision. Sometimes the cellular infiltrations are so extensive as to form distinct tumorous masses (Figs. 5 and 6). The liver of a leucemic fowl is often greatly enlarged, congested, and sprinkled with minute whitish spots (Figs. 7 and 8), or it may show a diffuse whitish yellow discoloration. A cross-section of the enlarged liver may be mottled in appearance and firm. In fowls having the acute form of the disease the liver may be greyish, soft, pulpy, and four or five times its normal size." (141)

"In the diseased specimen there is a decrease in number and change in shape of the red blood cells (a. erythrocyte, and b, erythroblast) and an increase in number and type of white blood cells (c. lymphocyte, and b, polymorphonuclear leucocyte)." (142)

Diagnosed by Blood Examination

"Because of the great variation in the appearance and distribution of leucemic lesions it is often necessary, before a diagnosis is possible, to examine not less than four live sick birds from a suspected flock. In certain flocks the evidence of leucemia has been so indefinite even in post-mortem findings as to delay positive diagnosis until blood smears could be made and histological sections examined." (143)

No Medicinal Remedy

"There is no known medicinal remedy for paralysis." (144)

No Cure

"There is no known cure for leucemia."
"Kill and burn all diseased birds." (145)

Infectious

It is regarded "as an infectious disease" and therefore radical measures must be used to eradicate it. (146)

Shooting In the Dark

"The avian leukosis complex, which includes fowl paralysis accounts for about half the total annual loss due to infectious diseases in poultry. Until research discovers the cause of this disease and the way it spreads, we are shooting in the dark in our efforts to control it." (264)

Different Manifestations of Leukosis

"The different strains of fowl leukosis agent vary in their action. Some cause stimulation of erythroblastic cells only; some have the ability to stimulate the granuloblastic cells; others under certain conditions are capable of producing sarcoma. The existence of agents capable of inducing fowl paralysis and lymphoid tumors as well as leukosis is an unsettled question. Fowl leukosis is not highly if at all contagious and the possibility that the disease agent is of spontaneous origin in the affected animal must be seriously considered. The disease is readily transmitted when the pathogenicity of the particular strain of agent in question has become established. The bile, urine, and feces of affected birds are either devoid of the agent or contain it in an inactive form. The agent can be demonstrated in most of the tissues of diseased chickens by inoculation of the material into other birds. Strong doses of roentgen rays do not destroy the activity of the agent. The agent is relatively resistant to drying, freezing, and to glycerin solutions. It is thermolabile and susceptible to inactivation by oxidation." (265)

Leukosis Complex

"One type affects the eye, causing loss of color in the iris, bulging of the eyeball, changes in the size and shape of the pupil, and sometimes partial or total blindness. Another, the visceral type, affects the internal organs—liver, lungs, heart, spleen, ovary, testicles; kidneys, intestines,—causing loss of flesh, weakness, and nonproductiveness. In still another type, the long bones become thickened and enlarged. In the blood type, there are alterations in the blood, the circulation, and sometimes the bone marrow (source of red blood cells) which may quickly endanger the life of the bird. A dozen or more lengthy scientific names have been applied to these various manifestations, all of which have features that are similar and also are suggestive of certain diseases of other animals and human beings." (266)

Hereditary Through the Egg

In 1928 Doyle of Indiana "advanced the idea that the condition was hereditary and that chicks hatched from eggs from flocks in which paralysis was present would have a tendency to develop paralysis." (147)

In 1938 workers in Montana reported, "The history of flock C supports the theory that fowl leukosis is transmitted through the egg. The history of flock D indicates that fowl leukosis may be transmitted through the egg." (148)

"Leucemia appears to be transmitted naturally by direct and indirect contact, and circumstantial evidence indicates that it may to a limited extent be carried in the egg." (149)

"There is considerable evidence that this disease is transmitted *through* the egg." (150)

"Since paralysis is a distinct, infectious disease, it can be controlled only by following methods which are effective for a disease of this type. The transmissibility through the egg must always be kept in mind. Since there is no test to detect the individual birds which may transmit paralysis to their offspring, the only dependable means of avoiding the disease is to avoid affected flocks as a source of eggs for hatching or breeding stock." (151)

The Only Remedy—Watch the Egg

"The only certain remedy for paralysis is to dispose of the entire flock in which the disease occurs and then establish a new flock on clean ground by obtaining eggs for hatching, baby chicks or breeding birds from a flock which has been entirely free from paralysis and the peculiar kind of eye disease which is associated with paralysis." (152)

How can one make sure that the eggs purchased or raised are free from disease?

INFECTIOUS AVIAN ENCEPHALOMYELITIS

"Infectious avian encephalomyelitis (epidemic tremor) occurs in chicks 1 to 2 days up to 2 to 3 weeks old. Fifty per cent or more of the chicks in a flock may be affected. Many are likely to recover, but others may continue to manifest some tremor symptoms for a time.

"The practice usually recommended is to finish surviving chicks quickly for early marketing as broilers or fryers. Under favorable living conditions, the recovered and slowly convalescing birds may mature and may become normally productive of eggs, and healthy chicks. They may, however, turn out to be carriers of the infection, which they may transmit to their offspring.

"The disease does not usually affect every hatch but may disappear during the hatching season only to return unexpectedly, recurring sporadically from time to time with varying degrees of severity.

"The disease is disseminated through contact among the brood. It may also be spread through contact in the incubator, and there is some scientific evidence to indicate that infection may be handed down from parent to offspring through the egg. In this way epidemic tremor may be broadcast to remote areas through the dispersal of an infected or exposed hatch of chicks. Fortunately some strains of chickens appear to possess more resistance to the disease than others." (267)

BLUE COMB DISEASE

A new disease in chickens not yet named is sometimes called "pullet disease" and sometimes "blue comb." It takes the heaviest, best type of birds enjoying the best housing and feed. (268)

FOWL CHOLERA

"The losses traceable to fowl cholera have stamped this disease as one of the more important poultry maladies in Illinois. The disease is not seasonal, but may break out in a flock any month of the year." (126)

Chronic Type Seldom Recognized

"The chronic type of fowl cholera remains in the flock for several weeks and usually is accompanied by diarrhea and a marked drop in egg production. In this type the symptoms are obscure and seldom recognized as those of fowl cholera." (127)

FOWL TYPHOID

"Fowl Typhoid: This disease is caused by a germ, is highly contagious and is very fatal to fowl. It may occur at any season of the year, but is more prevalent from October to April." (128)

PSITTACOSIS

This is a disease of fowls widely distributed among wild parrots and similar birds. In the past few years it has found its way into breeding places and pet shops, and so among human beings.

"The striking new development disclosed by Meyer is that a case of psittacosis (so-called parrot fever) in a human being has apparently been traced to chickens and 10 other cases have been traced to pigeons.

"Psittacosis was first discovered as a disease of birds of the parrot family and occasionally of other cage birds such as canaries and finches. The fact that it causes a peculiar type of pneumonia in human beings, reputed to be fatal in 20 per cent of the cases, has been known for a long time; but human psittacosis was a medical curiosity until over 750 cases occurred in 1929-30, and 600 more were recorded in subsequent years. As a result, embargoes on imported birds and other restrictive measures were put into effect in the United States. Some States maintain a permanent quarantine against birds of the parrot family. In an effort to stamp out the disease, California has instituted a system, described by Meyer, requiring testing of parrakeets in commercial aviaries and certification of the aviary.

"Psittacosis is caused by a virus and is highly infective; it can be spread, for instance, by particles of dust floating in the air. It can now be diagnosed by a blood test and also by an inoculation test with mice, which are very susceptible. These methods have been extremely useful in detecting carriers—apparently healthy birds that harbor and disseminate the virus.

"A few years ago it was proved by experiment that chickens are susceptible to the disease. Subsequently, a fatal case of human psittacosis was traced to a sick pigeon; then 9 other cases were traced to pigeons; and finally a test made in pigeon flocks in 5 states showed a surprisingly high percentage of positive reactions. The most recent discovery, already noted, was the isolation of the virus from 2 chickens on a poultry farm in the course of an investigation of a human case of the disease. It has also been isolated from 25 individual pigeons.

"How widespread is the infection among birds on farms? How do they acquire it? What is the risk to human beings? These, as Meyer points out, are among the pressing questions posed by the new discoveries." (269)

DISEASES OF FISHES

The fishes have not escaped the same increase of diseases as manifested in other forms of animal life. A few citations are given as examples of the trend of conditions among them.

Microscopic Organisms

"Many diseases of fishes are caused by small, usually microscopic organisms which are dependent upon the fish for their existence. Some of these microscopic organisms find congenial surroundings only in the body muscles or the internal organs of the fish. These organisms, known as endoparasites, are of little concern from the standpoint of treatment for there are no methods known at the present time for effectively combatting them, and all hope for the survival of the infected fish lies in a spontaneous natural recovery." (200)

A number of diseases in fish are given for which treatments are suggested, namely:

Several types of protozoan infections; ichthyophirius infections; gyrodactylus infections; copepod infections; bacterial infections; general infections; white fungus. In the same connection this statement is made: "Unquestionably, there are ailments of fish which are unknown as yet. Still more diseases are known but no satisfactory method of treatment has been evolved. However, in the case of the commoner diseases, the cause and a reasonably satisfactory cure are known. Although the commoner diseases are well known, very few of them present specific lesions visible to the unaided eye." (201)

Furunculosis

"Probably no disease of trout is more dreaded by fish-culturists than furunculosis, and with good reason. When once established it is very difficult to eradicate and almost invariably results in an exceedingly high mortality. The disease affects chiefly the various species of salmonoid fishes, but may also affect a large number of fresh-water and marine species. . . ."

"There is evidence that apparently healthy fish may act as carriers which greatly increases the difficulty of preventing the spread of the disease. In some instances furunculosis has run its course and apparently died out only to break out afresh at a later time. In such cases the bacteria are apparently carried over in healthy fish or in mud and debris in the ponds." (202)

Fish Parasites

"The association of meat-eating men and animals, as has long been known, results in the multiplication of the diseases of both. Man acquires the diseases of animals by eating their flesh and, through the pollution of streams by sewers, the infection is spread. This is especially true of the parasites of fish. A few years ago, a colony of Finns settled in the Lake Superior region. They brought with them from their European home dried fish, one of their food staples. Unfortunately, the fish was infected with the embryos of the tapeworm, a new variety not previously known in this country. The infection has spread throughout the Great Lakes until it has become very general. Many other parasites affect the fish of our inland seas.

"*The New York Times*, in calling attention to this great menace to life and health, says:

"'Many of the fish studied were so heavily infected internally that they gave the intestinal contents the appearance of being made up of about fifty per cent black pepper, while many others were seen in which it was difficult to see how it was possible for the heart and kidneys to function when so much of the host tissue had been replaced by parasite cysts.

"'The study also revealed that most of the birds that eat fish are carriers of one or more parasites that enter fish during part of their life cycle.'" (203)

Abundant Health

Fish Tapeworms

Man is subject to infection by the broad fish tapeworms of fresh-water fish. (270)

Fresh-water Fish

Man may be infected with parasites by eating fresh-water fish infected with the Chinese liver fluke (Clonorchis sinensis) and other similar parasites if the fish are eaten without sufficient cooking.

Dogs are prone to acquire these worms .

Other flukes that may be acquired from raw fish include Metagonimus and Heterophyes. (271)

Fish Infestation at Long Lake, Ely, Minnesota

"The walleyed pike measured from 21.2 to 28.8 cm. in length and harbored from one to twenty-six larvae. The average infestation was more than six larvae for each fish. The pickerel varied from 38.7 to 45 cm. in length and each harbored from four to twenty-six larvae. The average number of larvae for each fish was more than fifteen." (272)

Cancer in Fish

A few years ago official government reports on conditions in fish hatcheries recorded outbreaks among trout and Salmonoids of thyroid tumors which ran through the hatcheries like an epidemic. "In one case sixteen per cent of visible tumors in April increased to ninety-two per cent by the following August, with an accompanying heavy mortality."

The tumors were described as "typically those of goiter and cancer: . . . At the beginning it is a fish goiter, or is analogous to goiter in man. At the end it is fish cancer or is analogous to thyroid cancer in man. In both man and fish thyroid cancer begins with a goiterous enlargement. . . ." (204)

Eggs

He who has read the preceding pages on disease in animals and noted the frequent references to the egg as a carrier of disease must at least raise a question concerning the safety of using eggs as a human food. To those statements we wish here to add two more.

It is becoming increasingly difficult to secure eggs which are free from disease, as the following statements show.

"Pennington, to whose work we have referred, and Kossowitz,

of Vienna, have found that fresh eggs often contain molds, yeasts, and various other micro-organisms. Pennington found only twelve per cent of the eggs examined entirely free from bacteria. Kossowitz found most eggs sterile when first laid, but discovered that infection readily occurs through penetration of the shell by various bacteria if the eggs by careless handling are exposed to contamination." (205)

"All eggs are strongly open to suspicion. When hens are infected with white diarrhea, eggs, always contain the germs which produce colitis (Yissior). Eggs laid by sick hens should never be used, of course. Eggs usually become infected before they are laid. This is the chief reason for their poor keeping qualities. Germs also penetrate the shell, and thus set up putrefaction. Duck's eggs are more liable to infection than hen's eggs." (206)

"INSPECTED"

The most common disease in swine is trichinae with which every third American is already infested. There is no inspection of pork for this parasite,—inspection was discontinued in 1907 because it must be microscopic to be of any value.

Therefore they instruct us that all pork must be thoroughly cooked.

When slaughtered animals are inspected, "if the disease is found to be so slight as to render the undiseased portion of the carcass fit for food, the diseased area is removed, and the remainder is passed. It will be noted that such is the case in most carcasses retained." (9)

Here is a typical report of a meat inspector of a city health department:

Total number of carcasses inspected	19,877
Number of livers condemned	2,029
Whole carcasses condemned	5
Sick animals sold	2,024

These 2,024 animals from which diseased livers were removed were counted as fit for human food and were sold in the markets.

One author says that if the disease has not gone beyond the lungs, liver, and thoracic and pharyngeal lymphatics, the remainder of the carcass may be eaten.

But more.

"Only about sixty-five per cent of the cattle and swine, it is estimated, are slaughtered each year in establishments under Federal supervision." (8)

" 'Supervision' means 'inspection'; therefore, thirty-five per cent of the meat slaughtered is *not* inspected.

Therefore a noted writer on animal and human diseases, when starting to write a chapter on "Inspection" opens his article by saying that man's protection against infection when he eats meat will come from *thorough cooking.*

The same writer advises that eggs of tuberculous chickens are a grave danger to humans and that ordinary cooking does not destroy the disease producing organisms,—they must be "well done."

And so it goes all around the animal kingdom; everything must be pasteurized, cooked, and boiled, because of the extra microscopic animal life with which they teem which is a menace to the life of man. There is a growing number of people whose aesthetic sense rebels at a "diet of worms" even though they be "well done," and they welcome a cleaner, safer way of living.

PASTEURIZED MILK

It is freely granted that pasteurized milk is much safer than is the raw milk of today, and nothing printed here is intended to lessen interest in requiring it to be done, but our interest goes far beyond pasteurization to a cleaner, safer and more delightful way of living. To this end we introduce statements made by others about pasteurization, sterilization, and the non-use of dairy milk.

One state sends out a warning that the following diseases may be incurred from the milk: tuberculosis, undulant fever, scarlet fever, septic sore throat, staphylococcus, food poisoning, rabies, typhoid fever, bacillary dysentery, diphtheria, and infantile paralysis.

And then: "The final and most reliable safeguard against milkborne diseases is *pasteurization.*"

Another state warns,—"Because germs grow so rapidly in milk, the list of milkborne diseases is long, including typhoid fever, septic sore throat, scarlet fever, dysentery and enteritis, paratyphoid fever, diphtheria, undulant fever, infantile diarrhea, food poisoning, etc."

And then: "*Pasteurization* will always protect if it is properly applied."

And thus it is in every state.

Pasteurization is the *one protection* which is offered to us along with dirty and infected milk.

We are led to believe that though the cows may have had some deadly disease, their milk is "perfectly safe if pasteurized."

And so we trust the *pasteurization* process to defend the lives of our babies, our children, and ourselves. When a bottle of milk is left at the door, if it is labelled "Pasteurized" we regard it as "perfectly safe."

But let us look in the bottle and see what really is there.

There is not a uniform standard over the country concerning the number of bacteria allowed in milk; and, it is not fixed in any state and may change at any time. In Tennessee milk may lawfully contain the following numbers of bacteria:

Raw milk, when delivered, per c.c.	35,000
Milk before pasteurization, per c.c.	200,000
Pasteurized milk, when delivered per c.c.	50,000
A common 8 ounce glass contains 240 c.c. Therefore a common glass of pasteurized milk may lawfully contain, when delivered at your door .	12,000,000

Will the reader remember that this is *pasteurized* milk concerning which we are to rest at ease because it is "perfectly safe."

Not all milk contains the full number of bacteria allowed. As an example, a city in another state where the allowed count per c.c. is 30,000, reports that it took samples from 115 dairies. The average count found was 14,308. They found faulty pasteurization in 7 dairies, and faulty sterilization in 18. This is not an *annual* report, but a monthly one; and so it goes on month after month like this.

The report from the same city for a later month is as follows:

Standard pasteurized milk,—

Number of inspections 169

Number improperly pasteurized 2

Number improperly sterilized 22

Number showing high counts 36

Average bacteria allowed by law per c.c. 30,000

Average bacteria *found in the milk,* 50,487

These figures are for one c.c. of which there are 240 in a common 8 ounce glass which means each glass of pasteurized milk in that city actually contained 12,116,880 bacteria for the month reported.

In the same city the bacteria count allowed in the ice cream was 100,000 per c.c., and the number actually found in the samples taken averaged 258,334 per c.c. which in one 8 ounce glass would count 62,000,160.

Such conditions are common notwithstanding all of the regulations and the constant supervision given to dairies and milk distributors. Here is another example. In a city of 250,000 pop. the milk from 23 of the leading dairies was tested and it was found that in 21 of the 23 the milk was not properly pasteurized, but was being sold regularly to the public labeled "Pasteurized" and the buyers supposed it was "perfectly safe." How safe was it? Read and see.

A total of 287 samples was taken and tested for 12 different things, one of which was the number of leucocytes present. The officials fixed 800,000 cells per c.c. of milk as the maximum number to be allowed in the milk without discrediting it.

When we know that these white blood cells are in the milk because they were fighting infection in the udders of the cows, (most likely mastitis, treated elsewhere in this book) it seems that even as low a count as 800,000 would endanger the consumers of the milk. One c.c. is about 20 drops; 947 c.c. equal one quart. 800,000 cells per c.c. would be 18,940,000 in a glass of milk. Yet the report shows 51 samples of milk containing over the 800,000 allowed, and no sample was found free from these white cells, and, mind you, all of the 287 samples were *pasteurized* as sold to the people every day. These tests were not made by the city health department as a routine procedure but were made independent of the city milk inspection program by an authority from another state who was called in for that special purpose.

It is not supposed that the milk supply of that city is inferior to milk in other cities everywhere. (290)

"Approved Milk"

	Maximum number of bacteria per c.c.
(1 c.c. is about 20 drops. An 8-oz. glass holds about 240 c.c.)	
Pasteurized, certified	500
Raw, on Physician's Prescription only	10,000
Pasteurized when delivered to consumer	30,000
Before Pasteurization at Country Plant	150,000
Before Pasteurization, after shipment from Country Plant	400,000
Cream, Pasteurized, when delivered to consumer ..	100,000
Cream, before Pasteurization at Country Plant	250,000
Cream, before Pasteurization after shipment	500,000

City of New York Health Dept., 1944
Bureau of Food and Drugs
Bureau of Health Education
Revised August, 1944
Milk Supply Folder
30M-61544-114

The above is reprinted from a bulletin distributed by the health department of New York City, not as being different from other cities but as being a fair representative of all of them. The information about the c.c. is added.

But this is not all of the story. During any time that milk stands unrefrigerated, the bacteria multiply rapidly; they can *triple in one hour*.

If the milk which is represented and sold as having been pasteurized were all thoroughly and properly pasteurized, milk would be much safer than it now is. Even then it is not safe; it should be boiled.

Disease Germs Sometimes Survive Pasteurization

"Up to date baby specialists have become conscious of the dangers from disease in milk so that almost all of them recommend heating it to a much higher temperature than is attained during pasteurization. It is quite common these days for them to advise that the modified milk for a day's feeding be brought to the boiling point and kept there for twenty minutes." (275)

"Pasteurized milk has many of the most serious disease-producing germs killed by this process. It is said that there are six bad germs which may be present that pasteurization does not kill. That is why doctors suggest boiling babies' milk three minutes, as it tends to make it more sterile and safer." (292)

"Park and others have shown that milk of high bacterial content, even when pasteurized, is not a wholesome food for infant feeding. Without proper supervision, milk may contain the organisms of tuberculosis, undulant fever, septic sore throat, and numerous other serious transmissible diseases." (273)

Thomas G. Hull states that certain of the bovine streptococci can withstand a temperature of 143° F. for ninety minutes and some of them still live. (274)

Still another authority says, "Living staphylococci have often been recovered from market milk which has been pasteurized at 62° C. for 30 minutes. . . . The enterotoxin itself resists heating at 95° C. for 20 minutes. Thus, cows shedding staphyloccus in their milk, and milkers with staphyloccus infection of the hands are potentially dangerous, whether the milk is to be pasteurized or not." (293)

Farmers' Bulletin No. 1067, says, with regard to feeding milk to calves from tuberculous cows,—"To be safe for feed, milk from such cows should first be heated to a temperature of 145° F. and held there for at least 30 minutes, but as this method requires considerable attention to assure proper heating, boiling for a few minutes is considered a better plan. Page 7

Inasmuch as no one knows which milk is infected, and which is not, the rule has to apply to all milk.

If that is the only safe rule for calves, what should the rule be for human beings?

"Bacteria which may survive pasteurization are classified as follows: 1—Heat resistant non-spore-forming bacteria. 2—Thermophilic bacteria. 3—Streptococci. 4—Non-thermophilic spore-forming bacteria. Recently I submitted to the Gradwohl Laboratory 13 specimens of milk representing the different St. Louis dairies. These were cultured according to the United States Health Standards. Five of the specimens showed the presence of streptococcus viridons. Four showed acidophilus. One showed encapsulated streptococci, which failed to grow in cultures. One showed almost a pure culture of pneumococci-like organism. The cow is essentially an unclean animal. Efforts to sterilize the udder are unavailing. The skin cracks and becomes eczematous and the scabs fall into the milk. Mastitis is a frequent development. Despite all strenuous efforts and precautions, the best milk delivered from the dairies continues to show the presence of pathogenic bacteria. Milk is such a good culture medium that it is easily contaminated. It was largely implicated as a carrier in the great epidemics of typhoid and cholera that occurred in the days before pasteurization." (294)

Nearly half of his specimens were streptococcus viridons which produce a serious, often fatal, heart infection.

Dr. Soper summarized his paper thus:

"I conclude the tremendous incrimination of milk as a disseminator of infection as follows:

1. "All animals excepting the human, cease the use of milk as a food after weaning . . .

2. "As a result of his violation of a primary biologic law, man has been severely penalized by the host of infectious diseases that are disseminated by milk.

3. "The dairy cow, stimulated and bred to yield milk over a long period of time, develops hypertrophy of the mammary gland. She is frequently found to be infected with a low grade streptococcus mastitis. Efforts to disinfect the udder often cause a chronic eczema; crusts and scales fall into the milk.

4. "Milk is such a good culture medium that it is frequently contaminated by infectious agents not originating in the cow. 'Bacterial soup' is a good synonym for it.

5. . . . .

6. "Raw milk is unfit for human consumption.

7. "Pasteurized milk as it reaches the consumer usually contains pathogenic bacteria and is not to be relied upon as a safe food.

On the same point the California Farmer of Feb., 1948 carried an editorial commenting on the political aspects of pasteurization stated, "We have been told by agricultural college scientists, who do not think it politic to stick out their necks, that pasteurization does not kill all of the germs. In practical terms, the pasteurization of poor milk does not make it good milk." Page 173

Is Milk Cleaner Now Than Fifty Years Ago?

The answer usually given is, Yes. But is that correct? It must be remembered that to give a negative answer could not be popular and might be injurious to the one giving such an answer. A medical doctor, whose name we withhold, recently asked an agriculturist of wide experience in dairying if he thought pasteurized milk today is safer than raw milk of fifty years ago, and he replied emphatically that in his opinion the raw milk of fifty years ago was safer.

Pasteurizing Also Kills Lactic Spawn

"Pasteurizing has been devised to kill some four kinds of pathogenic germs. . . . The objection to pasteurization of milk is that it also kills the spawn of the beneficial lactic ferment. (295)

Other Milk Troubles

"In my experience of twenty years in treating allergy, milk has always been one of the most frequent reactors on skin testing, only house dust exceeding it in frequency. . . ."

"For two or three decades we in America have been under the pressure of an intensive drive for an ever-increasing consumption of milk. This has been pushed to such a point that recently a congressman introduced a bill into the Congress of the United States to appropriate enough money to furnish every child under 14 years of age a quart of milk daily. How much more intelligent would be a bill to furnish every child an adequate diet and to establish a commission to determine of what such a diet would consist!

"Through my office in these twenty years has passed a continuous stream of wheezy, itchy persons, many with stopped-up noses, many with chronic, recurring headaches, and others with various gastrointestinal complaints. A very large percentage of these persons have spent from one to many years trying to improve their health and increase their resistance to disease by an ever-increasing consumption of milk, only to find that milk is the chief, or one of the chief causes of their ill health.

"I am constantly impressed by the number of patients I see who date the onset of their allergic manifestations from the time or shortly after the beginning of a regime of intensive milk drinking, either for some stomach disorder or for the purpose of weight building. Then, too, I see many who have had little or no appetite over long periods of time and have fallen into the habit of drinking milk alone or with added egg at meal time instead of getting a regular meal. Many persons with little or no appetite can easily drink enough milk to maintain moderate weight and satisfy the conscience that they are not neglecting their health.

"Many of these milk drinkers sooner or later begin to have itchy, cracking, dry and red skins or stopped-up noses or wheezy chests or go to their physician for advice. The first thing the doctor tells them is that they are run down and need to build up their health and resistance, and for that purpose, of course, need to drink more milk. Thus the vicious cycle is intensified; more symptoms more milk, more milk more symptoms. The glaring coincidence of the increase of milk consumption and the increase of allergic manifestations cannot be overlooked.

"Many of our dietitians are not really dietitians, but milk drinking enthusiasts. If milk were suddenly taken away from them they would be entirely at a loss as to how to maintain weight alone, much less how to build it up. Many physicians as well as dietitians feel that milk has some occult quality which cannot be substituted.

"In any allergic syndrome of perennial occurence there is 40 per cent or better chance that milk plays a leading role in producing the symptoms." (277)

Milk Can Be Spared

"Dr. Irving S. Cutter, editor of a health column which appears daily in the Chicago Tribune, has received many letters from parents who said that the growth of their children was retarded until cow's milk was eliminated from their diet. The most frequent disorder is constipation, which gradually increases. There is often loss of appetite, fatigue, nervousness, colic, abdominal pain and vomiting, especially among infants. Iron tonics do not help. Skin eruptions may occur. In an effort to find out, without elaborate tests, the foods to which a child was allergic, he was asked what he did not like to eat. He promptly mentioned milk. When milk was no longer used, he became well. Dr. Cutter assures parents that cow's milk may be eliminated from a child's diet with safety. The minerals and vitamins it supplies may be obtained from other sources." (296)

"Thoroughly Sterilized"

An author who has never yet been found to be wrong summed it up this way:

"If milk is used, it should be thoroughly sterilized; with this precaution, there is less danger of contracting disease from its use." (278)

This calls for sterilization,—heat of 212 degrees where pasteurization is not more than 145 degrees. Sterilization does not remove all danger of disease from milk, but lessens it.

To drink raw milk today is unthinkable.

To use pasteurized milk is much safer.

To use sterilized milk is safer still.

To use soybean milk is safest of all.

The safest market dairy milk one can buy comes in sealed tin cans at the regular grocery store.

A Balanced Ration Without Milk

No doubt the reader has noted the prominent part milk plays in conveying animal diseases to man. In various sections of this book, will be found suggestions for securing a complete ration without milk.

Present Conditions Were Anticipated

Many years ago it was revealed that the present condition of animals would now obtain, and instruction was given for the guidance of those of today who understand the times and the meaning of these things, that they might know how to protect themselves from disease, and bear a message of good health to all whom their influence can reach.

These predictions and counsels are found in the writings of Ellen G. White, who wrote many books and articles on the subject of health. A few representative paragraphs are reproduced here.

"People are continually eating flesh that is filled with tuberculous and cancerous germs. Tuberculosis, cancer, and other fatal diseases are thus communicated." 1905. (207)

"Cancer, tumors, and pulmonary diseases are largely caused by meat-eating." 1909. (208)

"Cancers, tumors, and all inflamatory diseases are largely caused by meat-eating. From the light given me, the prevalence of cancer and tumors is largely due to gross living on dead flesh." (297)

The Significance

The reader is asked to consider the total combined effect upon the human organism of eating the several kinds of animal flesh and the various products derived from them, subject to conditions described in the reliable reports given in the preceding pages. If only *one* danger were present it might not be serious, but when such grave dangers appear so often in every kind of flesh and in every product derived from them, it seems to be time to stop and give serious thought to the whole subject.

The plan of getting a well-balanced ration direct from the products of the earth, when it is possible to do so, is of increasing interest, to say the least. That plan is explained in this book. The chapter you are now reading on "The Animal Kingdom A Reservoir of Disease" is an introduction to that subject, and it is hoped that every reader will be convinced that the use of animal flesh and animal products today is fraught with so much danger that it is time to investigate the better way of living.

WARNINGS

"The liability to take disease is increased tenfold by meat-eating." 1868. (209)

"Meat is the greatest disease breeder that can be introduced into the human system." 1898. (210)

"There is no safety in eating the flesh of dead animals, and in a *short time the milk* of the cows *will also be excluded* from the diet of God's commandment-keeping people. In a short time it will not be safe to use *anything* that comes from the animal creation." 1898. (211)

"Let the diet reform be progressive. Let the people be taught how to prepare food without the use of milk or butter. Tell them that the *time will soon come* when there will be no safety in using eggs, milk, cream, or butter, because *disease in animals is increasing* in proportion to the increase of *wickedness among men.* The time is near when, because of the iniquity of the fallen race, the whole animal creation will groan under the diseases that curse our earth." 1902. (212)

The Possession of Animals

"The curse of God is on the earth, the sea, the cattle, on the animals. There will soon be no safety in the possession of flocks and herds. The earth is decaying under the curse of God." 1898. (298)

COUNSELS

The Ideal Diet

"Grains, fruits, nuts, and vegetables constitute the diet chosen for us by the Creator. These foods, prepared in as simple and natural a manner as possible, are the most healthful and nourishing. They impart a strength, a power of endurance, and vigor of intellect, that are not afforded by a more complex and stimulating diet." 1905 (213)

Vigorous Health

"It is a mistake to suppose that muscular strength depends upon the use of animal food. The needs of the system can be better supplied, and more vigorous health can be enjoyed, without its use. The grains, with fruits, nuts, and vegetables, contain all the nutritive properties necessary to make good blood." 1905. (214)

Natural Foods Like Manna

"The light that God has given and will continue to give on the food question is to be to His people today what the manna was to the children of Israel. The manna fell from heaven, and the people were told to gather it, and prepare it to be eaten. So in the different countries of the world, light will be given to the Lord's people, and health foods suited to these countries will be prepared." 1909. (215)

Fortunate People

The warnings and counsels just quoted have been an inspiration to the writer for many years, and, with other writings from the same source, have been the guiding influence in study, in research, and in gathering and organizing the material now presented in this book. There is no other health literature in the world today written with such farsightedness, that is so penetrating, so accurate, and which so completely covers the subject of health in all of its ramifications. Fortunate are the people who are honored with its presence and blessed by its guidance.

BIBLIOGRAPHY

(1) "The Animal Kingdom—a Reservoir of Disease," by Karl F. Meyer, M.D., Director of the Medical Center at University of Calif., San Francisco, pages, 1, 2, 10, 27; published in the "Proceedings of the Institute of Medicine of Chicago," May-June, 1931, pages 234-261.

(2) Wisconsin Agricultural Experiment Station Bulletin No. 343, May, 1928.

(3) "Tuberculosis in Livestock," page 2. By A. E. Wright, Chief Tuberculosis Eradication Division, Bureau of Animal Industry, USDA Bulletin No. 1069, issued Nov., 1919, slightly revised July, 1939, Washington, D. C.

(4) Id., page II.

(5) Id., page 7.

(6) Id., page 8.

(7) Id., page 9.

(8) Id., page 4.

(9) Ibid.

(10) Id., page 1.

(11) Id., pages 6, 7.

(12) Id., page 2.

(13) "Udder Diseases of Dairy Cows," by Hubert Bunyea, veterinarian

and W. T. Miller, associate veterinarian Pathological Division, Bureau of Animal Industry, page 8. USDA Bulletin 1422, issued May, 1924, revised December, 1934.

(14) "Tuberculosis in Livestock," page 8. (See No. 3.)

(15) Id., page II.

(16) "Tuberculosis of Hogs," page 3. USDA Bulletin No. 781, by J. R. Mohler, Chief of the Bureau of Animal Industry and Henry J. Washburn, bacteriologist, Pathological Division, Bureau of Animal Industry, Washington, D. C. Issued May, 1917, revised August, 1939.

(17) Ibid.

(18) Ibid.

(19) "Tuberculosis in Livestock," page 1. (See No. 3.)

(20) "The Pathogenicity for Cattle of the Avian Tubercle Bacillus," by Wm. H. Feldman, D.V.M., M.S., Division of Experimental Medicine, and Alfred G. Karlson, D.V.M., M.S., Fellow in Comparative Pathology, The Mayo Foundation, Rochester, Minnesota, pages 115, 116. Reprinted from Proceedings Forty-third Annual Meeting of the U. S. Livestock Sanitary Association, Hotel Morrison, Chicago, Ill., Dec. 6-7-8, 1939.

(21) Condensed from U. S. Dept. of Agriculture Bulletin, No. 1069, of 1939, page 5. (See No. 3.)

(22) "Tuberculosis of Hogs," page II. (See No. 16.)

(23) Id., page 3.

(24) Id., page II.

(25) Id., page 2.

(26) Ibid.

(27) Id., page 9.

(28) "Tuberculosis in Livestock," page 15. (See No. 3.)

(29) "Tuberculosis of Fowls," by Robt. Graham and Frank Thorp, Jr., page 4. Cir. 354, Univ. of Ill., Urbana, Ill. Reprinted March, 1938.

(30) Ibid.

(31) Id., page 3.

(32) "Tuberculosis of Fowls," page 31. Wyoming Agricultural Extension Bulletin No. 2, April, 1929. Written by Cecil Elder and A. M. Lee.

(33) "Eradicating Tuberculosis," by Elmer Lash, veterinarian, Tuberculosis Eradication Division, Bureau of Animal Industry, page 2. USDA Leaflet No. 102, issued November, 1933.

(34) "Tuberculosis in Livestock," page 15. (See No. 3.)

(35) "Tuberculosis in Hogs," page 4. (See No. 16.)

(36) "Tuberculosis of Fowls," page 31. (See No. 32.)

(37) Id., pages 33, 35.

(38) Id., page 35.

(39) Id., page 36.

(40) Id., page 37.

(41) "Tuberculosis of Fowls," page 7. (See No. 29.) (Ill. Bulletin.)

(42) "Journal of the American Medical Association," March 18, 1939, page 1074, section on "Current Comment."

(43) "Tuberculosis of Fowls," page 32. (Wyo. Bulletin.) (See No. 32.)

(44) Id., page 44. (See No. 32.)

(45) Id., page 45.

(46) "Tuberculosis of Hogs," page II. (See No. 16.)

(47) Ibid.

(48) U. S. Dept. of Agriculture Special Bulletin.

(49) Paul A. Teschner, M.D., Director of Health Education, American Medical Association, in "Health," March, 1941, page 2.

(50) "Wisconsin Crusader," March, 1941, pages 8, 9.

(51) Wisconsin Agricultural Experiment Station Bulletin No. 343, May, 1928.

(52) "Brucellosis in Man and Animals," by I. F. Huddleston, D.V.M., M.S., Ph.D., page 51, 1939. Copyrighted and published 1934 by The Commonwealth Fund, 41 East 57th St., New York City, N. Y. Printed by E. L. Hildreth and Company, Inc. (I.F.H. is research Prof. in Bacteriology, Michigan State College.)

(53) Id., page 56.

(54) "Bang's Disease," by W. L. Boyd, page 3. Extension Bulletin, 209, University of Minn., University Farm, St. Paul, Minn., May, 1940.

(55) Id., page 3.

(56) "Brucellosis in Swine," by Robert Graham and Viola M. Michael, page 4. Circular 435, Univ. of Illinois, Urbana, Ill., May, 1935.

(57) Id., page 11.

(58) "Controlling Bang's Disease," by Gordon M. Cairns, Prof. of Animal Industry and J. F. Witter, Animal Pathologist, Maine Bulletin No. 279, June, 1940. From University of Maine, Orono, Maine. Page 3.

(59) "Answers to Questions Regarding Bang's Disease," by Robert Graham and Frank Thorp, Jr., from University of Illinois, College of Agriculture and Agricultural Experiment Station, Circular 360, Urbana, Ill. Revised Sept., 1938 (first published October, 1930). Page 2.

(60) "Bang's Disease," Extension Bulletin, No. 110, page 17, Michigan State College.

(61) "Infectious Abortion," page 6, Bulletin No. 201 from University of Wyoming, Laramie, Wyoming, May, 1934.

(62) Id., page 7.

(63) Id., page 8.

(64) "Brucellosis in Man and Animals," by I. Forest Huddleson. (See No. 52), from book cover.

(65) C. H. Clark, Veterinarian, Michigan State Department of Agriculture, in letter of Nov. 15, 1940, to the Haight Food School.

(66) "Health Briefs," Tenn. Dept. of Public Health, W. C. Williams, M.D., Commissioner, Vol. XII, No. 10, October 15, 1935.

(67) U. S. Dept. of Agriculture, Bureau of Animal Industry, Special Bulletin.

(68) "Brucellosis in Swine," page 11. (See No. 56.)

(69) "Bang's Disease," by W. L. Boyd, page 3. (See No. 54.)

(70) "Brucellosis in Man and Animals," by I. F. Huddleson, page 57. (See No. 52.) "Journal of the American Dietetic Assn.," June—July, 1941, p. 580.

(71) "Brucellosis in Swine," page 2. (See No. 56.)

(72) "Brucellosis in Man and Animals," by I. F. Huddleson, pages 57 and 58. (See No. 52.)

(73) Id., page 257.

(74) Id., page 90.

(75) "Bang's Disease," by W. L. Boyd, page 8. (See No. 54.)

(76) "Brucellosis or Bang's Disease of Farm Animals," page 9. Minnesota Bulletin 384, by C. P. Fitch and W. L. Boyd, from University of Minnesota Agricultural Experiment Station, University Farm, St. Paul, Minn., June, 1940.

(77) "Bang's Disease," by B. J. Killham, Extension Bulletin No. 110 (revised), August, 1936, from Michigan State College, Section of Animal Pathology, East Lansing, Michigan, page 7.

(78) "Bang's Disease," USDA Bulletin 1804, July, 1933, pages 4 and 11.

(79) Id., page 16.

(80) Id., page 8.

(81) "Infectious Abortion," page 9. (See No. 61.)

(82) "Bang's Disease," by W. L. Boyd, page 9. (See No. 54.)

(83) "Answers to Questions Regarding Bang's Disease," page 8. (See No. 59.)

(84) "Answers to Questions Regarding Bang's Disease," page 23. (See No. 59.)

(85) "Brucellosis in Man and Animals," by I. F. Huddleson, pages 55, 56. (See No. 52.)

(86) Id., page 55.

(87) Id., pages, 10, 11.

(88) "Bang's Disease," page 18. Bulletin 110 (revised), from Michigan State College, August, 1936.

(89) "Bang's Disease," page 4. (See No. 54.)

(90) Id., page 2.

(91) Id., page 12.
(92) "Brucellosis in Man and Animals," by I. F. Huddleson, page 257. (See No. 52.)
(93) "Bang's Disease," page 10, USDA Bulletin 1704, July, 1933.
(94) "Mastitis, Cause, Detection, and Control," Bulletin No. 225, June, 1936, published and distributed by Agricultural Extension Service, College of Agriculture, University of Maine, Orono, Maine, page 3. By J. F. Witter, Animal Pathologist.
(95) Id., page 14.
(96) Id., page 4.
(97) Id., page 5.
(98) Id., page 4.
(99) Id., page 8.
(100) Id., page 5.
(101) Id., page 10.
(102) Id., page 3.
(103) Id., page 8.
(104) "Mastitis," by C. S. Bryan, Extension Bulletin No. 165, July, 1936, Michigan State College of Agriculture and Applied Science, page 8.
(105) "Mastitis, Cause, Detection, and Control," page 9. (See No. 94.)
(106) Id., page 9.
(107) "Lumpy Jaw, or Actinomycosis," by John R. Mohler, Chief of Bureau, and Maurice S. Shahan, Associate Veterinarian, Pathological Division, Bureau of Animal Industry, pages 1, 2. USDA Circular No. 438, June, 1937, Washington, D. C.
(108) Id., page 9.
(109) Id., page 1.
(110) "Beef Cattle in Kansas," page 173. Kansas State Board of Agriculture Reports, Vol. LII, 211B. Quarter Begins Sept., 1934.
(111) "Lumpy Jaw, or Actinomycosis," page 2. (See No. 107.)
(112) "Anaplasmosis in Cattle," by George W. Stiles, bacteriologist, Pathological Division, Bureau of Animal Industry. USDA Circular No. 154, issued February, 1931, revised December, 1939, page 1.
(113) "Blackleg," by J. R. Mohler, Chief of the Bureau of Animal Industry; USDA Bulletin No. 1355, issued June, 1923, slightly revised October, 1930, page II.
(114) Ibid.
(115) "Pullorum Disease of Domestic Fowl," by L. F. Rettger and Wayne N. Plastridge, Bulletin 178, May, 1932, from Storrs Agricultural Experiment Station, Conn. Agricultural College, Storrs, Conn., page 109.
(116) "Pullorum Disease of Chicks," by Robert Graham, Chief in Animal Pathology and Hygiene, University of Illinois, Urbana, Illinois. Circular 432, March, 1935, page 3.
(117) "Pullorum Disease in Hens and Chicks," by H. L. Richardson, Extension Poultry Specialist, and Dr. J. F. Witter, Animal Pathologist, Bulletin 184 (revised), Sept., 1936, page 4. From University of Maine, Orono, Maine.
(118) "Diseases and Parasites of Poultry," USDA Bulletin No. 1652, issued January, 1931, revised May, 1939, from Washington, D. C., page 7.
(119) "Pullorum Disease of Domestic Fowl," page 126. (See No. 115.)
(120) "Diseases and Parasites of Poultry," page 7. (See No. 118.)
(121) "Pullorum Disease of Domestic Fowl," page 141. (See No. 115)
(122) "Pullorum Disease of Domestic Fowl," page 182. (See No. 115.)
(123) Ibid.
(124) "Pullorum Disease," by L. P. Doyle, Dept. of Veterinary Science, Perdue University Agricultural Experiment Station, Lafayette, Indiana. Leaflet No. 153 (second reprint, revised edition), Sept., 1939, page 2.
(125) "Pullorum Disease of Chicks," page 3. (See No. 116.)
(126) "Fowl Cholera," by Robt. Graham, Chief in Animal Pathology and Hygiene, page 4. Revision of Cir. 286 from Univ. of Illinois, Urbana, Illinois, December, 1935.
(127) "Fowl Cholera," page 4. (See No. 126.)
(128) "Common Diseases of Poultry," page 11. (Revised) Extension Circu-

lar No. 154, from Univ. of North Carolina, State College Station, Raleigh, North Carolina.

(129) Dr. Herbert R. Bird, University of Maryland, in Maryland Poultry Year Book, page 35, 1941. Published by Maryland State Poultry Council.

(130) 'Coccidiosis of Chickens," A. M. Lee and L. H. Scrivner, University of Wyoming. Wyoming Extension Service Circular No. 32, revised, March, 1936, page 2.

(131) "Leucemia of Fowls," by C. A. Brandly, Robert Graham, and V. M. Michael, page 3. Circular 467, University of Illinois, Urbana, Illinois, February, 1937.

(132) From "Nutrition as a Factor in the Incidence of Fowl Leukosis," by W. J. Butler, D. M. Warren and H. L. Hammersland, Montana Livestock Sanitary Board, Helena, Montana. Paper presented at the 75th annual meeting of the American Veterinary Medical Assn., New York, N. Y., July 5-9, 1938. Reprint from "Journal of the American Veterinary Medical Assn." Vol. XCIII, N. S. 46, No. 5, Nov., 1938, pp. 307-315.

(133) "Diseases and Parasites of Poultry," page 24. USDA Bulletin No. 1652, a bulletin which is revised and supersedes Bulletin 1337. Issued January, 1931, revised May, 1939, Washington, D. C.

(134) "Fowl Paralysis," A. M. Lee and L. H. Scrivner, page 3. Wyoming Extension Service Circular No. 31, revised March, 1936. From University of Wyoming.

(135) "Diseases and Parasites of Poultry," pages 24, 25. (See No. 133.)

(136) "Fowl Paralysis," page 6. (See No. 134.)

(137) "Fowl Paralysis," page 6. (See No. 134.)

(138) "Paralysis in Chickens," by L. P. Doyle, Dept. of Veterinary Science, Perdue University Agricultural Experiment Station, Lafayette, Indiana. Leaflet No. 146 (3rd reprint, revised edition), Nov., 1938, page 2.

(139) "Leucemia of Fowls," pages 10-13. (See No. 131.)

(140) Id., page 10.

(141) Id., page 9.

(142) Id., page 8.

(143) Id., pages 13, 14.

(144) "Paralysis in Chickens," page 6. (See No. 138.)

(145) "Leucemia of Fowls," page 14. (See No. 131) and "Fowl Paralysis," pages 8, 9. (See No. 134.)

(146) "Fowl Paralysis," page 4. (See No. 134.)

(147) Ibid.

(148) "Nutrition as a Factor in the Incidence of Fowl Leukosis," page 8. (See No. 132.)

(149) "Leucemia of Fowls," page 3. (See No. 131.)

(150) "Diseases and Parasites of Poultry," page 25. (See No. 133.)

(151) "Paralysis in Chickens," page 6. (See No. 138.)

(152) Ibid.

(153) "Anthrax," by W. S. Gochenour, senior veterinarian, Pathological Division, Bureau of Animal Industry, USDA Bulletin No. 1736, issued October, 1934 from Washington, D. C., page II.

(154) Id., page 1.

(155) Id., page II.

(156) Ibid.

(157) Id., page 1.

(158) Id., page 4.

(159) Id., page 6.

(160) Id., page 3.

(161) Id., page 2.

(162) "Foot-and-Mouth Disease," by John R. Mohler, Chief Bureau of Animal Industry, USDA Bulletin No. 666, issued April 22, 1915 and revised October, 1938, from Washington, D. C., page II.

(163) Id., page 1.

(164) Id., page 13.

(165) Id., page 2.

(166) Ibid.

(167) Ibid.

(168) Ibid.
(169) Ibid.
(170) Id., pages 4, 5.
(171) Id., page 5.
(172) Id., page 2.
(173) "Ohio Health News," State Dept. of Health Bulletin, December 1, 1937.
(174) "Hoosier Health Herald," February, 1928.
(174-a) "Ohio Health News," December 1, 1937.
(175) "Health," July, 1939, pages 10, 11.
(176) "Prevalence of Trichinosis in the United States," by Willi Sawitz, M.D., Parasitology Laboratory, Dept. of Tropical Medicine, Tulane University of Louisiana, New Orlean, La., page 7. Reprint No. 1915 from the Public Health Reports, Vol. 53, No. 10, March 11, 1938. U. S. Gov't. Printing Office, Washington, D. C., 1938.
(177) "Journal of the American Medical Association," March 18, 1939, page 1074, section "Current Comment."
(178) "Swine Erysipelas," page 4, by L. Van Es and C. B. McGrath, Dept. of Animal Pathology and Hygiene, University of Nebraska, Lincoln, Nebraska, August, 1936, Research Bulletin 84.
(179) Id., page 45.
(180) "Hog Cholera," page II, by M. Dorset, Chief Biochemic Division, and U. G. Houck, Chief Division of Hog-Cholera Control, Bureau of Animal Industry. USDA Bulletin No. 834, issued August, 1917; revised September, 1931, slightly revised July, 1939, Washington, D. C.
(181) Id., page 2.
(182) "Internal Parasites of Swine," by Benjamin Schwartz, Chief Zoological Division, Bureau of Animal Industry. USDA Bulletin No. 1787, issued November, 1937, Washington, D. C., page 6.
(183) Id., page 7.
(184) Id., page 8.
(185) Id., page 9.
(186) Id., page 9.
(187) Id., page 10.
(188) Id., page 12.
(189) Id., page 13.
(190) Id., page 16.
(191) Ibid.
(192) Id., page 17.
(193) Id., page 19.
(194) Id., page 26.
(195) Id., page 28.
(196) Id., page 31.
(197) Id., page 33.
(198) Id., page 39.
(199) Id., page 43.
(200) United States Department of the Interior, Fish and Wild Life Service, Bulletin 123033, 1-20.
(201) Ibid.
(202) United States Department of the Interior, Fish and Wild Life Service, Bulletin 123031, 11-1940.
(203) "Good Health," August, 1934, page 13.
(204) Report on "Thyroid Tumors in Salmonoids," by M. C. Marsh, in "Transactions of the American Fisheries Society," 1910.
(205) "New Dietetics," by J. H. Kellogg, M.D., page 433.
(206) "Good Health," May, 1937, page 149.
(207) "Ministry of Healing," by Mrs. E. G. White, page 313, 1905.
(208) Mrs. E. G. White, Vol. 9, page 159, 1909.
(209) Mrs. E. G. White, Vol. 2, page 68, 1868.
(210) "The Education Our Schools Should Give," 1898.
(211) "Counsels on Diet and Foods," page 411, 1898.
(212) Mrs. E. G. White, Vol. 7, page 135; "Counsels on Diet and Foods," page 349, 1902.

(213) "Ministry of Healing," page 296, 1905.

(214) "Ministry of Healing," page 316, 1905.

(215) "Counsels on Diet and Foods," page 269, 1909.

(216) George W. Stiles, Bacteriologist in Charge Branch Pathological Laboratory Division, Bureau of Animal Industry in 1942 Yearbook of Agriculture, U. S. Department of Agriculture pages 295, 296.

(217) 1942 Yearbook of Agriculture of U. S. Department of Agriculture page 304.

(218) Id., pages 305, 306.

(219) Id., page 306.

(220) Id., pages 22-24.

(221) Id., pages 5, 6.

(222) James H. Steele, Ohio Department of Health, Columbus, Ohio.

(223) N. C. Dysart.

(224) 1942 Yearbook of Agriculture, U. S. Department of Agriculture, page 3.

(225) Id., pages 105-107.

(226) J. Arthur Myers, M.D., Medical School University of Minnesota in an address before the veterinarians of the U. S. Livestock Association in annual convention.

(227) William H. Feldman, D.V.M., M.S., The Mayo Foundation, Rochester, Minn., in an address to the Medical College of Virginia, May 7, 1938, "Virginia Medical Monthly" January, 1939.

(228) George W. Stiles, Bacteriologist in Charge, Branch Pathological Laboratory at Denver, Colorado and John T. Lucker, Associate Zoologist, Zoological Division, Bureau of Animal Industry, 1942 Yearbook of Agriculture, U. S. Department of Agriculture, page 297.

(229) D. C. Lockhead, City Health Department, Rochester, Minn., "Proceedings of the U. S. Livestock Sanitary Association" December 2, 1942, page 75.

(230) 1942 Yearbook of Agriculture, U. S. Department of Agriculture, page 237.

(231) Id.

(232) Feldman, Hinshaw, and Mann in paper read before the annual meeting of the U. S. Livestock Sanitary Association December 2, 1942, Proceedings of Association, page 84.

(233) "Health Bulletin," Virginia Department of Health, March, 1942 and Georgia Health, December, 1942.

(234) Proceedings of the U. S. Livestock Sanitary Association, December, 1942, page 76.

(235) Id., December, 1941, page 21.

(236) C. H. Clark, Michigan State Veterinarian before U. S. Livestock Sanitary Association Convention, December, 1941, Report of Proceedings, page 121.

(237) See Thomas G. Hull in "Diseases of Animals Transmissible to Man" page 23.

(238) 1942 Yearbook of Agriculture, U. S. Department of Agriculture, page 42.

(239) Proceedings of the U. S. Livestock Sanitary Association, December, 1941, page 107.

(240) Carl F. Jordan, M.D., Iowa State Department of Health, before U. S. Livestock Sanitary Association Convention, December 2, 1942, pages 138-140.

(241) Proceedings of the U. S. Livestock Sanitary Association, December 2, pages 139, 140.

(242) H. M. Guilford, Wisconsin State Board of Health, before the annual convention of veterinarians, U. S. Livestock Sanitary Association, pages 78, 79.

(243) 1942 Yearbook of Agriculture, U. S. Department of Agriculture, page 732.

(244) H. M. Guilford, State Board of Health, Wisconsin, at annual convention of veterinarians, U. S. Livestock Sanitary Association.

(245) J. W. Jackson, M.D., Director Division of Communicable Disease in Indiana State Board of Health Bulletin, September, 1943, page 200.

(246) 1942 Year Book of Agriculture, USDA, page 42.

(247) Proceedings of the U. S. Livestock Sanitary Association, December 3, 1941, page 63.

(248) 1942 Yearbook of Agriculture, U. S. Department of Agriculture, pages 297, 298.

(249) See Thomas G. Hull, Ph.D., "Diseases Transmitted from Animals To Man," page 101.

(250) Id., pages 109, 119.

(251) 1942 Yearbook of Agriculture, U. S. Department of Agriculture, page 23.

(252) Proceedings of the U. S. Livestock Sanitary Association, December 2, 1942, page 35.

(253) Id., December 3, 1941, page 28.

(254) 1942 Yearbook of Agriculture, U. S. Department of Agriculture, page 375.

(255) 1942 Yearbook of Agriculture, U. S. Department of Agriculture, page 29.

(256) See Thomas G. Hull, Ph.D., "Diseases Transmitted from Animals To Man," page 121.

(257) 1942 Yearbook of Agriculture, U. S. Department of Agriculture, pages 36, 37.

(258) Id., page 301.

(259) Id., page 298.

(260) Proceedings of the U. S. Livestock Sanitary Association, December 4, 1940, page 33.

(261) See Thomas G. Hull, Ph.D., "Diseases Transmitted From Animals To Man," page 384.

(262) 1942 Yearbook of Agriculture, U. S. Department of Agriculture, page 80.

(263) Proceedings of the U. S. Livestock Sanitary Association, December 3, 1941, page 152.

(264) 1942 Yearbook of Agriculture, U. S. Department of Agriculture, page 3.

(265) Massachusetts Agricultural Experiment Station Bulletin No. 370, April, 1940, Transmissible Fowl Leukosis, by Carl Olson, Jr.

(266) 1942 Yearbook of Agriculture, U. S. Department of Agriculture, page 81.

(267) Id., page 997.

(268) Proceedings of the U. S. Livestock Sanitary Association, December, 1940, pages 153, 154, 155.

(269) 1942 Yearbook of Agriculture, U. S. Department of Agriculture, page 84, 85.

(270) See Thomas G. Hull, Ph.D., "Diseases Transmitted From Animals To Man," page 226.

(271) Id., page 227.

(272) From the Division of Experimental Medicine, The Mayo Foundation, Rochester, Minn., Reprinted from "Minnesota Medicine," April, 1938, Vol. 21, page 254.

(273) Proceedings of the U. S. Livestock Sanitary Association, December 3, 1941, page 62.

(274) See "Diseases of Animals Transmitted to Man," page 342.

(275) H. O. Swartout, M.D., "Health," June, 1934, page 31.

(276) See "Time," March 29, 1943.

(277) Marion T. Davidson, M.D., "Southern Medical Journal," Richmond, Va., February, 1942, pages 196-199.

(278) "Ministry of Healing," page 302.

(279) Thurman B. Rice, M.D., Indiana State Board of Health, "Health," June, 1942.

(280) William H. Feldman, D.V.M., M.S., Mayo Foundation, Rochester, Minn. in address to the Medical College of Virginia, May 7, 1938, in "Virginia Medical Monthly," January, 1939.

(281) "What is Known About Brucellosis," 1949, United States Livestock Sanitary Association.

(282) H. O. Swartout, M.D., in "Health," June, 1942.

(283) "What is Known About Brucellosis," 1949, United States Livestock Sanitary Association.

(284) Thurman B. Rice, M.D., Professor Bacteriology, Indiana University School of Medicine, Monthly Bulletin, Indiana State Board of Health, June, 1946, page 125.

(285) Thurman B. Rice, M.D., Editorial in Bulletin, Indiana State Board of Health, July, 1947, page 162.

(286) "What is Known About Brucellosis," 1949, United States Livestock Sanitary Association.

(287) "Good Health," October, 1941, page 149.

(288) "Time," December 8, 1947.

(289) "Hastings (Neb.) Tribune," October, 1948.

(290) "Providence Milk Supply Survey," October, 1949.

(291) "Good Health," August, 1946, page 121.

(292) Dietitian in "Life and Health," September, 1944.

(293) J. Howard Brown, Johns Hopkins School of Medicine, Bulletin, "Los Angeles County Medical Association," August 7, 1947.

(294) Horace W. Soper, M.D., F.A.C.P. of St. Louis, Mo., "Archives of Pediatrics," 60: 1-9, January, 1943.

(295) Lieut. Col. Edmund L. Zane, "Nutrition in Review," page 98. Report of the New York State Joint Legislative Committee on Nutrition, 1945.

(296) Editorial in "Good Health," June, 1944, page 85.

(297) Ellen G. White, "Counsels on Diet and Foods," page 388.

(298) Ibid., page 414.

Health and Tobacco

Tobacco has been named several times in previous chapters, as one of the injurious items in which people popularly indulge. Those references to it have paved the way for a more serious consideration of the subject.

I shall not undertake to cover the field of its effects. My library contains citations from fourteen hundred authors from fourteen countries concerning it. That mass of information has been condensed into a book with an extended bibliography which is available, and the reader is referred to it in case he desires more complete knowledge than this chapter provides, which will be only a summary.

All authorities agree that:

(1) Tobacco contains nicotine.

(2) The smoke contains carbon monoxide.

(3) These are deadly poisons.

(4) Tobacco is not a medicine.

(5) There is no food value in it except as sugar has been added in the process of manufacture.

(6) The only possible so-called benefits derived from its use arise through its poisonous properties. For instance, it is a narcotic, and therefore a small amount is a sedative, soothing and restful, and brings release from care, anxiety, and trouble, and in this way gives one kind of peace and contentment; not by solving problems, but by aiding one in forgetting them.

That common ground of agreement should give any one a good start toward a right conclusion concerning the use of tobacco. The popular concept is that tobacco is not very harmful and that a little will not hurt a person. I want to know how much poison it takes to make poison? I contend that any poison will inflict its injury to the extent it is used. May not the claim of the moderationist be based upon the fact that the harm develops so slowly that it is not readily discovered, rather than that no harm is done?

263

Scientific writers on the subject are noted for their conservatism —their slowness to conclude that it is harmful. I too, am conservative—slow to conclude that it is safe; I am conservative about the use of dangerous things rather than conservative about warning the public of their danger. We cannot over-safeguard the health; danger is always on the side of questionable indulgence.

PLANT EXPERIMENTS

Two parts of nicotine to a thousand of water will stop the growth of some kinds of plants.

Tobacco smoke will hinder the growth of certain seedlings.

ANIMAL EXPERIMENTS

The smoke of one cigarette will kill a rat, or a gold fish.

A turtle can wiggle his toes a week after his head is cut off, but one drop of nicotine on his tongue kills him in twenty-six minutes.

One-sixth of a drop of nicotine will kill a cat; one-half a drop to two drops will kill a dog, and eight drops will kill a horse in four minutes.

When guinea pigs or rabbits are subjected to tobacco-smoke-laden air their offspring are born dead or die soon after birth.

When a rooster is subjected to tobacco smoke the fertility of the eggs and the vitality of the chicks are lessened.

THE HUMAN BODY

The nicotine in one cigar, if injected into the veins of two men, will kill both of them.

There is more carbon monoxide in tobacco smoke than in automobile exhaust. He who smokes twenty cigarettes a day takes into his blood from one to five pints of carbon monoxide from them. This disables red blood corpuscles.

There are nineteen poisons in tobacco smoke.

The Brain

Tobacco lessens the power to think, understand and remember. It lowers the scholastic grades of students.

The Nerves

At first it excites the nerves, and then paralyzes them. The slight touch of this paralysis is the soothing, calming, sedative effect; this is its narcotic effect; this is how it "rests" the nerves. But a narcotic *always injures*.

The nerves at once temporarily lose a certain degree of accuracy and precision.

There may be dizziness, headache, migraine, irritability, jumpiness, trembling, anxiousness, insomnia, neuritis, sciatica, hysteria, paralysis, or atrophy.

Tobacco strikes at the "synapse," making it more difficult for messages to pass over the nerves both to and from the brain.

All of the five senses are operated by nerves, and when nerve efficiency is lessened, the senses are disturbed. There is a marked decrease in the ability to see and hear after one smoke. The loss may become permanent by heavy smoking.

The Heart

Disease of the heart takes more lives than any other. Heart failures are rapidly increasing and more people are dying younger in life—in the prime of life. All authorities agree that tobacco is a heart poison, yet many of these same authorities say that "A little won't hurt you," and they smoke and let you smoke. The result is that many of them and many of you die in the prime of life of heart failure.

Many of the pneumonia deaths occur because the heart has been weakened so it is not able to pull the patient through the crisis.

Arteries—Blood Pressure

It is very popular today to have hard arteries and high blood pressure. Tobacco is one of the leading causes of both. It immediately constricts the blood vessels throughout the body and so requires the heart to push harder to send the blood around its circuit. Then when the arteries become degenerated the walls thicken and this keeps the heart overworking till the end of life. A common way for life to terminate is with apoplexy.

When the arteries are constricted, the circulation of the blood is slowed and then the temperature of the extremities lowers a few degrees. This restricted circulation hampers the blood in carrying fresh oxygen and nutriment to the cells in the extremities and carrying away their wastes, and consequently many heavy smokers after a time suffer with dying tissue on hands or feet—Buerger's disease.

Digestion

It irritates the salivary glands and tonsils. It is a common cause of hyperacidity, which is a forerunner of ulcer, which may become a cancer.

The Liver

One of the dozen functions of the liver is to detoxicate the blood poisons when they pass through it. Such strong poisons as those in tobacco overwork the liver, lessen its efficiency, and may damage its structure.

The Throat

The throat, larynx, esophagus, and bronchi all are irritated. Smokers' sore throat, hoarseness, cough, laryngitis, pharyngitis, bronchitis, and catarrh are among the conditions to which tobacco contributes more or less.

The Lungs

The lungs provide an aborbing surface of one thousand square feet through which oxygen passes into the blood and wastes pass out of the blood to be exhaled. The smoke which lodges on this membrane hinders these two vital processes. Besides, its cells become less resistant to disease so that the smoker doubles his danger from tuberculosis. Then if he gets tuberculosis, his chance of recovery is cut in half.

Cancer

One of the most alarming diseases today is cancer. It is increasing rapidly. Many authorities contend that tobacco is *one* of the causes of cancer, particularly of the lip, tongue, mouth, esophagus, larynx, and lungs.

The Kidneys

The function of the kidneys has already been explained and how such poisons as tobacco injure their cells and contribute to Bright's disease.

The Glands

Some of the functions of these life activators have been related in former chapters, and the reader is asked to refer to them and consider how serious are the consequences when the glands cannot do their full duty.

Physical Efficiency

There is a temporary loss of muscular power from one smoke of from 10 per cent to 75 per cent. This is one reason why first class athletes ban its use. The athlete must consider the well-being of his entire body and mind as well as his muscular power.

LONGEVITY

Professor Raymond Pearl, of Johns Hopkins University, has shown that the death rate of heavy smoking men between ages thirty and sixty is double the death rate of non-smokers of those ages. Much information could here be given from life insurance statistics and other sources, but the above will suffice.

A RACE POISON

Many times the parent does not realize any injury in his body, but he passes it on to his posterity. When fathers smoke more babies are born dead or die in the first few years. The tobacco-using *father* violates the highest law of human existence—that we shall give our posterity our *best* without handicap. The injury to the future child is much greater when the mother smokes. Many babies born of cigarette smoking mothers have degenerated organs at birth.

MOTHERS

Women are the mothers of the race; they mould the character, shape life, and largely determine their destiny. When the world has needed a prophet or a prophetess, a Moses, Samson, Samuel, John the Baptist, or the MASTER among men, first a *mother* was prepared to bear, cherish, and train that life for its great mission.

Man has ever looked to womankind to hold to the ideals of purity, honor and nobility. The future of the world depends more upon the women than the men. When womankind abandons the lofty ideals which have been like a guiding star to each rising generation down through the ages, the world is doomed.

GOING UP IN SMOKE

We have read with much surprise
That some girls' schools advertise
A room in which a maid can smoke!
Has womanhood become a joke?
Its beauty and its sweetness—
Its glory and completeness—
   Going up in smoke?

Shall our mothers and our wives
Lose the freshness of their lives?
Ideals, romance, and love's bright sheen—
Shall they be choked with nicotine?
Are women's grace and pureness,
Stability and sureness
   Going up in smoke?

She whom Christ hath glorified
And His birth hath sanctified!
Shall babes drink poison at her breast
And breathe foul vapors while caressed?
Are all her love and worthiness,
Her sense of pride and motherliness
    Going up in smoke?

Shall the home life of the nation
Lose its strength and its foundation?
By habit gross and unrefined,
Be desecrated, undermined?
Are purity and piety
And virtue and sobriety
    Going up in smoke?

Shall our children, then, partake
Of this bane—who soon shall make
Our citizens, our nation's hope?
Shall they be crippled by this dope?
Are America's sedateness,
Her glory, strength, and greatness
    Going up in smoke?

           —*Mrs. B. W. Heinemann*

CHARACTER, MORALS

Tobacco blunts the conscience, the force within which says "No" to evil. To the extent that voice is stilled, wrong will rule the life and the world. In this crucial field of human poisons, the church is a dismal failure.

THE ADVERTISING

Money in the hands of conscienceless advertising experts is making the people believe that black is white, and very little is being done to offset it.

SELLING POISON WITHOUT WARNING

Strong agencies today are watching more and more carefully every line of foods to see that they are properly labeled and every ingredient revealed. If not, they cannot be sold. There is a growing tendency to consider it unlawful to label any food as a "health" food. Yet the strongest and most fatal poisons known to man are sold in every community to unsuspecting men and women, boys and girls, for a few cents without limit or restriction, and without skull and cross-bones being thereon—and nobody cares!

Saving and Losing Life

To save life we build great hospitals filled with elaborate, costly scientific equipment, and train doctors and nurses with the finest of skill and technique to operate them—not a germ is allowed in the operating room; serums and anti-toxins of every kind are provided; pharmaceutical preparations without number are on every hand; we call the doctor for every little ache or pain; railroad crossings go above or below the highway, or a falling gate is provided; safeguards are placed along the highways; police pilot pedestrians across the street; little children are especially guarded; factories, homes, office buildings, schools, and *all other* places are equipped with all manner of safety devices; great foundations with millions of money are doing continuous research in every possible field to discover any cause of disease (cancer included) and to find ways of prolonging human life; men pay great sums to have their lives "insured"; libraries of books, journals and pamphlets are published in the interest of health; the federal Government can spend billions of money on public health; when death stares in the face a single person will sometimes be willing to spend millions for life to be prolonged; and in the midst of it all the whole nation is slowly *smoking itself to death—and nobody cares!*

The money Americans spend every year for tobacco would be enough to run the government in ordinary times. We spend twice as much for tobacco as for education.

Yet this enormous monetary loss is nothing compared with the injury to body, character, and posterity.

Then after the user has thus done his worst, he throws down his match or burning stub and burns up the property of others in the city or country and so becomes the greatest fire hazard in the land.

Tolerance

When the beginner is learning to smoke it often makes him very ill, but after a few days of trying, the body ceases to rebel and he goes happily on his way. Nature's warning is stilled but the harm continues even though he suspects it not.

How to Stop Smoking

He who eats and drinks according to the Automatic Menu Planner in this book will gradually lose his desire for tobacco; the foods found there are anti-tobacco. For the first few days, live almost entirely on fruits and vegetables. Drink freely of water and fruit juices.

When tempted to smoke, eat an apple or an orange instead, and the smoke will not taste good. Continue doing so and living as recommended, and soon the appetite will lessen and finally dissappear. Find a strict vegetarian who smokes, if you can.

Do not try to "taper off"; it usually results in a long period of agony and fails at last. Remember what tobacco does to you. Read this chapter often and it will stiffen your will.

WHOSE RESPONSIBILITY

Who is responsible for the widespread use of tobacco by people of all ages and both sexes? There are many influences contributing to this, but back of all of them is a *master mind* at work to utterly destroy the human race.

Advertising is overpowering; newspapers, magazines, and billboards ding the "benefits" of tobacco into every mind; the movies extoll it; the radio repeats it to all the members of every household; and so the very air is permeated with the thought.

And what influences are equal to the task of turning back such a mighty tide of evil?

The home has well-nigh ceased to protest; and the home is the bulwark of the nation.

He who should be guarding the health of the home and the nation is himself smoking with the rest.

The church, Heaven's fortress in the world, has given way and largely gone to smoking.

The school seems to be the last stand. The law requires that the effects of tobacco be taught to the youth, and many educators are making a courageous fight to stem the tide; but they are losing ground. More and more teachers are smoking every year.

THE CHURCH

The ultimate source of saving educational influence is not the school or the hospital, but the church of the living God. Mere knowledge alone will not change the habits of life. Every physician who smokes knows that it is injurious, and if knowledge alone would debar, he would not smoke. There is only one sure remedy for the transgressions of life, and that is to be brought face to face with the fact that mankind has a Maker who designed each type of cell in the body, planned their functions, arranged their nutrition, gave and continues to give that mysterious thing we call life, and some day will call every person to account for the treatment meted to the "image" of his Maker. The acceptance of this truth gives vitality to the conscience which calls man to loyalty to his Maker. This becomes a stronger force in the life than the mere desire to be well, because duty to our Maker is higher than duty to ourselves.

But what is the church—the average church—doing about this matter of tobacco? Nothing! Anyone in the church can smoke who pleases, and nothing is said about it. Even some preachers smoke.

If every spiritual leader in all the churches of the land would take his stand in this matter and influence the people around him, it would help to stop this mighty curse.

If every church member in every denomination stood solidly against tobacco and used his influence to discontinue its use, much of the costly advertising would fall to the ground unheeded. But hardly anyone raises a protest. They have mostly lain down on the job, surrendered, capitulated to the enemy, as soldiers might turn traitors on Gibraltar.

And when the church, which is the fortress of heaven in the world, gives way, the world is overrun with evil.

If every man and woman in every religious organization in the land would take a firm stand; if every physician and nurse would be staunch and true and put forth every possible effort to educate all who come under their influence; and if every educator in all our institutions of learning would instruct all our youth, it would not be long until the mighty influences of the tobacco advertising campaigns would be like water on a duck's back—unheeded.

But they are not doing it, and so the race is headed for ruin unless the situation can be retrieved. The use of alcohol and tobacco is increasing by leaps and bounds. Degenerative diseases are cutting men and women down in the prime of life. Forty and on is now the dangerous age. Cancer is increasing at an alarming rate. The nerves and minds of men and women are giving way.

Some say the remedy lies in legislation. That is a false hope. You cannot get such laws, and if you could, they could not be enforced. Why not? Because too many people want tobacco, and because we live in a lost world, and the world is not to be rescued as a whole— we shall not be rescued by schools, ordinary hospitals, or by ordinary churches even, for these are doing only a partial work for humanity. We shall be rescued one by one by the acceptance of pure holy immortal principles! To make these principles plain is the object of this lesson.

If I have children to be educated and can select the school and teachers of my choice, I will select a school where no teacher smokes and where smoking is not allowed. The safest school is none too safe for my child.

If I am sick, nigh unto death, and have twenty-five years of life at stake, will I entrust that life to a physician who smokes? Or will I hunt for one who is free from the habit, and, therefore, in a position to thoroughly correct my physical habits; and one who will have a steady nerve and clear brain in case I need surgery?

If I have an eternity at stake and need a spiritual advisor to counsel me in securing an eternal existence, will I seek for one who smokes, or one whom I know to be himself keeping all the laws of the Most High and, therefore, in a position to give advice that will save me eternally?

If I am seeking for spiritual fellowship among God's true children, do you think I can find a satisfying fellowship in a church where two-thirds of the men and boys, many of the women and girls, and some of the preachers smoke? Never! Such have taken their stand against their Maker, and I am for Him. They are going in one direction and I in another. They and I can be friends, but we can have no spiritual fellowship. I will have to hunt for a church where no teacher, preacher, health lecturer, doctor, nurse, or member even is allowed to use tobacco, and where no member is retained who lives in open defiance of his Maker; there I will find sweet fellowship.

Health and Alcohol

Tobacco is a narcotic; so is alcohol. In the same group are marihuana, opium, morphine, heroin, and cocain. While their actions differ, they all are dangerous.

Much that was said in the preceding chapter on tobacco might be repeated in this one on alcohol. The degenerating effect on the organs is similar but may not be as serious. There is no doubt in my mind but that tobacco is doing more to destroy the vitality of human life than is alcohol. Alcohol makes a man into a greater nuisance in society and does it quicker than tobacco; its temporary influence on the brain and nervous system is immediate and disastrous; one glass of beer disqualifies a person for driving an automobile or bearing any other responsibility.

The user begins with what he calls "moderation" which he thinks is safe, but which ends in disaster.

A physician recently wrote me the following letter, which reveals the effects of moderate drinking upon the organs of the body:

A Striking Case of Moderate Drinking

"Here is a story that will interest you as a worker in the field of alcohol education. It is not heresay but an experience in my own medical practice.

"A prominent young man of this city died recently of 'moderate' drinking. He had never been 'drunk'—only 'happy'; but after three years of it he paid for it with his life. I was called at the last minute, but nothing could be done. He did not respond to any kind of treatment. I never knew why until I saw his body opened at the autopsy and viewed his organs. His heart was but a mass of degenerative fat instead of muscle. His liver was doubly enlarged, pitted and hardened and scarred—chronic alcoholic hypertrophic cirrhosis. His lungs appeared sclerotic, as did his kidneys, and were irregular and pale. His stomach and bowels were pale and fatty externally, but congested and reddened and thickened throughout the mucous membrane lining. His spleen and glands were swollen and congested. I had known him for twenty years and never knew that he drank. He was never ill, but told his wife, 'If I am ever sick, call Dr. Ritchie.' and so she did, but it was too late. When I arrived I worked with might and main and called another physician, but no therapy or heart stimulation or adrenalin had any effect. I have told you the reason. The last three years they said he had drank moderately but daily.

"The autopsy surgeon removed a piece of tissue from each of the above-named organs and sent these to the pathologist in charge of the laboratory of an accredited Class A Medical College. A microscopic study of these organs revealed the irreparable damage alcohol had done to the vital units or cells comprising these organs. No other cause for death could be discovered." (71)

THE DIRE CONSEQUENCES

To the extent that alcohol is used, the intellect is benumbed, the mind confused, the difference between right and wrong disappears the reason is paralyzed and dethroned, the will becomes impotent and loses the power to choose the right and resist the wrong; the power of habit becomes so strong that the will is overborne, enthralled, and degraded until the user has no power to break the snare. Everything depends on the right action of the will.

Slowly the conscience becomes dormant and there is no guide to moral conduct. The senses and all the noble powers of the mind are perverted, the moral perceptions are dulled so that corruption and debasement result. The animal passions are excited, sensual indulgence, licentiousness and adultery follow. The emotions degenerate —love to passion, joy to orgy, ardor to impatience, and courage to recklessness.

The brain becomes maddened, vice and crime of every description are multiplied, violence, strife, and bloodshed follow.

Delirium and insanity are sometimes the climax of what might have been brilliant careers. All of the fine ideals and aspirations of life are blighted. Love of the good, pure, and noble is destroyed. Thoughts of spiritual and divine things are extinguished. Man sinks to the level of the brute.

And then he passes his weaknesses on to succeeding generations. One writer has summarized the tragedy of the situation in these words:

"Liquor stupefies and defiles the user. But the evil does not stop here. He transmits irritable tempers, polluted blood, enfeebled intellects and weak morals to his children, and renders himself accountable for all the evil results that his wrong and dissipated course of life bring upon his family and the community. The race is groaning under a weight of accumulated woe, because of the sins of former generations. And yet with scarcely a thought or care, men and women of the present generation indulge in intemperance by surfeiting and drunkenness, and thereby leave, as a legacy for the next generation, enfeebled intellects, and polluted morals."

When it is realized that "the prosperity of a nation is dependent upon the virtue and intelligence of its citizens," it must be evident that we are headed for national ruin unless some saving influence be applied in a stronger way than is now operating. Most alarming of all is the rapid increase of drinking among women and girls.

Is Alcohol a Food?

One of the most specious, and therefore deceptive, arguments used to sanction the daily use of moderate amounts of beverages containing alcohol, is the claim that alcohol has a food value. For instance, the manufacturers of beer acclaim it as a food, and in this way beguile the ignorant into its use. They now prate about the minerals and vitamins in certain brands of beer, because it is known today that the human body cannot exist without minerals and vitamins. It is not possible, however, to embody in a poison like alcohol enough of these life-giving substances to make the concoction of value as a food, but it is possible to fool the public.

Still another claim has been made by its proponents for many years. They take certain statements to the effect that alcohol can be converted into heat and energy, and lead people to believe that these statements mean that alcohol is a food. They do this by disassociating these statements from others concerning its physiological actions, with which they belong, and which would give a balanced interpretation; and in this way they give a distorted or one-sided interpretation of the facts, which very easily deceives the unlearned and the unwary.

Thus it becomes necessary to do some very careful, thorough work to make known the true nature of alcohol.

The writer has gathered from many sources of authority, statements concerning the food value of alcohol, and concerning its physiological effects. These statements have been resolved into twenty-one points and placed in a column entitled "Alcohol." In a companion column, the relation of food to these twenty-one points has been stated as given by food authorities. The contrast between these two columns is strong enough to convince the truth seeker and to end all argument. The deception is unmasked. The numbers in parenthesis refer to bibliography at close of the chapter.

FOOD

1. Food is digested to make it ready for the body to use it. (1)

2. Food repairs the tissue. (7, 8)

3. Food provides energy.

4. Food maintains strength and endurance.

5. Food maintains the body's immunity or resistance to disease.

6. Food can be stored in the body for future use.

7. When the concentration of normal nutrient in the blood exceeds the rate of absorption by the body's demand, it is withdrawn from the blood by the liver and muscles, except in diabetes.

8. Food supplies elements which provide for oxidation.

9. Food oxidation increases with exercise, which is normal. (41)

10. Food assists in maintaining a natural temperature in the body.

11. Food properly includes water. (44) Although water is not a source of heat, energy, or repair, it is necessary to these processes, as it is essential to all life and life processes.

ALCOHOL

1. Alcohol passes unchanged into the blood and body cells. (2, 3, 4, 5, 6)

2. Alcohol damages tissue, and cannot repair it. (9, 10, 11, 12, 13)

3. Alcohol, it is claimed, can be oxidized (14) and produce energy (15, 16); but by hindering oxidation of food (17), hindering metabolism (18), and narcotizing nerves and cells, it lessens the amount of energy available to the body, so that the net result is a loss of energy. (19, 20, 21, 22)

4. Alcohol finally hastens fatigue and lessens endurance. (23, 24, 25, 26, 27)

5. Alcohol breaks down the body's resistance to disease. (28, 29, 30, 31, 32, 33, 34)

6. Alcohol cannot be stored. (35, 36, 37) The body gets rid of it as quickly as possible.

7. Alcohol is unlike food in that it cannot be withdrawn from the blood, as can food when the concentration is high. (38)

8. Alcohol hinders the oxidation of foods (39), and even hinders its own oxidation. (40)

9. Alcohol oxidation does not materially increase with exercise. (42)

10. Alcohol is claimed to produce heat by oxidation, but because it diffuses more heat than it produces, the net result is a loss of heat and a lowering of the body temperature. (This and No. 3 are the strongest claims (43) of the proponents of alcohol.)

11. Alcohol is said to be a dehydrant, which means that it draws water from the cells and tissues, lessening the amount of water available in the body and so hindering the life proc-

FOOD (Continued)

Water comprises about 70% of the weight of the body. The following percentages of water in various parts are given in medical books:

Tissue 70-90%
Muscle 75%
Blood plasma 92%
Red blood corpuscle 65%
Kidneys 80%
Liver 76%
Glands 80%
Brain gray matter 84%
Spinal cord 74%
Nerves 60%
Bone 40%
Saliva 99%
Gastric juice 99%
Pancreatic juice 98%
Liver bile 97%

Water is the chief constituent by weight of all of the secretions of the glands which are the life activators of the body. The life processes are dependent upon the presence of water in all parts of the body—in every cell. No cell, gland, or organ can function without it. In starvation an animal can survive after the loss of half of its protein, but it dies from the loss of one-fifth of its water. Therefore any substance which hinders the actions of water thereby hinders every life process to which water contributes.

12. Water allays thirst. (46)

13. Food contributes to normal mental functions.

14. Food contributes to normal physical functions.

15. Food's dominant action is to build up the body, and contribute to life. (52)

16. Food is essential to the life, growth, and development of the young.

17. Food can be used in quantities that will fully supply the needs of the body for heat, energy, and repair.

18. Food, as such, is in a natural state.

ALCOHOL (Continued)

esses. (45) This effect is present to the extent the alcohol is present. Alcohol is also a solvent and will dissolve or mix with many substances which water cannot dissolve, such as certain oils—castor oil, croton oil, and the volatile oils. It dissolves or disturbs a fat-like substance in the nerve cells called lipoid. (69)

12. Alcohol creates thirst. (47)

13. Alcohol paralyzes mental functions. (48, 49)

14. Alcohol paralyzes physical functions. (50, 51, 54)

15. Alcohol's dominant action is to destroy the body—to kill. (53, 54)

16. Alcohol hinders the life processes, and thus hinders the growth and development of the young. (55, 56, 57)

17. Alcohol, if used in quantities sufficient to supply the body's need for either heat or energy, is disastrous to the mechanism of the body. (58) If the quantity taken is so small as to do no damage, it has no food value. (59, 60) In order to get worth-while amounts of food, in this sense, from alcohol, one must swallow poisonous doses of the drug qualities.

18. Alcohol is a by-product of the decay of that which was food. (61)

FOOD (Concluded)	**ALCOHOL (Concluded)**
19. Food does not require an ever-increasing amount to produce the same effect.	19. Alcohol requires an ever-increasing amount to produce the same effect. (62, 63)
20. Food, when used, does not create a desire for an ever-increasing quantity. It satisfies a normal appetite.	20. Alcohol creates a desire that develops a craving which results in a "habit." It creates an unnatural craving. (64, 65, 66, 67)
21. Food is welcomed by the body, as a friend to all its parts and processes.	21. Alcohol is regarded as an intruder—an enemy and a poison—and the body seeks to eliminate (68) it as fast as possible in order to save the body from injury so far as possible.

The consideration of these points removes alcohol from being regarded as either a fuel or a food for the body. One authority has likened the fuel use of alcohol in the body to the use of sea water in running an engine. It may be attempted for a short time, but soon ruins the machinery.

For a complete treatise on the subject of alcohol the reader is referred to the book, "Health and Alcohol," which is a companion volume to "Health and Tobacco."

Is Alcoholism a Disease?

A recent teaching which has been highly developed in the last few years holds that it is, and sets forth the following propositions:

1—That alcohol is not the cause of alcoholism, but that human misery is the cause.

2—That alcohol is not the cause of alcoholism any more than the automobile is the cause of automobile accidents.

3—That the root of the trouble is in the man, not in the bottle.

4—That the man is maladjusted,—sick, and needs scientific medical treatment,—hospitalization under the care of specialists, and that his care in that way is a public responsibility.

5—That he should not be looked upon as one who has done any wrong, but as one who is a victim of a serious malady and needs to be helped.

6—That it is not wrong to drink; that alcohol is a necessity, and to drink moderately is quite all right.

7—That alcohol is not habit-forming, but is a food.

8—That alcohol in moderation has no harmful effects upon the human body.

9—That 95 per cent of those who drink are not harmed by it.

10—That only about 1 per cent become alcoholics, and that is not their fault but something happened to them in earlier years which gave them a wrong bent, or some present maladjustment now calls for alcohol in excess.

11—That the 95% should not be deprived of it because 1% become alcoholics.

12—That each person should be left to decide whether or not he will drink.

13—That if one chooses to practice total abstinence it should be entirely voluntary, and

14—That to require him to abstain is fundamentally wrong, and therefore

15—To prohibit the manufacture, advertising, sale, and drinking of alcoholic beverages is a wrong of first magnitude.

16—That all citizens, church people included, should unite in this new scientific approach to the alcohol problem.

17—That they should make provision for it and all work together for true temperance which is drinking in moderation by those who choose to do so.

Whose Program Is This?

This was one line of attack followed by the liquor industry when they were undermining prohibition, and it has been advocated with increasing subtility and effectiveness ever since. Manifestly if the industry is the sole source of this teaching, the very source will discredit it with many people, particularly church folk whom they are most anxious to reach and influence, and so kill total abstinence at its source. Therefore they seek helpers whom they can use to present these seductive principles under auspices which will be acceptable to all.

They know that the public generally, church people included, regard science almost with reverence, and that most people bow the knee to scientific teachers. To the point is a recent statement by Dorothy Thompson,—"It is safer today to take the name of God in vain than the name of science." Therefore a department of Yale University in New Haven, Conn., has become a scientific outlet for the presentation of these principles. It is known as "The Yale School of Alcohol Studies."

From Yale it can spread into the science departments of schools, great and small, throughout the land, and so reach other teachers, students, future teachers, parents, and parent-teacher associations. The National Education Association,—the teachers of America,— co-operates in the selection of teachers and school administrators to receive appointments to the Yale school. Yale is advocating that similar schools for the study of alcohol be set up from coast to coast. Already $150,000 has been given by seven distillers and a front organization with a good sounding name, to be used for the scientific study of alcohol at a renowned university in the state of New York.

Churches are invited to select leading workers to go to Yale under appointment, to take the studies. They are carefully taught "the scientific approach to the alcohol problem," and when they return they and their fellows feel that they have some advance information which should be shared with all, and their associates receive it with admiration and satisfaction. As an example, one preacher said, "This is the first really scientific training I have had in alcohol. I am going to change my lectures because of it . . . Up to now I declared alcohol was a poison, but the professors have about convinced me that it is a food."

As a result, entire churches are taking it on. State church temperance organizations are doing the same and turning their backs on prohibition, the work of the W.C.T.U. and all other dry forces. In certain instances great denominations, through their temperance departments are committed to it.

Such results begin when the church workers take time off from their "dry" work to attend a "wet" school, where they become engrossed with the so-called scientific intricacies of the alcohol problem and the glamour of "higher education." They are delighted with their advancement and forthwith turn their attention to the matter of salvaging the confirmed alcoholics (which too often is impossible), and become advocates of moderate drinking which makes more drunks to be taken care of, instead of continuing their divine mission of teaching total abstinence which is the sure preventative of alcoholism. Thus the light of the church is being extinguished. This, no doubt, is the chief purpose in all of these scientific studies of the alcohol problem,—divert the churches from the work of saving mankind to helping the liquor traffic to ruin them.

Several other strong organizations are operating under such names as Research Council on Alcohol problems, Committee for Education on Alcoholism, Committee on Alcohol Hygiene, etc. A great flood of propaganda is being circulated, some of which finds its way into church publications which would surprise those who read these lines. You are advised to examine your own church publications, and make a list of the articles which are at least tainted with some of the teachings on page one of this treatise.

A gigantic scheme has been devised and put into operation to thwart all attempts at the return of prohibition, and to undermine in the home, the school, and the church, the basic idea of total abstinence as the only safe course to follow.

One of the most subtle schemes goes under a name usually abbreviated into two capital letters, (A. A.). It enters the realm of religion and so easily enters into the membership of churches of all kinds. It is the organization to which the others turn for the rehabilitation of the alcoholics, and is in good standing with all of them, including the Yale school. It claims to direct the mind of the alcoholic to a supernatural power, but to what kind of a supernatural power it is hard to comprehend when one learns that there are infidels, atheists, and agnostics among their rescued alcoholics. One writer said, "It becomes evident that all this talk about God is mere camouflage." The organization is in good standing with the liquor industry. And why not, as they are heard to say in their meetings, "If alcohol helps you to have a good time, use it, but if you find it is beginning to get the best of you, do something about it."

They become missionaries for moderate drinking. They denounce abstinence in spite of the fact that under prohibition two hundred institutions for the care of alcoholics were forced to close for lack of patients. This, perhaps, is the most respected organization working on the basis that alcoholism is a disease.

Thus the forces of destruction disguised as "science" are capturing both schools and churches and through them the human race. What the outcome will be only God can foresee.

It is high time for every believer in God and lover of humanity to stand four-square on Holy Writ: "Wine is a mocker, strong drink is raging; and whosoever is received thereby is not wise. . . . At last it biteth like a serpent, and stingeth like an adder." Prov. 20:1, and 23:32

Let the battle cry everywhere be *"Total abstinence."*

The Last Stand—"Personal Liberty"

The last plea we hear made in defense of beverage alcohol is that of personal liberty—that we have a right to eat and drink what we please. People prate about living in a land where freedom is vouchsafed to all by the Constitution. They do not seem to understand that freedom does not impart the right to debauch one's self when it endangers the lives and property of others and the well-being of generations yet unborn. The drinker is a menace with his gun, fist and matches, to his wife, his child, and the public; he robs his family of support and their rightful heritage and casts them and himself as charges upon the public, and claims it as his sacred right—his "personal liberty."

That is not the kind of liberty our forefathers bought with their blood and wrote into the Declaration of Independence and the American Constitution. That is not the sort of liberty for which our glorious flag stands—to debauch one's self, shoot his fellow men, abuse his wife and make paupers of his children. These are not the principles symbolized by the world-famed Statue of Liberty in New York harbor. But rather our progenitors bequeathed to us the right to worship God as each individual may desire and to live in a land where all men are equal; civil and religious freedom are our heritage, not license to destroy the race.

The Law of the Land

This "personal liberty" plea became so popular that it swept away all law-restraining barriers. But should the law of the land make room for wrong because wrong is strong? Heaven has answered that question not only for America but for the whole world. Nearly six thousand years ago God gave His law of Ten Commandments for the guidance of the people of all nations as long as time shall last. Not once has He asked whether they are popular or not. Men may scorn them and treat them as if they are not there. Men may even say they have been repealed; but He does not repeal them, be they broken ever so often. If the last man on earth should say, "I will not keep them," they will still hang in the sky and will judge all mankind in the last great day. *Right cannot change.*

Likewise, the laws of physiology have not changed in the last six thousand years; they are the laws of life—the laws of God—and they cannot change. Should the American Constitution be repudiated, abandoned, and crumbled into dust, the human constitution will stand because it is the handiwork of God. Should civilized nations forsake their lofty ideals and the principles which have made them great, the laws of physiology discussed in this chapter and book will stand for aye; they are eternal; they are the laws of the Creator, and we shall meet them at His bar of justice some day.

THE YOUTH

I appeal to the youth to know physiology, which is yourself—and the laws of life upon which health of mind and body, usefulness and happiness depend. Guard and preserve your personal liberty. Alcohol makes slaves of its users. Abstinence preserves the highest form of personal liberty, both for ourselves and our fellows.

THE PARENTS

I appeal to parents to become informed concerning these principles of life and liberty. Make sure that your example is right. Throw a positive saving influence around your children.

It has been said that "the restoration and uplifting of humanity begins in the home. The work of parents underlies every other. Society is composed of families, and is what the heads of families make it. . . . The heart of the community, of the church, and of the nation, is the household. The well-being of society, the success of the church, the prosperity of the nation, depend upon home influences." (70)

THE EDUCATORS

I appeal to educators to teach these principles of physiology to all the students coming within the sphere of your influence, that they may be protected by knowledge within.

The Protectors of Health

I appeal to those who are set to guard the health of the community that this matter, which is fundamental to our individual and national welfare, be not neglected.

THE CHURCH

But most of all do I appeal to the church of the living God. The believers in the church must take up this work and be crusaders.

Do you say, we will leave this specific work for the scientists—the educators and the health workers—to do?

You cannot say thus. These laws of life are divine; they are the handiwork of the Creator; they are popularly violated. The church is Heaven's fortress in the world. The church is God's ambassador among men. She must teach His laws!

There are still other reasons why the church must take on the responsibility of this task. Listen a moment while I tell you.

The scientist may know all I have told you, and more, but he may wish to indulge. If so, there is no power on earth or in heaven to stop him.

The educator may know all I have told you, and more, but he may lack courage to take up the task of alcohol education.

The physician with all of his knowledge of medicine and physiology may yield to his own appetite or may even prescribe alcohol to his patients.

The lawyer and legislator may be too deep in politics to take a straight, honest stand in this matter.

The highest rulers may take their wine and the lowest peasants their beer, and the citizen may say, It does not matter.

But the Christian, who knows that he is made in the image of God and that his body is intended to be the temple of the Holy Ghost—he cannot indulge because he knows it is violating his Maker's will and destroys the image of the divine within him. There is a moral and spiritual force within him which says, Nay!

The work which I therefore call you, as citizens of a Christian land, to rise and do will not be done from convictions born of mere science or the knowledge of physiology (though we must have those), but rather by seeing back of science, back of physiology, God; and recognizing that our supreme duty in this, as in all other matters, is unto Him!

BIBLIOGRAPHY

(1) "Alcohol and the Human Body," Horsley and Sturge, page 182.
(2) "Alcohol and the Human Body," Horsley and Sturge, page 183.
(3) "Alcohol and Man," Haven Emerson, M.D., page 10.
(4) "Alcohol—Its Action on the Human Organism," Medical Research Council, pages 32, 119.
(5) "Journal American Medical Association," Editorial, No. 30, 1935.
(6) "What About Alcohol?" Emil Bogen, M.D., page 33.
(7) "Alcohol and the Human Body," Horsley and Sturge, page 182.
(8) "Alcohol and Human Life," C. C. Weeks, M.D., page 66.
(9) "Alcohol and the Human Body," Horsley and Sturge, page 183.
(10) "Alcohol and Human Life," C. C. Weeks, M.D., pages 65, 67, 75.
(11) "Alcohol, a Food, a Drug, a Poison" (leaflet), Haven Emerson, M.D., page 2.
(12) "Materia Medica, Pharmacology, Therapeutics, and Prescription Writing," Walter A. Bastedo, M.D., pages 394-397, 1933 edition.
(13) "Physiological Chemistry," Albert P. Mathews, Ph.D., pages 310, 311.
(14) Alcohol—Its Action on the Human Organism," Medical Research Council, page 2.
(15) "Alcohol and Man," Haven Emerson, M.D., pages 10, 11.

(16) "Alcohol—Its Action on the Human Organism," Medical Research Council, page 32.

(17) "Alcohol and Human Life," C. C. Weeks, M.D., pages 75, 81.

(18) "Alcohol and Human Life," C. C. Weeks, M.D., page 81.

(19) "Alcohol and Human Life," C. C. Weeks, M.D., pages 65, 59.

(20) "Alcohol, a Food, a Drug, a Poison" (leaflet), Haven Emerson, M.D., page 2.

(21) "Materia Medica," Walter A. Bastedo, M.D., pages 394-397.

(22) "Alcohol and Man," Haven Emerson, M.D., pages 11, 12.

(23) "The Truth About Alcohol as a Medicine" (pamphlet) J. H. Kellogg, M.D., page 14.

(24) "The Scientist Experiments with Alcohol," Williams and Stoddard, pages 10-14.

(25) "Alcohol and Man," Haven Emerson, M.D., page 47.

(26) "What About Alcohol?" Emil Bogen, M.D., page 42.

(27) "Effects of Alcoholic Drinks," Emma L. B. Transeau, page 33.

(28) "Alcohol and the Human Body," Horsley and Sturge, pages 204-207.

(29) "Effects of Alcoholic Drinks," Emma L. B. Transeau, page 59.

(30) "Narcotics and Youth Today," Robert E. Corradini, page 84.

(31) "Alcohol and Man," Haven Emerson, M.D., pages 54, 55, 180.

(32) "Alcohol and Man," Haven Emerson, M.D., pages 186, 187.

(33) "The Great Destroyer" (pamphlet) J. H. Kellogg, M.D., page 5.

(34) "The Truth About Alcohol as a Medicine," J. H. Kellogg, M.D., pages 4, 5.

(35) "Alcohol and Human Life," C. C. Weeks, M.D., page 69.

(36) "Alcohol—Its Action on the Human Organism," Medical Research Council, page 119.

(37) "What About Alcohol?" Emil Bogen, page 34.

(38) "Good Health," Dr. H. H. Mitchell, May, 1934, page 11.

(39) "Alcohol and Human Life," C. C. Weeks, M.D., pages 75, 81.

(40) "Alcohol and Human Life," C. C. Weeks, M.D., page 81.

(41) "Alcohol and Human Life," C. C. Weeks, M.D., page 81.

(42) "Alcohol and Human Life," C. C. Weeks, M.D., page 81.

(43) "The Alcohol Question," (pamphlet) Professor G. Von Bunge, page 5.

(44) "Physiological Chemistry," Albert P. Mathews, Ph.D., pages 310, 311.

(45) "Alcohol and Human Life," C. C. Weeks, M.D., page 75.

(46) "Alcohol and Human Life," C. C. Weeks, M.D., page 75.

(47) "Alcohol and Human Life," C. C. Weeks, M.D., page 75.

(48) "Alcohol and the Human Body," Horsley and Sturge, page 183.

(49) "Alcohol and Man," Haven Emerson, M.D., page 100.

(50) "Alcohol and the Human Body," Horsley and Sturge, page 183.

(51) "Alcohol and Man," Haven Emerson, M.D., page 100.

(52) "Effects of Alcoholic Drinks," Emma L. B. Transeau, page 2.

(53) "Effects of Alcoholic Drinks," Emma L. B. Transeau, page 2.

(54) "Materia Medica," Walter A. Bastedo, M.D., pages 398, 399.

(55) "Alcohol and Human Life," C. C. Weeks, M.D., page 67.

(56) "Alcohol, a Food, a Drug, a Poison" (leaflet), Haven Emerson, M.D., page 2.

(57) "What About Alcohol?" Emil Bogen, M.D., page 36.

(58) "Temperance Advocate," Toronto, Frank D. Slutz, January 25, 1935.

(59) "Material Medica," Walter A. Bastedo, M.D., pages 398, 399.

(60) "Alcohol—Neither Food Nor Medicine," (pamphlet) W. A. Evans, M.D.

(61) "What About Alcohol?" Emil Bogen, M.D., page 19.

(62) "Alcohol in Experience and Experiment," Cora Frances Stoddard, pages 21, 22.

(63) "Narcotics and Youth Today," Robert E. Corradini, pages 22, 24.

(64) "Christian Century," May 13, 1931, Prof. Samuel A. Mahood.

(65) "Alcohol—Its Action on the Human Organism," Medical Research Council, pages 119-121.

(66) "Alcohol in Experiment and Experience," Cora Frances Stoddard, pages 31, 32.

(67) "Why the Craving for Alcohol?" Dr. J. Glaig, Berlin, in "Scientific Temperance Journal, Summer," 1935.

(68) "Materia Medica," Walter A. Bastedo, M.D., page 381.

(69) "Alcohol and Man," Haven Emerson, M.D., page 68.

(70) "Ministry of Healing," page 349.

(71) I. S. Ritchie, M.D., 4146 Seventh Street, Riverside, California.

The Root of Intemperance

There are two ways of living. When the right way is followed, the body does not crave stimulants or narcotics; there is no desire for them. That is the plan set forth in this book. The other way is the popular way, and the foods and drinks consumed result, in many cases, in starting cravings which can be satisfied only with mild or strong stimulants and narcotics; if for mild ones, they, in time, lead to the stronger ones.

This chapter will reveal the manifold ways by which the appetites for tobacco, alcohol, and other narcotics are developed. Many of the primary steps in these experiences are usually overlooked, and therefore the reader should expect some very unusual information in this lesson.

Inasmuch as the cravings which are satisfied by alcohol, tobacco, and narcotics are often started by other things, manifestly, to deal with these appetites after they are developed and not eradicate the habits which constitute their source, is superficial and ineffective. Therefore the special object of this lesson is to study the interrelation between the different groups of common practices out of which these appetites grow.

It may seem to be somewhat revolutionary, but when you stop to think of the physical and mental condition of mankind today it is perfectly apparent that something revolutionary needs to be done.

This chapter is *so* revolutionary that I have elected, to a large extent, to ask other persons than myself to bear testimony to the principles involved, believing that the reader will be more easily convinced of the truth in the matter when a large number of people speak than when merely one person expresses his conclusions, even after much research. For this reason the reader is asked to pardon voluminous quotations. A book has been published bearing the same name as this chapter heading, in which a very large number of writers are represented. It is impossible to reproduce here more than a very few statements, and the reader should know that numbers of people could be heard where only one is quoted. Those who wish further information on any of the points discussed are referred to the complete book by the present author.

Group One, Irritating Foods

There are certain irritating foods which tend to develop a thirst which water does not quench, and which will be satisfied only with strong drink—something stronger than water.

The foods in this class include: Condiments and spices of all kinds, pepper, mustard, anything which is "hot" when it is cold, vinegar, excess of salt, excess of sugar.

From time immemorial the vendors of intoxicating beverages have ofttimes maintained a free lunch counter. The foods offered possessed enough food value to lure the hungry, but at the same time these foods carried other substances which tended to develop a thirst which water would not quench. An inventory of the free lunch reveals such foods as bologna sausage, liver sausage, cheese, codfish balls, pretzels, and potato chips. To these fried, freely salted highly spiced and seasoned foods will be added some form of grain such as crackers, rye bread or pumpernickel.

Concerning this sort of a free lunch offered in connection with the sale of alcoholic liquors, Haven Emerson, M.D., of Columbia University, a widely recognized authority, recently wrote the following in a personal letter:

"In answer to yours of May 15 let me say that articles used to stimulate thirst rather than to slake it are the common food of the free lunch counters. In general, persons with a well-balanced diet including sufficient fruits and vegetables are satisfied without recourse to alcoholic drinks."

"Neither of these statements can, however, be taken to mean that either the prevention or cure of alcoholism can be relied upon by dietary measures, although recovery from chronic alcoholism is certainly aided by a liberal use of fruits and vegetables as part of a balanced dietary."

Many writers—doctors, dietitians, and teachers—have recognized that irritating foods create a thirst for something stronger than water. Some of these writers have had many years of experience in treating alcoholic patients and have made numerous experiments with diet and have recorded their findings.

Perhaps the clearest statement of the kind that has come into my library from a physician was made by Daniel H. Kress, M.D., for many years connected with the Washington, D. C., Sanitarium. It is reproduced here.

How a Thirst Is Created

"From my own experience in the treatment of alcoholics, I am convinced that many may be cured if properly treated. The treatment if effective, however, must be directed toward the removal of the craving. Fruits, cereals, nuts, milk, and other products which are not irritating or stimulating will in time destroy all desire for alcoholic beverages. Again and again I have been forced to recognize that dietetic errors are in a large measure responsible for the craving which exists for alcohol. The irritation produced by irritating and stimulating foods and drinks calls for something that will afford temporary relief from the unpleasant symptoms associated with such irritation. Alcohol being a narcotic supplies this demand; and in the absence of alcohol the use of tobacco or cigarettes will afford temporary relief.

"The saloon keepers in former days observed that certain foods create a thirst that water will not quench. They kept a lunch counter for their patrons, but not because they had compassion on the unfortunate poor. If so, they would have fed the drunkard's wife and children. But with the saloon keeper it was a matter of business. The secret of the free lunch table could be discovered by taking an inventory of the food that was found upon it. It was not laden with juicy peaches, pears, oranges, etc. They knew that such foods would diminish their business. Upon that lunch counter were found highly seasoned foods, as sausage, pickled pigs' feet, smoked ham, mustard, pepper, and other irritating products. Experience taught the saloon keeper that these foods created a craving which led men to the bar for drink.

"The sad thing about this is that many a good, well-meaning wife and mother is supplying her husband and her sons with the same kind of food that was formerly found on the free lunch table in the saloon. Many a mother's prayer is in this way being neutralized.

"At a public gathering in England some years ago, Staff Captain Hudson, matron of the South Newington Inebriates' Home, in relating her experience in the treatment of inebriates after the adoption of a fruit, grain, and vegetable diet, said, 'Speaking generally, the benefits of this diet are incalculable. Lazy, vicious, bloated, gluttonous, bad-tempered women who had hitherto needed weeks and even months of nursing and watching, to my astonishment and delight, under this new treatment made rapid recovery.'

"For a number of years I have depended upon such foods in the treatment of inebriates, with gratifying results. From my experience of over forty years in the treatment of alcoholics I am convinced that when the relation that exists between what is served on our American tables and the use of alcohol is better understood and is given the attention that it deserves by physicians, ministers of the gospel, temperance advocates, and the makers of the home, the existing desire for alcohol will disappear, and with it will disappear much of the irritability, impatience, and domestic unhappiness which are chiefly responsible for the prevalence of divorce and crime.

"The temperance crusade of the future must begin in the homes of the American people. When this is done, there will be less need of state or national temperance crusades; and until it is done, the efforts of temperance workers will be hopelessly hindered. The hope of prohibition centers around the family circle and the home.

"Where are the mothers and housewives who by giving painstaking attention to the needs of the family table, and avoiding the use of rich, stimulating food, will strengthen our bulwarks of temperance? Mere public education can never accomplish this." (1)

"I have found that a diet free from unnatural irritants will always result in a decrease in the desire for both tobacco and alcohol. I have never yet discovered a drunkard or inebriate who was not passionately fond of spicy, highly seasoned foods and also of flesh foods. I have no doubt that one reason why these habits are so common is because dietetic errors are common." (2)

Dr. J. H. Kellogg Speaks

In a personal letter, John Harvey Kellogg, M.D., for nearly a lifetime medical director of the world-famed Battle Creek Sanitarium, gives his opinion of the statements by Dr. Kress, as follows:

"I think the statements made by Dr. Kress in his excellent paper are entirely dependable."

Arthur W. Spalding, known from coast to coast as an indefatigable worker in the interest of the home and family life, has written on this subject under the capturing head-line:

"Don't Raise Your Boy to Be a Drunkard"

"It is when we leave babyhood, and the child is made to share the diet of his elders, that we most commonly enter the school of training for drunkenness. Of course this is equally true for the adults; and if you want the basic reason for our recent dive into liquor, go to the American table. Coffee, tea, hot sauces, spices, pepper, ginger, mustard, vinegar, flesh foods, everything highly seasoned—what alimentary tract can harbor such a conglomoration, what blood receive its fever-forming products without being driven to the call for stimulants and narcotics? The irritants and poisons introduced by such a diet directly incite to the use of liquor.

"True, some thousands, possibly millions, of good people daily swallow these things and still do not drink alcoholic liquors. They have built up by other means a moral barrier to the imbibing of alcohol, and so far their dikes hold. But what a prodigality of moral power! You hear some of them say, 'I could drink as well as anybody, if I would let myself,' or, 'I like the taste of liquor, but I will not drink.' They are having to draw upon their reserves of will, of moral strength (which might be put to constructive rather than to purely defense use) to resist an appetite they are constantly feeding. Most of them yield to the tobacco habit and so narcotize their bodies and create a stronger demand for alcohol. Whosoever resists the power of alcohol, yet daily feeds himself with the creators of thirst, is to be likened to a foolish man who builds high his dikes to shut out the flood yet ever invites more floods to break them down. There is no necessity of a craving for alcohol, tobacco, or drugs. It is an unnatural craving. It can be bred out of the body by a correct, nonstimulating diet. Better still, in the child it can be absolutely prevented by a proper regimen."

"But it is not alone through the use of condiments, drugging beverages, and wrong foods that the tendency to stimulants is fostered. A diet deficient in the essential elements, or overbalanced in any one. creates conditions of unbalance and disease. Given a sufficient incentive or temptation, the individual with this deranged condition easily tips over into indulgence in surfeiting and drunkenness. An example is the inordinate use of sugar in many forms— piled upon breakfast cereals, stuffed in ice cream and candy, dished up in pastries. Refined sugar, whether in table form or confectionery, creates a hyperacid condition which invites stimulants; and indeed, sugar itself is quite capable, under certain not uncommon digestive conditions, of setting up a neat little distillery of its own within the body." (3)

In hunting for a wide variety of authors who have written upon this subject, the present writer found a statement made in 1883 by a layman who later wrote the book "Ministry of Healing," which has blessed thousands of lives. It is as follows:

A Thirst Which Water Does Not Quench

"Our tables should bear only the most wholesome food, free from every irritating substance. The appetite for liquor is encouraged by the preparation of food with condiments and spices. These cause a feverish state of the system and drink is demanded to allay the irritation. . . . The dishes are highly seasoned with salt and pepper, creating an intolerable thirst. . . . They irritate and inflame the delicate coating of the stomach. . . . Such is the food that is commonly served upon fashionable tables, and given to children. Its effect is to cause nervousness, and to create thirst which water does not quench. . . . Food should be prepared in as simple a manner as possible, free from condiments and spices, and even from an undue amount of salt." (4)

The Root of Intemperance

"But in order to reach the root of intemperance we must go deeper than the use of alcohol or tobacco. Idleness, lack of aim, or evil associations, may be the predisposing cause. Often it is found at the home table, in families that account themselves strictly temperate. Anything that disorders digestion, that creates undue mental excitement, or in any way enfeebles the system, disturbing the balance of the mental and the physical powers, weakens the control of the mind over the body, and thus tends toward intemperance. The downfall of many a promising youth might be traced to unnatural appetites created by an unwholesome diet.

"Those who accustom themselves to a rich, stimulating diet, find after a time that the stomach is not satisfied with simple food. It demands that which is more and more highly seasoned, pungent, and stimulating. As the nerves become disordered and the system weakened, the will seems powerless to resist the unnatural craving. The delicate coating of the stomach becomes irritated and inflamed until the most stimulating food fails to give relief. A thirst is created that nothing but strong drink will quench." (5)

The same writer, in the book, "Ministry of Healing," has directed attention to the fact that these

Foods Inflame the Stomach and Demand Stimulants

"In this fast age, the less exciting the food, the better. Condiments are injurious in their nature. Mustard, pepper, spices, pickles, and other things of like character, irritate the stomach and make the blood feverish and impure. The inflamed condition of the drunkard's stomach is often pictured as illustrating the effect of alcoholic liquors. A similarly inflamed condition is produced by the use of irritating condiments. Soon ordinary food does not satisfy the appetite. The system feels a want, a craving for something more stimulating." (6)

Again in "Ministry of Healing,"

How We Prepare the Way for Drunkenness

"Often intemperance begins in the home. By the use of rich, unhealthful food the digestive organs are weakened, and a desire is created for food that is still more stimulating. Thus the appetite is educated to crave continually something stronger. The demand for stimulants becomes more frequent and more difficult to resist. The system becomes more or less filled with poison, and the more debilitated it becomes, the greater is the desire for these things. One step in the wrong direction prepares the way for another. Many who would not be guilty of placing on their table wine or liquor of any kind will load their table with food which creates such a thirst, for strong drink that to resist the temptation is almost impossible. Wrong habits of eating and drinking destroy the health and prepare the way for drunkenness.

"There would soon be little necessity for temperance crusades, if in the youth who form and fashion society, right principles in regard to temperance could be implanted. Let parents begin a crusade against intemperance at their own firesides, in the principles they teach their children to follow from infancy, and they may hope for success.

"There is work for mothers in helping their children to form correct habits and pure tastes. Educate the appetite; teach the children to abhor stimulants. Bring your children up to have moral stamina to resist the evil that surrounds them. Teach them that they are not to be swayed by others, that they are not to yield to strong influences, but to influence others for good." (7)

GROUP TWO, STIMULATING FOODS

Stimulating food contributes to the development of an appetite for intoxicants.

The foods in this class are: Meat extracts, meat broths, beef tea, meat soups, raw meat in particular, all meats in general.

From Alexander Haig we take this paragraph showing the interrelation between meats, tea, and coffee.

"The animal foods in common use (meat, fish, fowl, game, and eggs) all contain uric acid or substances of the xanthin group which can be converted into it. The alkaloid of tea, coffee, chocolate and cocoa are also xanthins and are to be avoided." (8)

The table below is given to help the reader to appreciate how large are the amounts of these undesirable substances in the juices of flesh, and in tea and coffee, taken from "High Blood Pressure," by G. K. Abbott, M.D., page 48:

Uric Acid and Purines

	Grains per lb.
Hosp. Beef Tea (cooked 8 hours)	7.00
Meat Juice	49.70
Meat Extract	63.00
Tea	175.00
Coffee	70.00
Cocoa	59.00

Numerous authorities also recognize that these extractives of meat lead in the direction of *alcohol.* Dr. Fitch, a very noted authority, says:

Flesh-foods

"In cases of periodic alcoholism, in which there is no inordinate or indeed, as a rule, no desire whatever for alcohol between the attacks, a non-stimulating diet is believed by most authorities to be the best. Fruits, plainly cooked cereals, and vegetables should constitute the staple diet, according to Gilman Thompson, and animal food should be eaten only in moderation. There are those who hold that the consumption of meat in large quantities predisposes to drink, and that the proper treatment for those addicted to drink is to withhold meat as far as possible. Although undoubtedly great drinkers are often also large meat eaters, this is by no means universal. For example, in Australia, where probably more meat is eaten per capita than in any other part of the world, the favorite beverage and that most largely drunk is tea. Climate plays an important role in those countries in which meat and alcohol are the popular articles of diet. Nevertheless, a relationship apparently exists between the consumption of meat and alcohol, and it is perhaps sound advice to restrict the use of meat in those who are in the habit of drinking to their detriment." (9)

Dr. Fitch's citation that the Australians do not use much alcohol, but use much tea, confirms the idea that the tea will partially replace the alcohol, and so he strengthens our argument rather than weakening it.

We present another author who has written from the standpoint of curing the drink habit.

Vegetarianism and Alcoholism

"Speaking upon the relation between vegetarianism and total abstinence, Hon. Edvard Wavrinsky, a member of the Swedish parliament, a very active worker in the temperance cause, holding the office of International Chief Templar, said: "It is time that the friends of total abstinence duly appreciate and resort to the powerful ally they have in vegetarianism. If a drunkard can be induced to embrace the mild, healthful vegetarian diet, his desire for alcohol will at once be considerably reduced, and finally wholly fall off. He will feel somewhat lax in the beginning, lacking the excitement caused by flesh and alcohol; but soon he will feel his vitality increase, his outer and inner buoyancy return; and he will understand that under normal circumstances no stimulants are needed to keep the machinery of the body running.'

" 'Of course they who want to serve and elevate humanity must control themselves in food and drink. It does not suffice that we do not use the destructive, intoxicating liquors; we must go the whole length, and also work for the best food, since this stands in exceedingly close relation to temperance.' " (10)

All writers agree that meats contain stimulants, and many have pointed out the fact that these lead in the direction of alcohol. Several such are offered here.

Surely a diet that is anti-alcoholic after the appetite is established would be equally anti-alcoholic before the appetite is developed, and so be a preventive.

Meat Is a Stimulant

"Dr. Haig then shows that flesh, beef-tea, soups, meat-extracts, and other 'deadly decoctions of flesh,' are stimulants, quickly evolve quantities of force, and consequently produce a corresponding amount of depression. 'Stimulation is not force, but force renders a little more quickly available.'

" 'Hence it comes about that those who took alcohol on a flesh diet generally very soon give it up when they give up flesh, and smoke also very little, having no craving for any stimulants; while if what most meat-eaters say were true, that meat is very much better nourishment, it ought to be exactly the other way.' (11)

Meat and Tobacco

"The editor of the *London Clarion*, England, relating his own experience, said: 'I was a heavy smoker for more than thirty years. I have often smoked as much as two ounces of tobacco in a day. I don't suppose I have smoked less than eight ounces in a week for a quarter of a century. If there was one thing in life I feared my will was too weak to conquer, it was the habit of smoking. Well, I have been a vegetarian for eight weeks and I find that my passion for tobacco is weakening. I cannot smoke those pipes now. I have to get new pipes and milder tobacco, and am not smoking half an ounce a day. It does not taste the same.'" (12)

Evidently a non-flesh diet, consisting largely of fruits and vegetables, would constitute a mighty barrier against the development of the desire for alcohol.

The reader should keep in mind the balanced ration taught in this book, which is crystallized in the Automatic Menu Planner. The foods offered therein do not set up cravings for tobacco and alcohol but lessen them.

Group Three, Stimulating Drinks

Stimulating drinks are habit-forming and tend to create a craving for tobacco, alcohol and liquors in general, and for narcotics known as "dope." It should be remembered that alkaloids include morphine, cocain, nicotine, and caffeine. The drinks included in this class are: tea, coffee, coca-cola, cocoa, all caffeinated drinks.

"Coffee is a drug. Those who are addicted to its use are drug addicts. The people of the United States are among the largest users of coffee of all the people of the world. Its use is on the increase. From the standpoint of public hygiene the coffee question is worthwhile. It is much the most widespread form of drug addiction. Some people are certain that it harms them. The largest number enjoy their cup of coffee and they care not at all whether it harms them.

"Tea contains about twice as much caffeine as does coffee. "One to four grains of caffeine caused a slight tremor, six grains caused an appreciable unsteadiness of the hands, coming on about an hour after taking and increased for three hours. In order that no misunderstanding may arise, I should say that physiologists regard coffee, tea, tobacco and whiskey as drugs in the same sense that opium and cocain are. The craving for tea and that for whiskey, the hunger for a cigarette and that for a dose of morphine are of the same kind. Each comes of an inborn willingness to cheat in playing the game of life." (13)

Weak Drugs Lead to Stronger Ones

"Among the poisons which must be kept out of the body should be mentioned habit-forming drugs, such as opium, morphine, cocain, heroin, choral, acetanilid, alcohol, caffeine, and nicotine. The best rule for those who wish to attain the highest physical and mental efficiency is total abstinence from all substances which contain poisons, including spirits, wine, beer, tobacco, many much-advertised patent drinks served at soda-water fountains, most patent medicines, and even tea and coffee. . . . The natural tendency of drug craving is . . . from weak drugs to stronger ones." (14)

Tea and Vinegar Lead to Alcohol

"Dr. Hawkes found in Finsbury that the women and girls drank three or four pints of tea poison in the day, and their solid meals often consisted of pickles and vinegar. An enormous amount of dyspepsia is thus set up, often finally leading to alcoholism for relief. Many stint themselves terribly in order to afford more expense in personal adornment." (15)

Coffee Habit, Alcohol Habit, Morphine Habit

"Coffee, as everyone knows, produces a nervous excitement, which, if abused may lead to insomnia, hallucinations, troubles of the circulation, muscular innervation, to precordial distress and to dyspnoea. One may become caffeic just as one can become alcoholic, or a morphia maniac. . . . It ought to be especially forbidden to arthritics, or uratics, amongst whom it often causes gravel, to gastralgics, to dyspeptics and to those suffering from Bright's disease." (16)

Tea and Coffee Drunkards

"This country is full of tea and coffee drunkards. The most common drug in this country is caffeine. . . . Your children, innocent of any knowledge of its deleterious effects, consume it freely. They do this to their great physical and mental detriment. Coffee drunkenness is a commoner failing than the whiskey habit. The misuse of caffeine as a stimulant and as a beverage is more prevalent than the use of alcohol. Caffeine has a direct tendency to create Bright's disease. Caffeine is the essential alkaloid of coffee, as theine is of tea. Both are dangerous and detriments." (17)

Tea and Coffee Tendencies

"Under the head of stimulants and narcotics is classed a great variety of articles that, altogether used as food or drink, irritate the stomach, poison the blood, and excite the nerves. Their use is a positive evil. Men seek the excitement of stimulants, because, for the time, the results are agreeable. But there is always a reaction. The use of unnatural stimulants always tends to excess, and it is an active agent in promoting physical degeneration and decay.

"Tea acts as a stimulant, and, to a certain extent, produces intoxication. The action of coffee and many other popular drinks is similar. The first effect is exhilarating. The nerves of the stomach are excited; these convey irritation to the brain, and this in turn is aroused to impart increased action to the heart, and short-lived energy to the entire system. Fatigue is forgotten; the strength seems to be increased. The intellect is aroused, the imagination becomes more vivid.

"Because of these results, many suppose that their tea or coffee is doing them great good. But this is a mistake. Tea and coffee do not nourish the system. Their effect is produced before there has been time for digestion and assimilation, and what seems to be strength is only nervous excitement. When the influence of the stimulant is gone, the unnatural force abates, and the result is a corresponding degree of languor and debility.

"The continued use of these nerve irritants is followed by headache, wakefulness, palpitation of the heart, indigestion, trembling, and many other evils; for they wear away the life forces. Tired nerves need rest and quiet instead of stimulation and overwork. Nature needs time to recuperate her exhausted energies. When her forces are goaded on by the use of stimulants, more will be accomplished for a time; but, as the system becomes debilitated by their constant use, it gradually becomes more difficult to arouse the energies to the desired point. The demand for stimulants becomes more difficult to control, until the will is overborne, and there seems to be no power to deny the unnatural craving. Stronger and still stronger stimulants are called for, until exhausted nature can no longer respond.

"Great efforts are made to put down intemperance; but there is much effort that is not directed to the right point. The advocates of temperance reform should be awake to the evils resulting from the use of unwholesome food, condiments, tea, and coffee. We bid all temperance workers Godspeed; but we invite them to look more deeply into the cause of the evil they war against, and to be sure that they are consistent in reform.

"It must be kept before the people that the right balance of the mental and moral powers depends in a great degree on the right condition of the physical system. All narcotics and unnatural stimulants that enfeeble and degrade the physical nature tend to lower the tone of the intellect and morals. Intemperance lies at the foundation of the moral depravity of the world. By the indulgence of perverted appetite, man loses his power to resist temptation.

"Temperance reformers have a work to do in educating the people in these lines. Teach them that health, character and even life, are endangered by the use of stimulants, which excite the exhausted energies to unnatural spasmodic action.

"In relation to tea, coffee, tobacco, and alcoholic drinks, the only safe course is to touch not, taste not, handle not. The tendency of tea, coffee, and similar drinks is in the same direction as that of alcoholic liquor and tobacco, and in some cases the habit is as difficult to break as it is for the drunkard to give up intoxicants. Those who attempt to leave off these stimulants will for a time feel a loss, and will suffer without them. But by persistence they will overcome the craving and cease to feel the lack. Nature may require a little time to recover from the abuse she has suffered; but give her a chance and she will again rally, and perform her work nobly and well." (18)

"The use of tea and coffee is also injurious to the system. To a certain extent, tea produces intoxication. It enters into the circulation, and gradually impairs the energy of the body and mind. It stimulates, excites, and quickens the motion of the living machinery, forcing it to unnatural actions, and thus gives the tea-drinker the impression that it is doing him great service, imparting to him strength. This is a mistake. Tea draws upon the strength of the nerves, and leaves them greatly weakened. When its influence is gone and the increased action caused by its use is abated, then what is the result? Languor and debility corresponding to the artificial vivacity the tea imparted. When the system is already overtaxed and needs rest, the use of tea spurs up nature by stimulation to perform unwonted, unnatural action, and thereby lessens her power to perform, and her ability to endure; and her powers give out long before Heaven designed they should. Tea is poisonous to the system. Christians should let it alone. The influence of coffee is in a degree the same as tea, but the effect upon the system is still worse. Its influence is exciting, and just in the degree that it elevates above par, it will exhaust and bring prostration below par. Tea and coffee drinkers carry the marks upon their faces. The skin becomes sallow, and assumes a lifeless appearance. The glow of health is not seen upon the countenance.

"Tea and coffee do not nourish the system. The relief obtained from them is sudden, before the stomach has time to digest them. This shows that what the users of these stimulants call strength, is only received by exciting the nerves of the stomach, which convey the irritation to the brain, and this in turn is aroused to impart increased action to the heart, that we are the worse for having. They do not give a particle of natural strength." (19)

Intemperance Begins at the Table

"Intemperance commences at our tables, in the use of unhealthful food. After a time, through continued indulgence, the digestive organs become weakened, and the food taken does not satisfy the appetite. Unhealthy conditions are established, and there is a craving for more stimulating food. Tea, coffee, and flesh-meats produce an immediate effect. Under the influence of these poisons, the nervous system is excited, and, in some cases, for the time being, the intellect seems to be invigorated and the imagination to be more vivid. Because these stimulants produce for the time being such agreeable results, many conclude that they really need them, and continue their use. But there is always a reaction. The nervous system, having been unduly excited, borrowed power for present use from its future resources of strength. All this temporary invigoration of the system is followed by depression. In proportion as these stimulants temporarily invigorate the system, will be the letting down of the power of the excited organs after the stimulus has lost its force. The appetite is educated to crave something stronger, which will have a tendency to keep up and increase the agreeable excitement, until indulgence becomes habit, and there is a continual craving for stronger stimulus, as tobacco, wines, and liquors. The more the appetite is indulged, the more frequent will be its demands, and the more difficult of control. The more debilitated the system becomes, and the less able to do without unnatural stimulus, the more the passion for these things increases, until the will is over-borne, and there seems to be no power to deny the unnatural craving for these indulgences.

"The only safe course is to touch not, taste not, handle not, tea, coffee, wines, tobacco, opium, and alcoholic drinks." (20)

Mothers at Fault

"Many parents educate the tastes of their children, and form their appetites. They indulge them in eating flesh-meats, and in drinking tea and coffee. The highly seasoned flesh-meats and the tea and coffee, which some mothers encourage their children to use, prepare the way for them to crave stronger stimulants as tobacco. The use of tobacco and liquor invariably lessens nerve power." (21)

"The ill effects of excessive tea drinking are referable to its action upon the digestive and nervous systems and are cumulative."

"Tea precipitates the digestive ferments, retards the activity of digestion and may occasion gastric irritation and catarrh. Constipation usually results, and more or less flatulence (gas). The effect of the 'tea habit' on the nervous system is to overstimulate and then depress it, first producing restlessness, worry, and insomnia, and finally muscular tremors, sensory disturbances and palpitation. Tea should be avoided in dyspepsia, gastric irritability from any cause, constipation, anemia, insomnia, nervousness and gastric catarrh. A case of multiple neuritis caused by drinking between two and three pints daily of strong tea has been reported by Spratling and I have met with one or two similar cases. In a recent report upon insanity, in Ireland, tea is mentioned as a contributing factor." (22)

Coca-Cola Leads Toward Drug Addiction

"The investigations which we made in connection with the coca-cola case indicated very clearly that many drug addicts had in the early stages of their disease drunk large quantites of coca-cola." (23)

Coca-Cola Is Pernicious

"It is not necessary here to discuss the end effects of the coca-cola habit; it is serious, and is especially harmful to children and youth. The cause of the habit is the caffeine in the mixture. It is not pertinent to discuss the small amount that one glass may contain, or that the civilized world drinks tea and coffee freely. The coca-cola habit is pernicious." (24)

Spurious Happiness

David Starr Jordan of Stanford University, classes alcohol, opium, tobacco, kola, tea, and coffee together as drugs which give happiness when happiness does not exist, and which destroy to the same extent they give happiness. Their function is to force the nervous system to lie. "As a drop of water is of the same nature of the tea, so in its degree is the effect of alcohol, opium, tobacco, cocaine, kola, tea, or coffee." "Each of them, if used to excess, brings, in time, insanity, incapability, and death. With each of them the first use makes the second easier. To yield to temptation makes it easier to yield again. The weakening effect on the will is greater than the injury done to the body."

GROUP FOUR, TOBACCO LEADS TOWARD ALCOHOL

The use of tobacco tends to create an appetite for alcoholic beverages—and to lead toward morphine and cocain.

"Men who have had the drinking habit have almost invariably been first addicted to tobacco. Out of seven hundred convicts in New York state prison, who were examined a few years ago, six hundred were confined for crimes committed while under the influence of liquor, and five hundred said they were led to drink by tobacco." (25)

Cigarette Fiends Often Become "Dope" Fiends
Alcoholics Are Usually Smokers

"Also many cigarette fiends become later 'dope' fiends, and young men who were wont to take too much alcohol were also frequently very hard smokers, mostly of cigarettes. In other words, the use of tobacco in young boys and the over-use in young men is conducive to bad morals in all lines, and the greatest disturbance to mental efficiency seems to occur in those who use cigarettes." (26)

Alcoholic May Turn to Tobacco, Tea, Coffee, or Other Drug

"With prohibition it is a question whether the individual who has this strong desire for alcohol will get and take some other drug, or whether he will become a hard smoker, or an excessive eater of sugar or an excessive drinker of coffee or tea. At any rate, he is likely to develop some abnormal excessive habit. The advantage of prohibition is that the young individual cannot well acquire the taste or desire for alcohol. The future lessening of crime by prohibition that prohibits cannot at the present time be forecasted." (27)

No Alcohol or Tobacco to Morphine Patients

"All these patients need iron, and they may need organic extract treatment. Sometimes they develop a very great appetite, and the amount of food that they take should be regulated. All alcohol should be withheld from these morphine addicts, and they should be cured of the tobacco habit, as each one of these habits stimulates other habits, and the better they are cured of all habits, the less likely are they to return to the morphine habit." (28)

GROUP FIVE, PAINKILLING REMEDIES HARMFUL, AND LEAD TOWARD DOPE

This section deals with pain-killing remedies, hypnotics, habit-forming nostrums, and many "patent medicines," from two standpoints:

(1) The direct harm done by them to the body;

(2) Their tendency toward the use of more pronounced narcotics.

In this class are: Cough cures, sleeping powders, headache powders, soothing syrups, certain cathartics, aspirin.

There is a strong element of danger in the use of all pain relievers, whether they be opium, morphine, cocain, heroin, or their derivatives, or hashish made from the loco weed, cigarettes made from the Mexican marihuana, or the plain everyday sleeping powders, headache-powders, soothing syrups, or aspirin so commonly used for the relief of pain and many other things.

One writer has said:

"Drugs given to stupefy, whatever they may be, derange the nervous system." (29)

That is a guiding principle.

In other words, all drugs which numb the nerves, by doing so, injure the nerves, and so derange the nervous system.

I feel constrained to speak a few words of caution concerning the use of aspirin, headache and sleeping-powders, and other "patent" medicines.

"Patent Medicines"

"Among the addicts are many who were started on their road to addiction through the use of such 'patent medicines' as cough cures, cathartics, headache powders, and soothing syrups. If the reader is using a 'patent medicine,' he should examine the label carefully to find out whether it contains morphine, heroin, cocaine, laudenum, or paregoric. . . . If the reader is using a 'patent medicine' containing any of these drugs, he is started on the sure road to addiction, for thousands upon thousands have gone this way before." (30)

"Almost one-tenth of the cases of (drug) addiction are traceable to the use of 'patent' medicines." (31)

Let us consider a statement by the leader of the White Cross work for the state of California, in a very enlightening little book on drug addiction—"Battling the Wolves of Society":

"Patent medicines have always been and still are a prolific cause of drug addiction. The various nostrums for hay fever, asthma, colds, consumption, etc., contain opium, morphine, codeine, or other narcotic drugs. Some treatments for the tobacco habit have been found to contain dope." (32)

"Many of the popular nostrums called patent medicines, and even some of the drugs dispensed by physicians, act a part in laying the foundation of the liquor habit, the opium habit, the morphine habit, that are so terrible a curse to society." (33)

The Way Aspirin Kills

"The way aspirin kills is by deadening pain. Make no mistake about pain. It is unpleasant but beneficient. It is a red flag set up by nature to warn us that something has gone wrong. Aspirin pulls down that flag and makes people think that everything is all right—till often it is too late to make it right.

"Thousands and thousands are dying every year from pneumonia, tuberculosis, and heart disease for no other reason than that aspirin lulls them into a false sense of security. It conceals the symptoms; it waves aside the sore throat, the slight cough, the headache, as a thing of no consequence till it gets a grip that no medical skill can break." (34)

"I am copying from 'Pharmacotherapeutics,' a standard book on drugs:

" 'Aspirin, although commonly well borne in moderate doses, is distinctly depressant to the heart. Great cardiac weakness and a tendency to collapse may follow the administration of a dose representing less than half the quantity of sodium salicylate previously and subsequently well borne by the same patient. Children are particularly subject to this cardiac depression; thus in a girl of twelve years with scarlatinal arthritis, alarming symptoms were caused by nine grains of aspirin given in the course of fifteen hours, although there was no evidence of endocarditis of pericarditis, and recovery of cardiac vigor ensued on withdrawal of the drug. The cardiac depression may not be immediately evident; but continued resort to aspirin may so weaken the heart, that in an emergency, or under the additional depression of an acute infection, as influenza or pneumonia, it fails to respond. Death may thus be an indirect effect of aspirin poisoning. Moreover, an aspirin habit is easily set up by its use for relief of recurrent headaches and neuralgic pains." (35)

Headache Powders and Aspirin

"Dr. Wiley, when connected with the government as chemist, referring to headache powders, said: 'Hardly a day passes that I do not receive from some part of the country the report of a death from taking headache powders. Every such preparation sold contains large quantities of either acetanilid, phenacetin, antipyrin, or caffeine, all of which affect the heart more or less. No physician would think of prescribing more than one or two grains of these drugs; but the headache powders contain from four to six grains. Many people afflicted with headache get accustomed to taking these powders for relief. Instead they should go to a physician, find out what causes the headache and follow the prescription given for permanent relief.

"Dr. Wiley continues: 'If I had my way, the sale of these powders would be prohibited. They are poisonous to a person with a weak heart and are likely to result in death at any time. Most of these powders are sold with instructions to take a second dose in case relief is not immediate. No physician would give such drugs with these instructions.

"Many have become acquainted with the dangerous nature of the drugs named, and have abandoned their use, but other drugs have come into prominence. Among these is aspirin. No other drug is more widely advertised than is aspirin, and reputed to be harmless. Doctor Eggleston, of the department of pharmacology in Cornell University Medical School, has this to say of aspirin:

" 'I believe that the worst charge I can bring against aspirin is that it is indirectly responsible for thousands of deaths which are ascribed in our mortality tables to pneumonia, tuberculosis, heart disease, and others almost as prevalent and deadly.'

"Apsirin weakens the heart at a time when recovery from diseases of a febrile nature depends entirely upon keeping the heart fit. Again and again I have had patients come to me in a serious condition, resulting from the free use of aspirin." (36)

Seven million pounds of aspirin are consumed in one year in the United States.

Headache Relievers

"Proprietary remedies for the relief of headache are legion. Practically without exception, however, these potent pain-relievers (aspirin excepted) are based upon a 'coal-tar' derivative most commonly acetanilid but sometime acetphenetidin, antipyrin, or pyramidon with, more rarely, lesser known derivatives of these usually in association with caffeine, an aromatic and sometimes an alkaline, such as sodium bicarbonate.

"Their essential action is to relieve pain and to reduce body temperature. . . . They all are recognized as being habit-forming and in some degree narcotic in their action.

" 'Bromo-Seltzer' contains the definitely harmful and habit-forming drug, acetanilid. The latter is recognized by authorities as partaking in some respects of the character of a narcotic.

"Acetanilid is a highly potent drug, one profoundly capable of causing serious health impairment, and the use of which has been held as directly responsible for more than a few deaths. In support of this the following authoritative testimony is presented from "Legal Medicine and Toxicology" by Peterson and Haines:

" 'It has a similar narcotic action in certain forms of headache. . . . With small doses the red blood corpuscles remain intact, but the large doses destroy the cells and free the methemoglobin, which may lead to hematuria, nephritis and jaundice. . . . The most frequent source of poisoning from acetanilid has been its use as a remedy for headache. . . . A definite acetanilid habit is recognized; maniacal excitement has followed the sudden withdrawal of the drug.'

"And what has been said concerning acetanilid applies in at least some degree or respect to the other drugs named. In short, there is no such thing as a perfectly safe headache remedy of the coal-tar derivative type." (37)

Conclusion

It is better to suffer a little than to incur the danger of contracting a body-and-soul-destroying habit. The pain is a divine messenger warning us that we have violated the inexorable law of life, and it is calling us to mend our ways. By stilling the warning voice with a pain deadener, we correct no wrong but deceive ourselves into continuing our heedless course of deranging the nervous system. It is like removing the red light without removing the danger.

I do not say that no pain deadener should ever be used, but I do say that we American people are doping ourselves with these things, becoming addicts to them, and in doing so are fast destroying ourselves. It is time that we call a halt and use these dangerous drugs only under the advice of a competent and conscientious physician, and then only in cases of extreme pain.

Group Six, the Drug Habit

This section presents the "Drug Addict"—the "Dope Fiend"—and his horrible, hopeless condition from which there is no known deliverance outside of the power of Divinity.

Six ways by which people get started on the road to drug addiction, are given by Narcotics Education Association, Bulletin No. 2, May, 1923:

"*First*: Through the use of 'patent medicines' and self-medication to obtain relief from sickness, pain, fatigue, or mental strain.

"Among the 'patent medicines' may be listed cough cures, cathartics, headache powders and soothing syrups.

"*Second*: By taking narcotic drugs prescribed by physicians.

"*Third*: By inheriting addiction.

"*Fourth*: Through gratifying the craving for alcohol by substituting addiction drugs.

"*Fifth*: Through idle curiosity.

"*Sixth*: By taking drugs to tide them over some strenuous mental or physical period."

Concerning the second, Clyde L. Eddy, vice-president of the American Pharmaceutical Association, says:

"Most persons become addicted as the result of having opiates administered to them by family physicians. A patient suffering from the after-effects of an operation is given morphine over a period of a few weeks or months, and addiction results. Hundreds of addicts can trace their addiction directly to unfortunate efforts to relieve themselves of headaches or nervousness by the use of nostrums. Not a few veterans of the recent war are confirmed opiate addicts as the results of having morphine administered to them while recovering from wounds. Given the right condition—a painful illness, an operation or an automobile accident resulting in sufficiently painful injuries—and any one of us might easily be one of the addicted millions, twelve months, or for that matter as many weeks from now." (38)

The International Narcotics Association has sent out the following warning:

"The continued use of these drugs (morphine, heroin, and cocain) for thirty days will establish addiction in the strongest individual. In very nervous and susceptible persons the use of them for a period of ten days places the user well past the danger point of becoming a confirmed addict." (39)

Closing Summary

What does this lesson mean to us?

Behold the list of "roots" from which intemperance comes:

1. Spices, condiments, pickles, and other irritating foods.
2. Meats and their extractives, which contain stimulants.
3. Tea, coffee, cocoa, coca-cola and other caffeinated drinks.
4. Tobacco.
5. Remedies with alcohol content.
6. Alcohol.
7. Pain alleviators.
8. Narcotics—"dope."

The scheme of this series of indulgences was designed by a *master mind* to completely *ruin the human race*. How many are the victims? Who has escaped? It is appalling! It is baffling! How many "temperance" people are free from the bondage of these habits?

How wide-spread and sweeping should be the reform? How great is our task? Who will take hold of it? This situation calls for the unflagging toil of those who are willing to make the greatest sacrifice in the interest of humanity in the name of the Master. But before we can lead others to abandon bad habits we ourselves must be free from them.

"Ministry of Healing," page 130, presents the seriousness of the situation in these words:

"The body is the only medium through which the mind and soul are developed for the upbuilding of character. Hence it is that the adversary of souls directs his temptations to the enfeebling and degrading of the physical powers. His success here means the surrender to evil of the whole being."

Let us respect the will of our Creator as He has expressed it in the laws of life He has fixed in our bodies for our guidance and happiness, and remember that "Ye are the temple of God. . . . If any man defile the temple of God, him shall God destroy."—*Paul* (40)

Then let us take up the task of revealing these great truths to all the people around us and do all we can to change their course from the downward path to the one that leads up to life, joy, peace, happiness and usefulness.

The "Roots" of Intemperance

The Progressive Effects of
irritating and stimulating foods and drinks, tobacco, alcohol, pain alleviators, habit-forming nostrums, and narcotics—"dope" From health to sickness, misery, and death

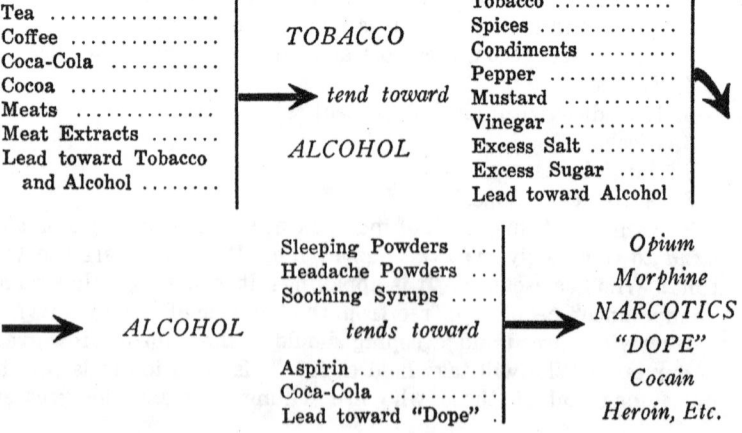

Tea		Tobacco ....
Coffee	*TOBACCO*	Spices ....
Coca-Cola		Condiments ....
Cocoa		Pepper ....
Meats	→ *tend toward*	Mustard ....
Meat Extracts		Vinegar ....
Lead toward Tobacco	*ALCOHOL*	Excess Salt ....
and Alcohol		Excess Sugar ......
		Lead toward Alcohol

		Sleeping Powders	*Opium*
		Headache Powders ...	*Morphine*
→	*ALCOHOL*	Soothing Syrups	*NARCOTICS*
		tends toward	*"DOPE"*
		Aspirin	*Cocain*
		Coca-Cola	*Heroin, Etc.*
		Lead toward "Dope" .	

BIBLIOGRAPHY

(1) "Signs of the Times," February 6, 1934.
(2) D. H. Kress, M.D., in "Tobacco and the Cigarette Habit from the Medical Viewpoint," a pamphlet, page 10.
(3) "Health," June, 1934, Page 10.
(4) Mrs. E. G. White, "Review and Herald," No. 44, 1883.
(5) "Education," pages 202, 203.
(6) "Ministry of Healing," page 325.
(7) "Ministry of Healing," page 334.
(8) "Uric Acid," by Alexander Haig, page 884.
(9) "Dietotherapy," by William Edward Fitch, M.D., page 529.
(10) Quoted in "Temperance Torchlights," by Matilda Erickson, page 201.
(11) "Strength and Diet," by Hon. R. Russell, pages 363, 364.
(12) D. H. Kress, M.D., in "Tobacco and the Cigarette Habit From the Medical Viewpoint," a pamphlet, page 11.
(13) Dr. W. A. Evans, for many years Health Commissioner of Chicago, Ill.
(14) "How to Live," by Fisher and Fisk, pages 78, 79. 15th Ed.
(15) "Strength and Diet," by Hon. R. Russell, page 45. Published by Longmans, Green and Co., 39 Paternoster Row, London, New York, Bombay.
(16) "Diet and Dietetics," by Armand Gautier, page 272.
(17) Dr. Harvey W. Wiley, former chief of the Bureau of Chemistry of the United States.
(18) "Ministry of Healing," pages 325, 326, 327, 335.
(19) Mrs. E. G. White, Volume 2, page 64.*
(20) Mrs. E. G. White, Volume 3, pages 487, 488.
(21) Mrs. E. G. White, Volume 3, pages 488, 489.
(22) "Practical Dietetics," by W. G. Thompson, M.D., Cornell University Medical College, page 250.
(23) H. W. Wiley, in a letter to J. W. Hopkins, April 19, 1912.
(24) "The Principles of Therapeutics," by Oliver T. Osborne, M.A., M.D., page 216. W. B. Saunders Co., Philadelphia and London, 1921.
(25) Quoted in "Tobacco Under the Searchlight," by Will H. Brown, page 147. The Standard Publishing Company, 1925, Cincinnati.
(26) "The Principles of Therapeutics," by Oliver T. Osborne, M.A., M.D., page 726.
(27) "The Principles of Therapeutics," by Oliver T. Osborne, M.A., M.D., page 711.
(28) "The Principles of Therapeutics," by Oliver T. Osborne, M.A., M.D., page 722.
(29) Mrs. E. G. White, "How to Live," Sec. 3, page 57.
(30) Bulletin No. 2, May, 1923, Narcotic Education Association.
(31) From "Fifty Facts About Narcotics," published by International Narcotic Association, Los Angeles, California.
(32) "Battling the Wolves of Society," page 43.
(33) "Ministry of Healing," page 127.
(34) "Health," June, 1934, published monthly by New Hampshire State Board of Health.
(35) "Life and Health," magazine, "Question Box," December, 1933.
(36) "Life and Health," magazine, January, 1934, from the pen of Dr. D. H. Kress.
(37) "Health," July, 1934, monthly bulletin of the New Hampshire State Board of Health, Charles Duncan, M.D., Secretary.
(38) "Literary Digest," August 25, 1923.
(39) "Fifty Facts About Narcotics," published by International Narcotic Association, Los Angeles, California.
(40) I Cor. 3:16, 17.

---

*Mrs. E. G. White wrote a series of books known as Volumes 1-9.

The Right Use of the Mind

The world is filled with a confusing variety of teachings concerning the use of the mind. Systems of psychology of every variety are on every hand, varying all the way from simple thinking to mysticism. The reader is asked, while reading this chapter to lay all these teachings aside, and think simply and carefully of the principles here presented.

THE POWER OF MIND OVER MATTER

The Mind Is King

"The brain is the capital of the body, the seat of all the nervous forces and of mental action. The nerves proceeding from the brain control the body. By the brain nerves, mental impressions are conveyed to all the nerves of the body as by telegraph wires; and they control the vital action of every part of the system. All the organs of motion are governed by the communications they receive from the brain." (1)

The mind is placed in the body as the seat of government, as the king over a kingdom, which is real, governed by laws which are inexorable, which if obeyed bring blessing but if transgressed bring pain, sickness, and death. The mind is to know these laws and enforce them.

All other parts of the body are to work under its guidance—receive orders from it. The brain is the guiding, compelling force of the body. It is in direct contact with all parts of the body through a system of nerves over which electric currents pass to and from the brain carrying orders out and receiving information which they bring to the brain.

The brain is said to be like four quadrillions of dynamos, and that the electric distribution system of the human body is more intricate, delicate, and vastly greater than all the lines of communication on the earth.

The brain of a cat contains enough electricity to run a small radio—it has been done.

When oxygen was added to a solution of proteins from calf brains, it glowed for a few seconds like a weak electric light bulb. Thus the light locked up in a brain was made to shine in a dark room. Men now have a "brain meter" by which they measure the electric activity of the brain. (2)

MECHANICAL GENERATOR DRAWS ELECTRICITY FROM THE AIR

A mechanical electrical generator collects electricity from the earth and atmosphere and sends it out over wires to such places as the wires go. This is accomplished by the turning of the generator. Man has no "wheels" in his head, but yet there are means for generating the current and sending it out over the nerves which means are just as real as the turning of the generator.

THE BRAIN GETS ITS ELECTRICITY FROM THE AIR

Dr. George Crile, of the Cleveland (Ohio) Clinic, has written a book, "The Phenomena of Life," devoted to expounding his views concerning the origin of electricity in the body, and its functions. He holds "oxidation" to be its primary source (page 17). This agrees with a statement published in 1868 by a layman many years before any scientist knew there were electric currents in the human body. The statement follows: "Air is the free blessing of heaven calculated to electrify the whole system." (3) It also agrees with work done at the Harvard School of Public Health by Professor Yaglou and associates. They determined the number of electrified air particles (ions) per cubic foot of air in a room and then watched their reduction after thirty-four people came into the room. They found that in twenty minutes only one-fifth of the ions remained. The same reduction occurred with only seven people in the room. No amount of window ventilation could restore the ions while the people remained in the room, and one hour's time was required for the normal amount of ions to be restored after the people left the room. (4)

It is understood that when breathing pure air, the respiratory system retains from 15 to 40 per cent of the ions. (5) Another reports a retention of from 60,000 to 150,000 ions at each breath.

Koller also says these ions have an affinity for oxygen, (6) while other research workers have said that the red blood corpuscles which carry oxygen are so heavily charged with electricity that their combined charge would light a 25-watt bulb enough so one could read by its light for five minutes. (7)

All evidences go to show that in some way oxygen and electricity are tied together in their work.

Koller says the air is constantly flowing toward the earth, that approximately 50 per cent of the volume of soil is air; the air is ionized in the soil and comes out from the soil recharged. (8)

These scientific discoveries strongly impress the advantages of living out of doors and in close touch with nature as much as possible, and that when we must be inside of buildings, health demands a constant free circulation of fresh air. Additional value is also seen in deep breathing and in breathing exercises, and in erect posture without which proper breathing is impossible.

The Brain Governs the Body Electrically

Electrically speaking, the brain serves as the dynamo and the nerves as the wires. What causes the currents to go? How is this power of mind over matter exercised?

Many years ago (1903) an author wrote: "The electric power of the brain, promoted by mental activity, vitalizes the whole system." (9) Thinking generates the current. It is sent out by the act of decision enforced by the power of the will. First we think, then we decide, and then the will produces the action. That is how everything in life is done. Science has said:

"Through every person's arms, legs, tongue, and brain, electrical impulses are continually flashing, varying according to his thoughts."

"A simple hook-up of electrical apparatus will amplify these 'thought waves,' and record them on paper."

"A month ago Dr. Hallowell Davis and his colleagues at Harvard University were proving to the Federation of American Societies for Experimental Biology that electrical waves in the brain indicated mental activity. Last week, Dr. Louis William Max, New York University psychologist, harnessed a dreamer to the apparatus, and made records of dreams, which were shown before the New York Academy of Sciences." (10)

Electricity and Life

It has been abundantly shown that life cannot exist apart from electricity; that this is true of plants, animals, and man; it is even true of the existence of matter itself, which seems to be composed of electricity.

In the body it has been shown by Dr. Crile that each cell is a bi-polar battery-like mechanism, the inner part having a positive charge and the outer part a negative charge, and that the existence and function of the cell and its ability to resist disease depend upon the constant passing of electricity from one part to the other; that the development of current in the cell depends upon oxygen; that when the oxygen is shut off, the electric activity ceases and death occurs; that when ether, or chloroform are injected into a cell, it ceases to use oxygen, and life ceases. When death ensues, he says that the energy which was locked within the molecule returns again to the atmosphere from whence it first came. Thus he says, "Electricity keeps the flame of life burning in the cell." This is, perhaps unknowingly, a scientist's way of describing the source of the life which the Creator maintains within the cells of man moment by moment.

On this point, the author of "Education" wrote: We "need to understand the deep truth underlying the Bible statement that with God 'is the fountain of life.' Ps. 36:9. Not only is He the originator of all, but He is the life of everything that lives. It is His life that we receive in the sunshine, in the pure sweet air, in the food which builds up our bodies and sustains our strength. It is by His life that we exist, hour by hour, moment by moment. Except as perverted by sin, all His gifts tend to life, health and joy." (11)

On the subject of "life" the author of "Education" wrote as follows in 1872:

"God endowed man with so great vital force that he has withstood the accumulation of disease brought upon the race in consequence of perverted habits, and has continued for six thousand years. This fact of itself is enough to evidence to us the strength and electrical energy that God gave man at creation. It took more than two thousand years of crime and indulgence of base passions to bring bodily disease upon the race to any great extent. If Adam, at his creation, had not been endowed with twenty times as much vital force as men now have, the race, with their present habits of living in violation of natural law, would have become extinct." (12)

ELECTRICITY AND HEALTH

In view of these discoveries it must be apparent that to artificially tamper with the electric currents of the body could be fraught with danger, and that for it to be of value the worker should know and follow the electrical laws of cells, of health and disease. This is a vast mostly unexplored field. A few principles have been learned. One point concerning disease was stated many years ago by the writer already quoted:

"The electric power of the brain, promoted by mental activity, vitalizes the whole system, and is thus an invaluable aid in resisting disease." (13)

Contrariwise,

"If your mind is impressed and fixed that a bath will injure you, the mental impression is communicated to all the nerves of the body. The nerves control the circulation of the blood; therefore the blood is, through the impression of the mind, confined to the blood-vessels, and the good effects of the bath are lost. All this is because the blood is prevented by the mind and will from flowing readily, and from coming to the surface to stimulate, arouse and promote the circulation. For instance, you are impressed that if you bathe you will become chilly. The brain sends this intelligence to the nerves of your body, and the blood-vessels, held in obedience to your will, cannot perform their office and cause a reaction after the bath. There is no reason in science or philosophy why an occasional bath, taken with studious care, should do you anything but real good. Especially is this the case where there is but little exercise to keep the muscles in action, and to aid the circulation of the blood through the system. Bathing frees the skin from the accumulation of impurities which are constantly collecting, and keeps the skin moist and supple, thereby increasing and equalizing the circulation." (14)

ELECTRICITY IN EVERY LIVING THING

"By the aid of a recently perfected instrument which can measure an electrical current as small as one two hundred thousandth of a volt, Yale scientists have shown by many thousands of tests that every living thing generates electricity in quantities that can be measured. Each species appears to produce its own special pattern of electrical effects, and every variation that occurs in the processes of living organism is reflected in changes in the electrical pattern. By the aid of this new means of studying life processes, the need of which has long been recognized, it is believed that many new and important facts will be in due time discovered." (15)

ELECTRICAL CHARGES OF BACTERIA

"The minute electrical charges borne by bacteria in solution have been measured by a method developed at Cornell Medical College by Prof. Harold A. Abramson. The amount of the charge has been found to vary in different kinds of bacteria, and by this means the various types of microbes, causing pneumonia, and even the virulent and non-virulent forms of the diptheria bacillus, may be differentiated." (16)

Research workers are now beginning to learn what parts of the body carry negative and what parts positive charges of electricity, and something about the diseases which occur when normal electrical conditions are disturbed. The glomeruli of the kidneys and the tissue in the tonsils carry a positive charge. Certain bacteria carry negative and others positive charges. (17)

LISTENING TO LIFE PROCESSES

Dr. George W. Crile, when Director of the Cleveland Clinic and the Cleveland Clinic Hospital, publicly stated:

·"Man is a mechanism run by electricity and chemical reaction —a machine made up of twenty-eight trillion electric cells. Every one of these twenty-eight trillion cells is a tiny wet battery, with negative and positive poles. The greater the difference in electric potential—the difference between positive and negative—the greater the energy. Electricity keeps the flame of life burning in the cell and the flame—oxidation—supplies the electricity used in operating the animal.

"The medical man of the future will 'tune' in on the living body as one does now on the ordinary radio. By 'listening in' to the short waves transmitted by the various organs, he will hear the symphony played by the living organism and will determine the rhythms of the 'dance of life' . . . Long before there is any outward evidence of disease, the physician-radio-engineer of the future will thus be enabled to tell by the 'reception' of the 'life waves' whether they are playing a melody of health or signalling an S.O.S." (18)

THE EFFECT ON HEALTH

One worker has found that positive electric ions introduced by air into the body produce feelings of fatigue, dizziness, headaches, roaring in the ears, and nausea, while after inhaling negative ions of high concentration for an hour in most cases a feeling of exhilaration is produced. (19) In a study of two hundred cases of high blood pressure there was a permanent improvement in eighty per cent of the cases by frequent inhalations of negative ions. (20)

Here let it be remembered that there are positive and negative elements in foods—that the elements which make a food acid-forming take on a positive charge and the alkalies a negative charge.

Normal Program, Normal Health

Man ought by this time to begin to understand that nature possesses a very delicately arranged balance of all elements and forces, and that when we disturb any of these balances, abnormal conditions must arise, and that if we would maintain or restore normalcy in the body we must have normal balanced rations, pure fresh air, sunshine, exercise, rest, and all the other factors which make up normal life and living.

THE MIND IN ACTION

"The minds of thinking men labor too hard. They frequently use their mental powers prodigally, while there is another class whose highest aim in life is physical labor. The latter class do not exercise the mind. Their muscles are exercised, while their brains are robbed of intellectual strength; just as the minds of thinking men are worked, while their bodies are robbed of strength and vigor by their neglect to exercise the muscles. Those who are content to devote their lives to physical labor, and leave others to do the thinking for them, while they simply carry out what other brains have planned, will have strength of muscle, but feeble intellects. Their influence for good is small in comparison to what it might be if they would use their brains as well as their muscles. This class fall more readily if attacked by disease, because the system is vitalized by the electrical force of the brain to resist disease.

"Men who have good physical powers should educate themselves to think as well as to act, and not depend upon others to be brains for them." (21)

Everyone knows that he who is determined NOT to be sick is less likely to be than he who expects to be sick; the mind vitalizes the cells.

A discouraged army cannot win the battle, but an army will win against heavy odds if the soldiers believe they can and are determined to do so. In that case each man is a likeness of each cell in the body which is vitalized by the mind with the idea of keeping well.

The Power of the Will

"The power of the will is not valued as it should be. Let the will be kept awake and rightly directed, and it will impart energy to the whole being, and will be a wonderful aid in the maintenance of health. It is a power also in dealing with disease. Exercised in the right direction, it would control the imagination, and be a potent means of resisting and overcoming disease of both mind and body. By the exercise of the will-power in placing themselves in right relation to life, patients can do much to cooperate with the physician's efforts for their recovery. There are thousands who can recover health if they will . . . Often invalids can resists disease, simply by refusing to yield to ailments and settle down in a state of inactivity. Rising above their aches and pains, let them engage in useful employment suited to their strength. By such employment and the free use of air and sunlight, many an emaciated invalid might recover health and strength." (22)

The Emotions

Dr. Crile has said that the emotions—worry, fear, hate, and jealousy—affect every cell in the body. Some organs are stimulated; others are inhibited; all are disturbed; waste products are increased; foundations of certain characteristics of human diseases are laid. (23)

Another noted author has said: "The relation that exists between the mind and the body is very intimate. When one is affected, the other sympathizes. The condition of the mind affects the health to a far greater degree than many realize. Many of the diseases from which men suffer are the result of mental depression. Grief, anxiety, discontent, remorse, guilt, distrust, all tend to break down the life forces, and to invite decay and death."

"Disease is sometimes produced, and is often greatly aggravated by the imagination. Many are lifelong invalids who might be well if they only thought so. Many imagine that every slight exposure will cause illness, and the evil effect is produced because it is expected. Many die from disease, the cause of which is wholly imaginary." (24)

Therefore it is of first importance that the mental attitudes be right.

Furthermore, if one is to have abundant health, he must find and know the great Burden Bearer who can assuage human grief, relieve anxiety and discontent, take away remose and guilt by pardoning transgression, and so lift these loads off the mind. The fullness of health cannot be enjoyed while the mind is weighted with woe. A health message cannot be complete until the remedy for these ills is found.

And the reverse is equally true. "Courage, hope, faith, sympathy, love, promote health and prolong life. A contented mind, a cheerful spirit, is health to the body and strength to the soul. 'A merry heart doeth good like a medicine!'" (25)

THE WHOLE BEING INVOLVED

The entire life must be brought into the right way of living. We must know what is right and then do it. This includes the physical, moral and spiritual phases of human life.

We need to confess and forsake our sins in all three realms, and then trust everything to God. This is necessary to good health.

The program begins with the mind because the mind is the king. This excellent counsel is found in Holy Writ: "Whatsoever things are true, whatsoever things are honest, whatsoever things are just, whatsoever things are pure, whatsoever things are lovely, whatsoever things are of good report; if there be any virtue, and if there be any praise, think on these things." Phil. 4:8.

Think right concerning the physical, mental, and spiritual phases of life; speak right concerning them to your fellows; and then live that way. These principles do not belong exclusively to any cult or church but are found in the Book which has been given for the guidance of all people.

EXAMPLES OF A DISTURBED BODY FROM A DISTURBED MIND

Shame fills the cheeks with blood.

Fear drives it away.

Excitement quickens the heart beat.

Grief brings tears from the tear glands. (How many other glands may also be disturbed?)

Great shock to the mind will draw the blood from the head and so cause fainting.

Worry will stop digestion.

Emotion will stop the work of the stomach and the intestines.

Nausea can be produced by some disgusting sight.

Emotion can increase the sugar in the blood and urine like diabetes.

Fright or excitement can cause cold perspiration to come from the sweat glands all over the body.

Anger sends blood to the head and makes the face red.

Patients given fake sleeping powders often sleep soundly after taking them.

Medical students sometimes "get" the diseases about which they study.

A lady developed attacks of hay fever when merely a rose was brought into her room. One day her physician brought in an artificial rose, and the usual symptoms followed. He then showed her that the rose was made of paper, and the symptoms speedily disappeared.

If you fear your food will hurt, it probably will. If we become introspective, it can undo all the benefits of our efforts to secure health.

Relaxation of Mind and Body

> The bow that's always bent will quickly break;
> But if unstrung 'twill serve you at your need.
> So let the mind some relaxation take
> To come back to its task with fresher heed.
> —*Phaedrus' Fables*

Relaxation is one of the most urgent needs of modern life. It is preliminary to rest. Rest begins with the mind. In order for the body to secure proper rest, the mind must be at rest. Rest must first be mental. The mind should be at ease, calm and reposed. Many people in this age maintain a constant nervous tension which is very destructive of vitality. There should be at least periods of entire relaxation and repose. The Orientals could teach us Occidentals many valuable lessons in this matter.

One who is highly nervous should take a few minutes during the day for complete relaxation. In fact, he should train himself to do his work with a calm, serene state of mind rather than under a nervous tension. By so doing he will live many years longer.

Not only are periods of rest and relaxation good for the body and mind; they are also uplifting and ennobling, if we lift our thoughts above the sordid things of earth.

Grenville Kleiser has said:

"Cultivate silence and stillness. You grow your best thoughts in times of solitude and meditation. To continue to grow and accumulate useful ideas, you must have frequent periods of mental and physical relaxation." "Beware of the modern tendency to hurry and waste. The time you give to quiet and intelligent meditation will repay you well. Cultivate quietness, poise and deliberateness. When you are still and receptive you can best hear the voice of God and learn His will." (26)

AMUSEMENT IS NOT RELAXATION

It should also be borne in mind that amusement is not relaxation, nor a substitute for it, but may be, indeed, opposite to it. Many amusements excite the nerves and lead to greater tensity rather than to relaxation. Some other means should be sought by which to find relaxation. Perhaps you are saying, How can we relax? We have tried and failed! That makes me think of a little skit I read the other day, which runs like this:

RELAXED

My work just worried me today,
I'm simply overtaxed;
Right now I'm all worked up and tense,
I'm trying so to be relaxed.
—*"The Cheerful Cherub"*

Doesn't that express it? But relaxation does not come in that way, nor from wishing for it. Would you like to know how to find repose? I will tell you.

HOW TO FIND REPOSE

It is a state of mind by which you have decided to lay aside for the time the things which trouble you, and take a little time to rest and recoup your vital forces. Just as we learn to take on responsibility, so we must learn to lay it off, temporarily. One of the helpful things to do is to close your ears to life's annoyances and open them to the voices of nature. The patter of rain on the roof, the rustle of leaves by a gentle breeze, the murmur of a babbling brook, the songs of birds, the smell of grass and earth and flowers, the odor of pines, honey and fruits, the waving of fields of grain, are some of Nature's many voices calling us to relaxation and repose. But the mightiest influence of all is a clear conscience, a knowledge of having lived each day in the interest of humanity and the service of God; for, having done our duty we may rest in the kind care of Him who watches over all.

STIMULANTS

Stimulants cannot take the place of rest and relaxation. Dr. A. N. Donaldson has expressed it in these words:

"The restoration of vital force depends upon relaxation of mind and body. The present system is to call upon 'reserve' energy, stifling the cry of fatigue by coffee, tea, beef extract, coca-cola, and other stimulants—'refreshing drinks'—to supply more 'go.' We borrow from the future, and repay in a sanitarium, in an asylum, or in a mausoleum. Rest is the essence of cure whether it be in nerves, heart, colon or bones. Rest, with an environment that will direct the mind toward the work and workings of the Great Physician—that is fundamental therapy." (27)

Rest is often the therapy needed to increase the mysterious vital forces which carry on the wonderful life processes, from digestion down through the list of every organ and gland and their functions. In many instances a few days' rest in bed would be of great benefit. It is claimed that quiet rest in bed is ninety percent efficient for sleep.

As a general principle, whenever pain is present, rest is indicated as one of the primary procedures.

A DAY OF REST

The fundamental necessity of periods of rest is evidenced by the act of the Creator in establishing the seventh day of every week as a day of rest in the routine life of all mankind. This day of rest is therefore not only a religious privilege and duty, but a physiological necessity in order to maintain the highest physical and mental efficiency. He who disregards this necessity, in doing so suffers a loss of fitness for his work, and will diminish his happiness and cut short his days of usefulness.

Ponder these beautiful lines from Janet Hegbie, entitled:

SLEEP

"O you who give new lives for old,
Who heal, and never ask for gold—
Kind Sleep, receive and make afresh
This flagging mind and weary flesh.
"At nightfall, as the shadows do,
My cares grow tall and threatening, too,
I doubt the cause for which all day
I wore the golden hours away,
And as I stumble to my bed
The beauty of the world seems dead.
"O best Physician, I resign
This treachery tainted heart of mine,
Which, like a sword, I prithee make
All bright once more before I wake;
Anoint these eyes, too weak to stare
Straight up and see the glory there;
Oh, steep my soul in seas of dew
And make me clean and brave and new."

MENTAL ATTITUDE NOT A SUBSTITUTE FOR FOOD

Notwithstanding the truth of all these principles, the control of the emotions, the will, and mind, will not take the place of right food—of vitamin B1 for the nerves and phosphorus for the nerves and brain—but this mental attitude is to be added to the use of right foods. This chapter does not take away or lessen the force of the preceding ones but is an addition to them. All of these principles are necessary to good health. Even the brain itself must be fed good food if it is to function normally. The force of the will cannot take the place of food.

THE KING CORRECTED

The mind rules over the body. The mind must recognize the existence of the body (not regard it as a phantom), and must know the laws governing the body—the rules of life—the laws of physiology and the Ten Commandments—and must enforce them. Sickness comes from failure to do so; that is being made abundantly plain in this book.

The change from sickness to health must begin in the mind; it must start with learning the rules of life and understanding the mistakes of the past. The mind must first be convinced. People need to change their habits, but they will never change their habits until they first change their minds.

And so I have been working to change your minds to recognize the importance of whole grains, natural foods, raw foods, balanced meals; and to see the harm of using flesh, tea, coffee, spices, soda, baking powder, sugar, cakes, pies, pudding, ice cream, cookies, tobacco, alcohol, etc., etc.

But Johnnie may say, "I don't like spinach!" He can if he will change his mind and try. Mother may say, "I cannot get along without my coffee," but she can if she will make up her mind and try. Father or brother may say, "I must have my cigarette," and so it goes! No one can change until he changes his mind and comes to a definite decision, and in doing that the battle is more than half won.

The Right "Mind Cure"

The change of mind that produces a change of habits is the right kind of "mind cure." All health-seeking should begin here.

To study the laws of health is a science. To keep them in obedience to the Creator is true Christian science. To deny the existence of the body with its organs and their laws in order to deny the reality of sickness is not science and is a repudiation of the Author of all things and of laws governing all. Such a teaching makes obedience unnecessary. It demands only a change of mind without a change of life. True Christianity and true science demand a change of mind that it may produce a change of life. And the optimism associated with the truth is far more wonderful than that associated with error. It is that we are to know the right way of living, live that way, confess to God our departures therefrom, and then confidently trust all our cares and affairs to the Author of the Truth. Optimism belongs linked with truth, not with error.

Mental Health Philosophies

There are many health philosophies offered the people today. The popular ones hold that man is innately good; that within him reside the elements of goodness and powers which will relieve him of sickness and trouble, and bring him the desires of his heart. Such teachings do not recognize that man is a transgressor, and that his transgressions are the primary cause of his troubles, and that they must have his first attention; they do not recognize that the kind ministrations of a forgiving God are necessary to our healing and restoration, without which man cannot achieve the longings of his heart. And so-called "mind cure" that is popular is weak in its call for obedience to the laws of life.

Perhaps the most dangerous of all mental philosophies is that in which one mind is asked to surrender to another human mind. That is the devil's substitute for surrender to God; it is the devil's plan to ruin his victim. The will should be yielded only to the maker thereof.

"It is not God's purpose that any human being should yield his mind and will to the control of another, becoming a passive instrument in his hands. No one is to merge his individuality in that of another. He is not to look to any human being as the source of healing. His dependence must be in God. In the dignity of his God-given manhood, he is to be controlled by God himself!" (28)

This, now, is the ideal completed. The mind is a king which knows the laws of the realm and enforces them. It is to choose every thought and direct every word and act.

The king, in turn, is to be surrendered to the great mind on high, who is the Great King over it, that He, through the human mind, may have complete charge over every detail of life—of every thought, and word, and act.

That is the right use of the mind.

BIBLIOGRAPHY

(1) Mrs. E. G. White, Vol. 3, page 69.
(2) "Good Health," March, 1935, page 91.
(3) Mrs. E. G. White, Vol. 1, page 701.
(4) Reported in the journal, "Heating, Piping, and Air Conditioning," October, 1931, pages 865-869.
(5) Lewis R. Koller, Ph.D., Research Laboratory, General Electric Co., Schenectady, N. Y., in "Journal of the Franklin Institute," November, 1932, page 559.
(6) Same as No. 5, page 553.
(7) Dr. Lawrence S. Moyer and Dr. Harold Abramson of the Biological Laboratory, Cold Spring Harbor, Long Island, N. Y., in "Literary Digest," July 4, 1936, page 17.
(8) Same as No. 5, pages 544, 555.
(9) "Education," page 197.
(10) "Literary Digest," June 1, 1935.
(11) "Education," pages 197, 198.
(12) Mrs. E. G. White, Vol. 3, pages 138, 139.
(13) "Education," page 197.
(14) Mrs. E. G. White, Vol. 3, pages 69, 70.

(15) J. H. Kellogg, M.D., "Good Health," Feb., 1937, page 49.
(16) "Science Snap-Shots," "The Literary Digest," for October 27, 1934, page 19.
(17) Reported in "Good Health," Feb., 1938, page 51.
(18) "Micro-Dynamics," by F. S. Ellis, B.Sc., (E.E.) Research Engineer, Director Ellis Research Laboratories, Inc. Published by Ellis Research Laboratories, Inc., 400 North Michigan Avenue, Chicago, Illinois.
(19) Lewis R. Koller, Ph.D., in "Journal of the Franklin Institute," November, 1932.
(20) Lewis R. Koller, Ph.D., in "Journal of the Franklin Institute," November, 1932.
(21) Mrs. E. G. White, Vol. 3, pages 157, 158.
(22) "Ministry of Healing," page 246.
(23) "Phenomena of Life," pages 184-190. "Man the Unknown," by Alexis Carrel, pages 102, 144-146. "How to Live," by Fisher and Fisk, pages 122-131. "Food, Nutrition and Health," by McCollum and Becker, pages 82-85.
(24) "Ministry of Healing," page 241.
(25) "Ministry of Healing," page 241.
(26) "Good Health," January, 1934.
(27) "Signs of the Times," April 26, 1932.
(28) "Ministry of Healing," page 242.

Health Habits and Character

CHARACTER

"There is nothing truly great in man but character."

"No one can eventually fill the positions in the community that he ought to fill, and which he hopes to fill, unless his character is spotless." (1)

"He most lives who thinks most, feels the noblest, and acts the best." (2)

A true philosophy of life "does not ignore the value of scientific knowledge or literary attainments; but above information it values power; above power, goodness; above intellectual attainments, character. The world does not so much need men of great intellect as of noble character. It needs men in whom ability is controlled by steadfast principle." (3)

"It is character, not position, that decides future destiny." (4)

In the first chapters of this book, the body, its functions, and needs were studied in detail, in search of health.

It is now in order to consider the highest function of both mind and body in the formation of character.

As the body and mind are inseparable in their work, so health habits and character development are inseparable.

"Whatever injures the health, not only lessens physical vigor, but tends to weaken the mental and moral powers. Indulgence in any unhealthful practice makes it more difficult for one to discriminate between right and wrong, and hence more difficult to resist evil. It increases the danger of failure and defeat."

LIFE

Life consists of experiences secured through the combined exercise of the physical, mental, and spiritual powers—the body, mind, and spirit. The harmonious development of these three, prepares one for this life and for eternity.

327

The physical powers find their expression largely through the five senses—seeing, hearing, tasting, smelling, and feeling, under the direction of, and through coordination with, the mind.

THE SENSES

The greatest satisfactions of life are not obtained from the exercise of mere physical strength, but through the proper use of the five senses.

The highest and noblest aspirations of life are gained through the enjoyment of the senses under the direction of the mind, which in turn is guided by the eternal principles of right.

CHOOSING THE CHARACTER

The mere possession of the five senses does not constitute character, but the daily proper use of them develops character. This is the field where man's priceless endowment, the power of choice, is exercised for weal or woe. The daily decisions made by the mind concerning the use of these senses shape the character and determine the destiny. Habits are formed through their exercise, and the sort of habits formed depends upon the kind of experiences chosen by the mind for the five senses to enjoy, and therefore the use or misuse of these senses will largely determine the nature of the character being developed.

SELF-CONTROL

To make the right choice in the use of the senses, two things are indispensable. The first is knowledge of their proper use; the second is self-control. Concerning this, one writer has said—

"Real glory springs from the conquest of yourself; and without that, the conqueror is but the veriest slave."

"It is not enough to have great qualities, you should also have the management of them."

"He who has mastered himself will be stronger than his passions, superior to his circumstances, higher than his calling, and greater than his speech."

"No one can call himself educated until every voluntary muscle obeys his will." (5)

"It is a great thing to have brains, but it is vastly better to be able and willing to command your brains confidently under all circumstances." (6)

The world needs men today who are masters of, not salves to, circumstances; and the mastery of self is fundamental to the mastery of life's problems.

Self-control is exercised and habits are formed through the use of the five senses, and the habits that are formed wherein the sense of taste is involved are very strong and some of them are very destructive. The reason follows.

THE KING OF SENSES

Man's physical life is maintained by food, and he was given the sense of taste that he might receive pleasure from the experience of putting into his body the things which would prolong his existence.

It being more important that he eat and sustain life, than that he see, or hear, or smell, or touch, these senses become servants to the sense of taste, and are largely engaged in occupations which will produce the chief necessity of life—food.

Because the satisfaction of the appetite in the proper use of food to sustain life is a first necessity to existence, it affords the greatest opportunity for perversion; and therefore from the dawn of human history it has been man's great weakness, and the source of the most subtle temptations, which work for his greatest degradation; it is the most vulnerable point at which to attack him.

And, like as the other senses contribute of their powers in securing food to sustain life, so, when the taste becomes perverted, these other four senses are likewise diverted from their natural uses and become slaves to the appetite to provide the indulgences it craves.

The sense of taste can be satisfied with things which will upbuild body, mind, and soul, or it can be indulged with things which will destroy them all.

THE MIND

The use or abuse of the sense of taste, in conjunction with the other senses as helpers, will build up or undermine the mental powers with the reasoning faculties, the power of choice, and the will.

THE SPIRITUAL LIFE

When the mental powers are weakened it becomes difficult or impossible for the mind to perform its highest function in the contemplation and acceptance of spiritual ideals and opportunities.

The mind allies the finite with the infinite. Therefore anything that dulls its perceptions or disturbs its normal action, to some extent lessens man's ability to comprehend divine ideals and objectives, or to lay hold of infinite power to achieve them.

For these reasons a full spiritual experience cannot be found unless by self-control the use of the five senses is yielded to the wishes of their Author. This is one of the requisites of spiritual growth, and a most vital one.

One author of note has said, "The body is the only medium through which the mind and the soul are developed for the upbuilding of character. Hence it is that the adversary of souls directs his temptations to the enfeebling and degrading of the physical powers. His success here means the surrender to evil of the whole being." (7)

Therefore the most vital spot in human experience and existence is the proper use of the sense of taste in maintaining health, in the preservation of strong mental powers, and in laying the foundation for the character, which finds its highest exercise in a spiritual experience. The use or abuse of the appetite can aid in upbuilding or in destroying all.

Furthermore, not only can the mental powers be weakened, the character undermined, and the spiritual powers prostituted, but the persistent violation of the laws of life through the misuse of the senses, the leader of which is the taste, places one in open antagonism to the Author thereof and so enters the realm of loyalty; for how can a person claim to be loyal to his Maker when he persists in any indulgence which is contrary to his Maker's will as expressed in the laws of life which he has established within the body?

THE APPLICATION

The object in stating here the foregoing principles which are fundamental to character development is that they be considered in connection with the health habits already mentioned in this book, a few of which will now be considered one by one. Let it be first noted that anything which disturbs the brain or nerves disturbs the mind, has an effect upon the thinking, and so influences character. Each of the following items, experiences, or conditions influence the mind and so affect the character in some specific manner.

Alcohol deadens the nerves and the brain, weakens the will, blunts the conscience, and arouses the animal instincts. It is habit-forming.

Tobacco is a narcotic to nerves and brain, weakens the will, and blunts the conscience. It is habit-forming.

Tea, coffee, and cola drinks injure the nerves, interfere with the function of the brain, weaken the will, and are habit-forming.

Cocoa is in the same class as coffee but is weaker and is not habit-forming.

Spices irritate the nerves.

Pain-killing remedies deaden the nerves and the brain to some extent.

"Dope"—the derivatives of opium, and similar preparations—injures the nerves and the brain cells.

Sour stomach makes clear thinking very difficult and the best thinking impossible.

Constipation, by causing toxins to be absorbed into the blood, contributes to a dull mind.

Worry has a disastrous effect on both nerves and mind.

Minerals, vitamins, air, sunshine, exercise, rest, and other things, build up nerve vitality, strengthen the mind and aid in securing a normal mental poise. When nerves are undernourished because these elements are lacking, the individual becomes nervous, easily irritated, fretful, cross, and impatient. This condition seriously mars his relation to his family, his friends, and to God. This condition is destructive to health, to character, and to spirituality.

Manifestly the need is for (a) knowledge, and (b) self-control.

The items just mentioned are all involved in forming merely the "good moral character" apart from any definitely spiritual experience; but the best character develops from roots which run deeper yet; it comes through loyalty to the Author of the laws involved in all these matters of health and habits.

Two Kinds of People

Certain people wish to learn the principles of healthful living merely for health reasons, and others desire to have the use of their strength directed by principles which are understood only when man recognizes his obligations to his Maker. If this lesson is to really cover the subject of "Health Habits and Character" it must add this higher viewpoint to the lower, to follow which may be termed "the higher order of living."

A Dangerous Viewpoint

Among church people a dangerous attitude is often taken. The sick either are not well-informed concerning health principles, or they are unwilling to follow them and cease their injurious habits, and consequently they seek for miracles of healing instead of reforming their habits.

Miracles have their place in the church, but their place is very definite and clearly defined. Four points should be well understood and properly related, in the following order:

1. Obedience to life's laws
2. The use of natural remedies and treatments
3. Surgery in case of necessity
4. Miracles as a last resort

If we seek for a miracle from Him whose laws we ignore, that is to scorn Him whose blessing we seek. That is not faith, but is presumption; it is not loyalty, but is rebellion; that is not consistency, but is hypocrisy. Before a miracle is sought, obedience should be rendered, rational treatment employed, and surgery used if indicated; all we can do with the means Heaven has provided should be done before seeking for miracles.

The Gospel of Health

If there is a God, and if the laws of nature are His, it follows that His desire must be that we know and keep His laws, and it is inevitable that He be working to that end. Consequently, if He has a Gospel being proclaimed in the earth, it must include this because these laws of life are an expression of His desires. The Gospel must have within it the "Gospel of Health."

Miracles and Obedience

Those who seek Heaven to bestow a miracle should do it in a consistent way. They should:

1. Believe and follow the Scriptures.
2. Know and observe the laws of health.
3. Use all possible means as He has specified to aid nature, such as treatment and surgery if needed, but no poisonous drugs, and then
4. Submit and say, "If the Lord wills."

Someone may ask, "Why say, if the Lord wills?" Because it may not be His will that everybody recover. If you are surprised, remember that the apostles who healed so many all died at last.

It may not be His will that we recover but it is His will that we keep His laws whether we get a miracle or not. The call to obedience is absolute and is of first importance because disobedience is disloyalty, and loyalty develops character. Miracles are of relative importance and are given only upon conditions.

CHRIST'S MIRACLES

You may ask, "Why then did the Master heal everybody so promiscuously? I answer, "To prove His divinity" (John 20:30, 31). And you ask, "Why not have the miracles now to prove His divinity?" I answer, "It is not necessary now to prove His divinity."

His divinity is established, we passed that point nineteen hundred years ago. You say, "But science questions that." Yes, I know. You say, "Most of our preachers are Modernists and they question His divinity." Yes, I know. You say, "Atheism scoffs and there are but few people who believe His divinity." Yes, I know all that and yet I repeat, it is not needed now to prove His divinity for that was accomplished nineteen hundred years ago, as you will see presently.

Christ's Achievements of Three and a Half Years

Dr. Sherwood Eddy says:

"Men are usually made by their environment, limited by the circumstances of their lives. In some strange way Jesus transformed and transcended the limitations of His life.

"His race was probably the most hated and persecuted, the most bigoted and provincial in the world. Yet, though a Jew, He becomes the one universal man, uniting Orient and Occident, appealing equally to East and West. In Him there is neither Jews nor Gentile, bond nor free, male nor female. He becomes the symbol of unity and universality.

"His family was that of a peasant carpenter, yet for all time He gives a new infinite content to the words 'father,' 'son' and 'brother.' He widens the thoughts of the family to a universal communion of love, a commonwealth of mankind.

"Let us note how He transcends His time and place. He had less than three years of public life in which to do His work in the world; less than any other world leader. Socrates taught for some forty years; Plato for fifty; Aristotle had a long life and filled libraries with his learning. Jesus seems to outlive time and founded an eternal kingdom. His place was a little, conquered, Jewish province in despised Galilee, as small as an American or English county, yet He embraced the world in His thought and plan.

"He was no moralist, and yet He stands supreme in the moral sphere. It is He who creates the world's highest moral standard.

"He was no professional religionist or priest, yet He stands supreme in the realm of religion.

"He was no writer, yet He is more quoted than any other author in history, and His words are repeated to the very ends of the world. They are being read today in a thousand languages and tongues, and form the one universal Book of humanity. No man has ever laid down his life in Africa to translate Aristotle, Kant, or Hegel, nor any other great leader of thought, but hundreds have died to carry the words of Jesus to the ends of the world. More than two hundred languages have been reduced to writing in order to embody His life-giving message.

"He was no architect, yet the Carpenter of Nazareth has somehow become the Master builder of time. The great cathedrals were erected for His worship—St. Sophia, St. Peter's, St. Paul's, Milan, Cologne, and Amiens; Canterbury and Westminster, and the masterpieces of architecture were reared in His praise.

"He was no artist, yet the works of the great masters were dedicated to Him. Fra Angelico, Raphael, Leonardo da Vinci, Michael Angelo, and the greatest of the old masters seems to attain their highest under His inspiration.

"He was no poet, yet He made poetry the possession of the common people. He lends a new rhythm to life and teaches the human heart to sing. Dante, Shakespeare, Milton, Browning, Tennyson, Whittier, and a host of great writers with a spiritual message are inspired by Him.

"He was no musician, yet Haydn, Handel, Beethoven, Bach, Wagner, Mendelssohn, often reached their highest in the hymns, symphonies, and oratories in His praise.

"He had no home, yet He creates the Christian family and secures its sanctity and its safety through a new conception of marriage. Before the degeneracy of Greece and Rome, the bestiality of paganism, the sensuality in some of the ethnic religions, and the growing laxity of modern divorce, He holds up the highest ideal conception of marriage, not as legalized licentiousness, but as what 'God hath joined together.' It is an original relationship divinely ordained.

"He had no wide human opportunity of culture or travel. He was no versatile Greek nor cosmopolitan Roman, no citizen of Athens, or Alexandria, but lived His life in the isolation of village farmers and fishermen. Yet no one in all history has such strange power of self-identification with all mankind—with the suffering, the poor, the sinful, with little children, with men in all walks of life, in all times, in all nations. All claim Him as theirs, and seek to vindicate their position by appeal to His standards.

"Who then is this? Can we deny that God was in Him in some unique way? Was He a mere village carpenter? Or in truth the Christ of Humanity? As we ask Him, with His judges and persecutors of old, 'Art Thou the Christ, the Anointed of God?' He answers clearly and simply, from the depth of His consciousness 'I AM.' And as He questions us like Simon Peter, 'Who do you say that I am?' are we not constrained to reply with Simon, 'Thou art the Christ, the Son of the living God'? As we feel the influence of His life upon us shall we not rise up at His call, 'Come and follow Me'? Not in abstract reasoning or empty theory, but in actual experience, as we seek to follow Jesus' way of life, we shall find Him indeed the supreme manifestation of God." (8)

Everybody Honors Christ

You need not tell me He was not divine for He has put His stamp on the whole world for all time. The Declaration of Independence was dated July 4, A.D. 1776, which means "in the year of our Lord." This means 1776 years after Christ.

An atheist announces a lecture; he has to date his appearance "in the year of our Lord" whether he wants to or not.

The Events of Today

Every social or friendship letter is dated in His name. Society thus recognizes Him.

Every business letter, telegram, check, invoice, receipt book entry, bank deposit, is dated in His name. Business acknowledges Him.

Thus men acknowledge that He lived and that He is the dominant figure of all time.

You cannot buy or sell a piece of land, a house, or an automobile without acknowledging Him. Every piece of personal property, every home, every piece of real estate is a witness to His Divinity.

You cannot pass a law in city, state, or nation, and make it legal, or execute any sort of legal document, without affixing thereto "in the year of our Lord." He is thus acknowledged to be higher than all the laws of earth.

You cannot hold an election of any earthly ruler or petty officer without doing it "in the year of our Lord." Every earthly potentate thus bows to Him.

And who does this? Every person! Whether he be Christian, Modernist, Hebrew, scientist, atheist or infidel. Why do they do it? Because they must do it. He compels it. They cannot help doing it. Thus He manifests His power over them, and thus they acknowledge His power over them.

So much for the things being done today; but there is still more to be said.

History

He has divided the history of the world into two parts with His cross between. All time is reckoned from His cross—from it forward, and from it backward. This makes the cross the center of all time, of all events, and of all history. Every act of man since the cross that has been recorded in the annals of history is written in His name, and every deed of mankind before the cross that is written in history is said to have been done so many years B.C., before Christ.

Therefore all that man has ever done, or is doing is recorded in such a way as to honor His name.

These things witness to the fact that He towers above all mankind and their doings, He dominates the world and compels them to acknowledge Him even while they are denying Him.

How has this come to be? Could any man thus compel all mankind to honor him? These things witness that He is the Master.

You cannot tell me that this has come about by accident, or that it has been fixed by human thought and hands. Nobody ever did that before or since. No man could thus divide all history and stamp everything that ever was done or ever will be done with his name. No mere man could thus compel all classes to do him honor, even against their wills. This could only be done by Him who is over all mankind, who is DIVINE! His divinity has been established once for all time and it does not need to be done again.

The Apostles and His Divinity

After His ascension His followers continued His work. With the early church the testing message was the acceptance of Jesus as the Messiah of prophecy, and His miracles were often cited as one of the proofs, and they were repeated in the ministry of the disciples as further proof.

The Present Time

Those were events of nearly nineteen hundred years ago. Now the emphasis is not concerning matters which He established at His first coming, but on things He will establish at His second coming. The next time, He comes not to submit Himself to men and be put to death, but to establish His kingdom and put out of existence every opposing force.

The Climax of History

On every hand I meet people from various religious beliefs and sundry walks of life who are wondering what is coming next. They look upon the earth and observe the changing unstable conditions, the rapid downward trends, the increasing animosity among nations which modern means of communication and transportation have brought so close together that all are neighbors, and they feel that some portentous event impends, that conditions are becoming intolerable, that the world cannot stand much longer, and that there is no hope for mankind except in the return of the Son of Man which has been the goal of all Scripture, both Old and New.

The basis of citizenship in His kingdom, like every nation of this world, is loyalty—obedience—if you please. There can be no other. He will save and take into His Kingdom those whom He finds obeying Him. Therefore the emphasis now must be on obedience, whether there be any miracles or not. He is seeking after loyalty among all mankind—loyalty in the spiritual realm, and loyalty in the physical realm. Health education and heart education thus unite to produce perfect loyalty. This sort of emphasis placed on the necessity of knowing and keeping the laws of health for the sake of both health and character is at once sensible, scientific, and religious.

Deceptive Miracles

You may ask, What about the miracles of which we hear and read today? I reply, If they are done among those who are doing the will of God the best they know and are in harmony with divine specifications, well and good. But, if miracles appear among those who are against any expressed will of God, beware!

Can there be counterfeit miracles? Read your Bible. There always have been; there always will be; there are now. Their purpose is to deceive the people concerning the will of God. The Master said that in the closing days of earth's history counterfeit miracles would deceive, if possible "the very elect" (Matt. 24:24). Their purpose is to deceive the people concerning doctrine, truth, and loyalty.

The common belief is that miracles can be performed only by divine power, and therefore when any miracle is done, the people believe that the doctrines taught in connection with it must be the truth. But this is not the way to determine what is truth. The miracles which will almost deceive "the elect" will have deceptive power because they are associated with error, and the people will believe the error because it is accompanied by miracles. The presence of a miracle does not prove that the doctrines associated with it are the truth, but rather, the sort of doctrines taught will reveal whether the miracle is from above or beneath. Miracles cannot be a proof of the correctness of the doctrines taught, but the doctrines taught prove whether the accompanying miracles are of God or of Satan.

POPULAR HEALERS

If a "healer" influences you to ignore any of the laws of health or any of the Ten Commandments, shun his miracles. The people who receive such miracles conclude that it is not necessary to keep the laws of the Creator, either physical or the Ten Commandments, and they will never change their ways and reform; they will become established in error by such miracles. That is Satan's scheme to abolish loyalty to God and to ruin the human race, even while some of them think they are serving Him.

IF CHRIST WERE HERE

If Christ were here He would teach obedience to His own laws. If He has any ambassadors here, they will do the same. Therefore an individual who is willfully violating the laws of health should not expect a miracle from God; and a "healer" or preacher who is not teaching and observing the laws of health need not expect miracles from God.

Furthermore, a church that does nothing about teaching its members and disciplining them concerning the use of alcohol, tobacco, tea, coffee, and other health habits need not expect miracles from God. Sincere penitence, which brings pardon, will inspire loyalty to Him who forgives. A church that is fully representing God will teach the laws of God, both spiritual and physical.

THE NEED OF THE WORLD TODAY

Inasmuch as Christ is not now seeking to establish His divinity but is making preparation to establish His kingdom, the test or deciding factor is not miracles but obedience—loyalty.

A COMPLETE INTERPRETATION OF CHRISTIANITY

The need of the world today, among all nations, creeds and churches, is a complete interpretation of Christianity. We have a confusing array of creeds and churches, but I would have you know that there are not several kinds of Christianity, but only varying degrees of it. I am working in the interest of a complete interpretation of the Gospel. Nothing less will meet the need of this closing hour of earth's history.

Anyone who seriously ponders the conditions in the world today —social conditions, economics, physical and mental degeneracy, the increase of cancer and other degenerative diseases, the relation of nations to each other, the relation between capital and labor, the criminality of youth, the prevalence of life-destroying habits, the decadence of the home and of morals, the lack of honor among nations, the mad rush for pleasure, the decadence in religion both in the power of the pulpit and the empty pews, the corruption of politics, etc., etc., cannot fail to see that the world is fast getting into a condition for which there is no human help—God Must Take Charge. And then—

"The kingdoms of this world will become the kingdom of our Lord and of His Christ, and He shall reign for ever and ever."

BIBLIOGRAPHY

(1) "Character—A Moral Text-Book," page 28, by Henry Varnum, published by Hinds and Noble, 31 West 15th Street, New York, N. Y.

(2) P. J. Bailey, Festus Book XV (International Encyclopedia of Prose and Poetical Quotations) by Wm. S. Walsh. Published by John C. Winston Co., Philadephia, Pa.

(3) "Education," page 225, by Mrs. E. G. White. Published by Pacific Press Publishing Co., Mountain View, California.

(4) "Christ's Object Lessons," by Mrs. E. G. White, page 123. Published by Pacific Press Publishing Co., Mountain View, California.

(5) "Character—A Moral Text-Book," page 61, by Henry Varnum.

(6) "Character—A Moral Text-Book," page 75, by Henry Varnum.

(7) "Ministry of Healing," page 130, by Mrs. E. G. White, published by Pacific Press Publishing Co., Mountain View, California.

(8) "Facing the Crisis," pages 31-46, quoted in "Review and Herald," August 12, 1926.

(9) "Ministry of Healing," page 128.

PART II

Side-Lights on Miscellaneous Subjects

The subjects in Part I are arranged in the right order to be easily understood. Some of them were not developed as fully in Part I as they should be, and therefore additional information is given in Part II. Part I is visualized by 850 colored slides for those who use it as a teaching or lecture text.

These additional comments are not in any sense exhaustive concerning any subject, but are offered as extra helps. They have been gathered from a wide range of sources. The entire grouping has never appeared in any one book before. The aim is to bring into the compass of one book the very best and most helpful information to be found anywhere.

Need of Education in Health Principles

"Education in health principles was never more needed than now. Notwithstanding the wonderful progress in so many lines relating to the comforts and conveniences of life, even to sanitary matters and to the treatment of disease, the decline in physical vigor and power of endurance is alarming. It demands the attention of all who have at heart the well being of their fellow men.

"Our artificial civilization is encouraging evils destructive of sound principles. Custom and fashion are at war with nature. The practices they enjoin, and the indulgences they foster, are steadily lessening both physical and mental strength, and bringing upon the race an intolerable burden. Intemperance and crime, disease and wretchedness, are everywhere.

"Many transgress the laws of health through ignorance, and they need instruction. But the greater number know better than they do. They need to be impressed with the importance of making their knowledge a guide of life.

"Too little attention is generally given to the preservation of health. It is far better to prevent disease than to know how to treat it when contracted.

"It is the duty of every person, for his own sake, and for the sake of humanity, to inform himself in regard to the laws of life, and conscientiously to obey them. All need to become acquainted with that most wonderful of all organisms, the human body. They should understand the functions of the various organs and the dependence of one upon another for the healthy action of all. They should study the influence of the mind upon the body, and of the body upon the mind, and the laws by which they are governed." (1)

Seven Essentials to Good Health

To build and maintain the maximum of health, it is necessary to see that every habit is correct and every law of life observed. These may be summarized under these heads:

1. A proper diet
2. Fresh air day and night in abundance.
3. Regular exercise
4. Systematic rest—relaxation, repose and sleep
5. A good supply of sunshine
6. Strict cleanliness
7. A right mental attitude, which includes obedience to and trust in the Creator

These rules of hygiene are interwoven more or less in this book, but in addition a section of this book has been given to a few of the most choice statements of others that can be found bearing upon these essentials to health.

Air and Breathing

Air is life's first necessity. One may live for many days without food, and for a few days without water, but for only a few moments without air.

Air purifies the blood, contributes to the production of heat and energy, and conveys electrical energy with which to vitalize every organ of the body.

That it may accomplish these things the air must be kept in motion, be pure and fresh and abundant at all times and in all places, day and night; the sitting, walking, and working posture should be correct, and deep, full, abdominal breathing should be practiced.

"Exercise and the growth of cells develop lactic acid which is then broken down into carbon dioxide and water and much of it is converted back again into carbohydrate, which process requires oxygen. In case of excessive exercise a great deal of lactic acid is made and much oxygen is required to handle it. This means faster breathing. If breathing is hampered or the circulation of the blood slow, lactic acid accumulates, which is 'acidosis' or weariness." (2)

The following comprehensive, forceful statements concerning air have been arranged from the writings of the author of "Ministry of Healing":

"In order to have good blood, we must breathe well. Full, deep inspirations of pure air, which fill the lungs with oxygen, purify the blood. They impart to it a bright color, and send it, a life-giving current, to every part of the body. A good respiration soothes the nerves; it stimulates the appetite, and renders digestion more perfect; and it induces sound, refreshing sleep." (3)

"Air is the free blessing of Heaven, calculated to electrify the whole system. Without it the system will be filled with disease, and become dormant, languid, feeble." (4)

"Air, air, the precious boon of Heaven, which all may have, will bless you with its invigorating influence, if you will not refuse its entrance. Welcome it, cultivate a love for it, and it will prove a precious soother of the nerves. Air must be in constant circulation to be kept pure. The influence of pure, fresh air is to cause the blood to circulate properly through the system. It refreshes the body, and tends to render it strong and healthy, while at the same time its influence is decidedly felt upon the mind, imparting a degree of composure and serenity. It excites the appetite, and renders the digestion of food more perfect, and induces sound and sweet sleep." (5)

Mr. X "breathes only from the top of his lungs. It is seldom that he exercises the abdominal muscles in the act of breathing. Stomach, liver, lungs, and brain are suffering for the want of deep full inspirations of air, which would electrify the blood and impart to it a bright, lively color, and which alone can keep it pure and give tone and vigor to every part of the living machinery." (6)

"The lungs should be allowed the greatest freedom possible. Their capacity is developed by free action; it diminishes if they are cramped and compressed. Hence the ill effects of the practice so common, especially in sedentary pursuits, of stooping at one's work. In this position it is impossible to breathe deeply. Superficial breathing soon becomes a habit, and the lungs lose their power to expand. . . . Sufficient room is not given to the lower part of the chest; the abdominal muscles, which were designed to aid in breathing, do not have full play, and the lungs are restricted in their action." (7)

"Thus an insufficient supply of oxygen is received. The blood moves sluggishly. The waste, poisonous matter, which should be thrown off in the exhalations from the lungs, is retained, and the blood becomes impure. Not only the lungs, but the stomach, liver, and brain are affected. The skin becomes sallow; digestion is retarded; the heart is depressed; the brain is clouded; the thoughts are confused; gloom settles upon the spirits; the whole system becomes depressed and inactive, and peculiarly susceptible to disease." (8)

"The effects produced by living in close, ill-ventilated rooms are these: The system becomes weak and unhealthy, the circulation is depressed, the blood moves sluggishly through the system because it is not purified and vitalized by the pure, invigorating air of heaven. The mind becomes depressed and gloomy, while the whole system is enervated; and fevers and other acute diseases are liable to be generated. Your careful exclusion of external air, and fear of free ventilation leaves you to breathe a corrupt, unwholesome · air which is exhaled from the lungs of those staying in these rooms, and which is poisonous, unfit for the support of life. The body becomes relaxed; the skin becomes sallow; digestion is retarded, and the system is peculiarly sensitive to the influence of cold. A slight exposure produces serious disease. Great care should be exercised not to sit in a draught or in a cold room when weary, or when in a perspiration. You should so accustom yourself to the air that you will not be under the necessity of having the mercury higher than sixty-five degrees." (9)

"Those who have not had a free circulation of air in their rooms through the night, generally awake feeling exhausted and feverish, and know not the cause. It was air, vital air, the whole system required, but which it could not obtain. Upon rising in the morning most persons would be benefited by taking a sponge bath, or if more agreeable, a hand bath, with merely a washbowl of water. This will remove impurities from the skin. Then the clothing should be removed piece by piece from the bed, and exposed to the air. The windows should be opened, the blinds fastened back, and the air allowed to circulate freely for several hours, if not all day, through the sleeping apartments. In this manner the bed and clothing will become thoroughly aired, and the impurities will be removed from the room." (10)

"Many labor under the mistaken idea that if they have taken cold, they must carefully exclude the outside air, and increase the temperature of their room until it is excessively hot. The system may be deranged, the pores closed by waste matter, and the internal organs suffering more or less inflammation, because the blood has been chilled back from the surface and thrown upon them. At this time, of all others, the lungs should not be deprived of pure, fresh air. If pure air is ever necessary, it is when any part of the system, as the lungs or stomach, is diseased. Judicious exercise would induce the blood to the surface, and thus relieve the internal organs. Brisk, yet not violent exercise in the open air, with cheerfulness of spirits, will promote the circulation, giving a healthful glow to the skin." (11)

"In the construction of buildings, whether for public purposes or as dwellings, care should be taken to provide good ventilation and plenty of sunlight. Churches and school rooms are often faulty in this respect. Neglect of proper ventilation is responsible for much of the drowsiness and dullness that destroy the effect of many a sermon and make the teacher's work toilsome and ineffective." (12)

"In the building of houses it is especially important to secure thorough ventilation and plenty of sunlight. Let there be a current of air and an abundance of light in every room in the house. Sleeping-rooms should be so arranged as to have a free circulation of air day and night. No room is fit to be occupied as a sleeping-room unless it can be thrown open daily to the air and sunshine. In most countries bedrooms need to be supplied with conveniences for heating, that they may be thoroughly warmed and dried in cold or wet weather." (13)

God's Gift, the Air

Now, is there anything that freer seems
　　Than air, the fresh, the vital, that a man
Draws in with breathings bountiful, nor dreams
　　Of any better bliss, because he can
Make over all his blood thereby, and feel
Once more his youth return, his muscles steel,
　　And life grow buoyant, part of God's good plan!

Oh, how on plain and mountain, and by streams
　　That shine along their path; o'er many a field
Proud with pied flowers, or where sunrise gleams
　　In spangled splendors, does the rich air yield
Its balsam; yea, how hunter, pioneer,
Lover, and bard have felt that heaven was near
　　Because the air their spirit touched and healed!

And yet—God of the open!—look and see
  The millions of Thy creatures pent within
Close places that are foul for one clean breath,
Thrilling with health, and hope, and purity;
  Nature's vast antidote for stain and sin,
Life's sweetest medicine this side of death!
How comes it that this largess of the sky
Thy children lack of, till they droop and die?
                              —*Richard Burton*

Exercise

Exercise quickens and increases the circulation of the blood. This contributes to a more rapid and efficient purification of the blood because it passes oftener through the lungs and kidneys and skin where it is relieved of its poisonous wastes.

After exercise all of the organs and all of their cells carry on metabolic processes better because of the fuller supply of fresh purified blood.

Because of the better supply and quality of blood, all healing processes are hastened. This increase in circulation tends to relieve any existing congestion. It improves the digestion.

Thus the reader can readily see that exercise promotes the well-being of the body in many ways.

The following quotations are from the author of "Ministry of Healing":

"Action is a law of our being. Every organ of the body has its appointed work, upon the performance of which its development and strength depend. The normal action of all the organs gives strength and vigor, while the tendency of disuse is toward decay and death. Bind up an arm even for a few weeks, then free it from its bands, and you will see that it is weaker than the one you have been using moderately during the same time. Inactivity produces the same effect upon the whole muscular system." (14)

"Inactivity is a fruitful cause of disease. Exercise quickens and equalizes the circulation of the blood, but in idleness the blood does not circulate freely, and the changes in it, so necessary to life and health, do not take place. The skin, too, becomes inactive. Impurities are not expelled as they would be if the circulation had been quickened by vigorous exercise, the skin kept in a healthy condition, and the lungs fed with plenty of pure, fresh air. This state of the system throws a double burden on the excretory organs, and disease is the result." (15)

"By active exercise in the open air every day, the liver, kidneys, and lungs also will be strengthened to perform their work."

"Without physical exercise no one can have a sound constitution and vigorous health; and the discipline of well-regulated labor is no less essential to the securing of a strong, active mind and a noble character." (16)

"The chief if not the only reason why many become invalids is that the blood does not circulate freely, and the changes in the vital fluid, which are necessary to life and health, do not take place. They have not given their bodies exercise nor their lungs food, which is pure, fresh air; therefore it is impossible for the blood to be vitalized, and it pursues its course sluggishly through the system. The more we exercise, the better will be the circulation of the blood. More people die for want of exercise than through over-fatigue; very many more rust out than wear out. Those who accustom themselves to proper exercise in the open air, will generally have a good and vigorous circulation. We are more dependent upon the air we breathe than upon the food we eat. Men and women, young and old, who desire health and who would enjoy active life, should remember that they cannot have these without a good circulation. Whatever their business and inclinations are, they should make up their minds to exercise in the open air as much as they can." (17)

"Exercise aids the dyspeptic by giving the digestive organs a healthy tone. To engage in severe study or violent physical exercise immediately after eating, hinders the work of digestion; but a short walk after a meal, with the head erect and the shoulders back, is a great benefit." (18)

"Invalids should not be encouraged in inactivity. When there has been serious overtaxation in any direction, entire rest for a time will sometimes ward off serious illness; but in the case of confirmed invalids, it is seldom necessary to suspend all activity." (19)

"The sick should be taught that it is wrong to suspend all physical labor in order to regain health. In thus doing the will becomes dormant, the blood moves sluggishly through the system, and constantly grows more impure. Where the patient is in danger of imagining his case worse than it really is, indolence will be sure to produce the most unhappy results. Well-regulated labor gives the invalid the idea that he is not totally useless in the world, that he is, at least, of some benefit. This will afford him satisfaction, give him courage, and impart to him vigor, which vain mental amusements can never do." (20)

"In order for men and women to have well-balanced minds, all the powers of the being should be called into use and developed. There are in this world many who are one-sided because only one set of faculties has been cultivated, while others are dwarfed from inaction. The education of many youth is a failure. They overstudy, while they neglect that which pertains to the practical life. That the balance of the mind may be maintained, a judicious system of physical work should be combined with mental work, that there may be a harmonious development of all the powers." (21)

"The exercise of the brain in study, without corresponding physical exercise, has a tendency to attract the blood to the brain, and the circulation of the blood through the system becomes unbalanced. The brain has too much blood, and the extremities too little." (22)

"Those who have broken down from mental labor should have rest from wearing thought; but they should not be led to believe that it is dangerous to use their mental powers at all. Many are inclined to regard their condition as worse than it really is; this state of mind is unfavorable to recovery, and should not be encouraged." (23)

"And a portion of the time each day should have been devoted to labor, that the physical and mental powers might be equally exercised." (24)

"Ministers, teachers, and students do not become as intelligent as they should in regard to the necessity of physical exercise in the open air. They neglect this duty, which is most essential for the preservation of health. They closely apply their minds to books, and eat the allowance of a laboring man. Under such habits, some grow corpulent, because the system is clogged. Others become lean, feeble, and weak, because their vital powers are exhausted in throwing off the excess of food; the liver becomes burdened and unable to throw off the impurities in the blood, and sickness is the result. If physical exercise were combined with mental exertion, the blood would be quickened in its circulation, the action of the heart would be more perfect, impure matter would be thrown off, and new life and vigor would be experienced in every part of the body." (25)

"Those who have overtaxed their physical powers should not be encouraged to forego manual labor entirely. But labor to be of the greatest advantage, should be systematic and agreeable. Outdoor exercise is the best; it should be so planned as to strengthen by use the organs that have become weakened; and the heart should be in it; the labor of the hands should never degenerate into mere drudgery.

"When invalids have nothing to occupy their time and attention their thoughts become centered upon themselves, and they grow morbid and irritable. Many times they dwell upon their bad feelings until they think themselves much worse than they really are, and wholly unable to do anything.

"In all these cases, well directed physical exercise would prove an effective remedial agent. In some cases it is indispensable to the recovery of health. The will goes with the labor of the hands; and what these invalids need is to have the will aroused. When the will is dormant, the imagination becomes abnormal, and it is impossible to resist disease." (26)

"When the weather will permit all who can possibly do so ought to walk in the open air every day, summer and winter. But the clothing should be suitable for the exercise, and the feet should be well protected. A walk, even in winter, would be more beneficial to the health than all the medicine the doctors may prescribe. For those who can walk, walking is preferable to riding. The muscles and veins are better enabled to perform their work. There will be increased vitality, which is so necessary to health. The lungs will have needful action; for it is impossible to go out in the bracing air of a winter's morning without inflating the lungs." (27)

"Walking, in all cases where it is possible, is the best remedy for diseased bodies, because in this exercise all the organs of the body are brought into use. Many who depend upon the movement cure, could accomplish more for themselves by muscular exercise than the movements can do for them. In some cases, want of exercise causes the bowels and muscles to become enfeebled and shrunken, and these organs that have become enfeebled for want of use will be strengthened by exercise. There is no exercise that can take the place of walking. By it the circulation of the blood is greatly improved." (28)

"Such exercise would in many cases be better for the health than medicine. Physicians often advise their patients to take an ocean voyage, to go to some mineral spring or to visit different places for change of climate, when in cost cases if they would eat temperately, and take cheerful, healthful exercise, they would recover health, and would save time and money." (29)

"Exercise in a gymnasium, however well conducted, cannot supply the place of recreation in the open air." (30)

Rest

"Rest strengthens labor and labor sweetens rest."—*Varnum.*

These paragraphs will not deal with rest as a treatment, though it is a very important one, but will consider it principally as a rule of hygiene.

Activity exhausts the resources of the body faster than they are restored and this makes periods of rest and relaxation necessary to make it possible for the body to catch up and restore itself to its normal condition. This has been well stated by Dr. Clark as follows:

"Everything in animal life requires, among other fundamentals, that there be exercise and rest following each other in regular order; and anything that disturbs the proper relation or proportion between them disturbs the health and efficiency. For example the brain cell, after a day's work, becomes exhausted; but after a night in sleep, it is refreshed and ready to resume its normal work. This can be easily demonstrated with the microscope. After work, the nerve cell is shrunken in size and the little granules in its protoplasm disappear. After rest, they are again plump and the granules restored. This change takes place regularly in our nerve cells daily, following work and rest."

"The same is true of the heart. Its regular beat occupies about seven-tenths of a second; that is, three-tenths for contraction, three-tenths for dilation, and one-tenth for rest. Whenever anything happens to the heart to deprive it of this one-tenth-second rest in every beat, it shows it in decreased efficiency, and flies the flag of distress at once, asking for rest." (31)

Rest should be preceded by exercise, or it will be indolence, which is a frequent cause of disease. Exercise makes the rest necessary.

"In a hygienic life there must be a certain amount of actual rest. Every bodily power requires rest after exertion. The heart rests between beats. The muscles require relaxation after every contraction. The man who is always tense in muscle and nerve is wearing himself out." (32)

"A very hot bath, lasting only a minute, or even a hot footbath, is restful in cases of general fatigue. The most restful of all is a neutral, tepid bath, the temperature about body-heat (beginning at 97 or 98 degrees and not allowed to drop more than five degrees and continued as long as convenient).

"The wonderful nervous relaxation induced by neutral baths is an excellent substitute for sleep in case of sleeplessness, and often induces sleep as well. Neutral baths are now used not only in cases of insomnia and extreme nervous irritability, but also in cases of acute mania. When sleep occurs in a neutral bath, it is particularly restful. A physician who often sleeps in the bathtub expresses this fact by saying that 'he sleeps faster there than in bed.'

"Sleep may also be induced by monotonous sounds, or lack of sound, or the monotonous holding of the attention. Keeping awake is due to continued change and interruption or arrest of the attention.

"Exercise taken in the afternoon will often promote sleep at night in those who find sleep difficult. Slow, deep rhythmic breathing is useful when wakeful, partly as a substitute for sleep, partly as an inducer of sleep.

"Sleep is Nature's great rejuvenator, and the health-seeker should avail himself of it to the fullest. Our sleep should not only be sufficient in duration but also in intensity, and should be regular.

"The number of hours of sleep generally needed varies with circumstances. The average is seven to nine. In general one should sleep when sleepy and not try to sleep more. Growing children require more sleep than grown-ups. Parents often foolishly sacrifice their children's sleep by compelling them to rise early for farm 'chores,' or in order to sell papers, or for other 'useful' purposes.

"One's best sleep is with the stomach practically empty. It is true that food puts one to sleep at first, by diverting blood from the head; but it disturbs sleep later. Water, unless it induces bladder-action during the night, or even fruit, may be taken without injury before retiring. If one goes to bed with an empty stomach, he can often get along well with six or seven hours' sleep, but if he goes to bed soon after a hearty meal, he usually needs from eight to ten hours' sleep.

"It has already been pointed out that sleeping outdoors is more restful than sleeping indoors." (33)

Sunshine

The sun seems to be the mother of all nature's processes, the source of all energy, and necessary to all life and growth. The vitamins are the product of sunlight. Sunshine is antiseptic. Scientific research and experiments have taught us wonderful lessons in the value of sunlight, which would require volumes to relate. It has become an important factor in the treatment of several maladies.

However, these paragraphs are not intended to cover the use of sunlight as a treatment, but to give a few simple rules to prevent sickness. Sunlight as a treatment should be taken under the guidance of a physician.

The following quotations from the author of "Ministry of Healing" are comprehensive, practical, and easy to understand and follow:

"Life in the open air is good for body and mind. It is God's medicine for the restoration of health. Pure air, good water, sunshine, the beautiful surroundings of nature—these are His means for restoring the sick to health in natural ways. To the sick it is worth more than silver or gold to live in the sunshine or in the shade of the trees." (34)

"In buildings, many make careful provision for their plants and flowers. The greenhouse or window devoted to their use is warm and sunny; for without warmth, air and sunshine, plants would not live and flourish. If these conditions are necessary to the life of plants, how much more necessary are they for our own health and that of our families and guests!" (35)

"If we would have our homes the abiding-place of health and happiness, we must place them above the miasma and fog of the lowlands, and give free entrance to heaven's life-giving agencies. Dispense with heavy curtains, open the windows and the blinds, allow no vines, however beautiful, to shade the windows, and permit no trees to stand so near the house as to shut out the sunshine. The sunlight may fade the drapery and the carpets, and tarnish the picture-frames; but it will bring a healthy glow to the cheeks of the children." (36)

"Shade trees and shrubbery too close and dense around a house are unhealthful; for they prevent a free circulation of air, and shut out the rays of the sun. In consequence of this, dampness gathers in the house. Especially in wet seasons the sleeping rooms become damp, and those who occupy them are troubled with rheumatism, neuralgia, and lung complaints which generally end in consumption. Numerous shade trees cast off many leaves, which, if not immediately removed, decay, and poison the atmosphere. A yard beautiful with trees and shrubbery, at a proper distance from the house, has a happy, cheerful influence upon the family, and if well taken care of, will prove no injury to health. Dwellings, if possible, should be built upon high and dry ground. If a house is built where water settles around it, remaining for a time, and then drying away, a poisonous miasma arises, and fever and ague, sore throat, lung diseases, and fevers will be the result." (37)

"The guest-chamber should have equal care with the rooms intended for constant use. Like the other bedrooms it should have air and sunshine, and should be provided with some means of heating to dry out the dampness that always accumulates in a room not in constant use. Whoever sleeps in a sunless room, or occupies a bed that has not been thoroughly dried and aired, does so at the risk of health, and often of life." (38)

Cleanliness

"A great amount of suffering might be saved if all would labor to prevent disease, by strictly obeying the laws of health. Strict habits of cleanliness should be observed. Many, while well, will not take the trouble to keep in a healthy condition. They neglect personal cleanliness, and are not careful to keep their clothing pure. Impurities are constantly and imperceptibly passing from the body, through the pores, and if the surface of the skin is not kept in a healthy condition, the system is burdened with impure matter. If the clothing worn is not often washed, and frequently aired, it becomes filthy with impurities which are thrown off from the body by sensible and insensible perspiration. And if the garments worn are not frequently cleansed from these impurities the pores of the skin absorb again the waste matter thrown off. The impurities of the body, if not allowed to escape, are taken back into the blood, and forced upon the internal organs. Nature, to relieve herself of poisonous impurities, makes an effort to free the system. This effort produces fevers, and what is termed disease. But even then, if those who are afflicted would assist Nature in her efforts, by the use of pure, soft water, much suffering would be prevented. But many, instead of doing this, and seeking to remove the poisonous matter from the system, take a more deadly poison into the system, to remove a poison already there." (39)

"Most persons would receive benefit from a cool or tepid bath every day, morning or evening. Instead of increasing the liability to take cold, a bath, properly taken, fortifies against cold, because it improves the circulation; the blood is brought to the surface, and a more easy and regular flow is obtained. The mind and the body are alike invigorated. The muscles become more flexible, the intellect is made brighter. The bath is a soother of the nerves. Bathing helps the bowels, the stomach, and the liver, giving health and energy to each, and it promotes digestion." (40)

"If every family realized the beneficial results of thorough cleanliness, they would make special efforts to remove every impurity from their persons, and from their houses, and would extend their efforts to their premises. They are not awake to the influence of these things; there is constantly arising from these decaying substances an effluvium that is poisoning the air. By inhaling the impure air, the blood is poisoned, the lungs become affected, and the whole system is diseased. Disease of almost every description will be caused by inhaling the atmosphere affected by these decaying substances.

"Families have been afflicted with fevers, some of their members have died, and the remaining portion of the family circle have almost murmured against their Maker because of their distressing bereavements, when the sole cause of all their sickness and death has been the result of their own carelessness. The impurities about their own premises have brought upon them contagious diseases, and the sad afflictions which they charge upon God. Every family that prizes health should cleanse their houses and their premises of all decaying substances." (41)

"Every form of uncleanliness tends to disease. Death-producing germs abound in dark, neglected corners, in decaying refuse, in dampness and mold and must. No waste vegetables or heaps of fallen leaves should be allowed to remain near the house, to decay and poison the air. Nothing unclean or decaying should be tolerated within the home. In towns or cities regarded perfectly healthful, many an epidemic of fever has been traced to decaying matter about the dwelling of some careless householder.

"Perfect cleanliness, plenty of sunlight, careful attention to sanitation in every detail of the home life, are essential to freedom from disase and to the cheerfulness and vigor of the inmates of the home." (42)

Sugar

How The Body Uses Sugar

Sugar is a very important element in nutrition, but its nature and use are little understood by most people. Concerning it there is popular misunderstanding and confusion. The easy way to understand the matter is to begin with sugar as it is found in normal, healthy blood, where, for every thousand parts of blood, one part must be sugar,—the substance the body cells burn to produce heat and energy for use by all parts of the body. About sixteen ounces of sugar is so used daily in the body of a person weighing 154 pounds doing normal work.

This blood sugar is derived from certain kinds of food. The body can convert a portion of the protein and fat intake into this sugar (glucose), but the larger part of the body's supply is secured from starch and sugar. (160)

Storage of Sugar

When taken in three meals to provide for 24 hours' need, the supply is not uniform or steady enough; there is apt to be either a "feast" or a "famine." Too large amounts would accumulate in the blood at one time unless there were some way to regulate it. For this reason temporary storage is provided in the skin, muscles, and liver. The liver stores sugar in a "compressed" form called "glycogen," and on demand from the blood it releases it again as glucose for use as needed. When it is stored in the skin no chemical change takes place in it as it is simply an outflow from the blood stream and an inflow back into it which is called storage by "inundation." The storage of glucose in the cells is called storage by "segregation" which is more complicated than storage by "inundation." Shortage in the cells and release from them is thought to be under the control of the nervous system in cooperation with glands of internal secretion.

Sugar and the Kidneys

This concentration of sugar in the blood fluctuates from 100 milligrams of sugar in 100 cubic centimeters of blood to 180 milligrams. When it exceeds 180 milligrams the kidneys release the excess into the urine and it is lost from the body. The level at which the kidneys release the sugar is called the "threshold."

The constant handling of large excesses of sugar by these kidney cells is held by some writers to be one cause of kidney cell damage. (161)

Sugar and the Pancreas

Sugar is rapidly absorbed from the digestive tract into the blood and if large amounts are eaten at a time so that it enters the blood faster than the body can use or store it, the result will be a "high tide" of sugar in the blood. It is said that in this case the pancreas secretes a larger amount of insulin than it normally does. If this is continued over a considerable period until the cells of the pancreas are depleted, diabetes could result. (162)

Sources of Sugar

The term "sugar" is applied to several types of sweet substances, some of which are excellent food while others are irritants to the digestive tract while being prepared to go into the blood stream. It is important that we know the difference between the helpful and harmful types.

Simple Sugar

First we will consider the form of sugar as it is found in normal blood as used in the body. It is known as a "simple" or "single" sugar called a "monosaccharide" because it is the simplest form in which sugar is found and cannot be further broken down. This is the form in which sugar passes from the small intestine into the blood.

The chemist says every molecule of this sugar is made of 24 atoms,—6 atoms of carbon, 6 of oxygen, and 12 of hydrogen, associated together. He diagrams a representative molecule as follows; C means carbon, O is for oxygen, and H is hydrogen:

```
        H—C—O
        H—C—O—H
    H—O—C—H
        H—C—O—H
        H—C—O—H
        H—C—O—H
        H
```

GLUCOSE, DEXTROSE, AND GRAPE SUGAR (Group 1)

There are three groups of these single sugars, of which this is the first to be discussed.

These sugars are used by the cells to produce heat and energy as already explained, but if they are held too long in the digestive tract they will be attacked by fermentive bacteria which derive energy for their growth by the partial oxidation of sugar. The chief products of this fermentation are carbon dioxide and alcohol which will be a curse to the body instead of the blessing as was intended.

These sugars come from the juices of fruits and the saps of plants; even the starch of seeds, roots, bulbs, stems and leaves, like cereals, potatoes, mature peas and corn, ripe apples and bananas, is broken down by the saliva, pancreatic juice and the intestinal juice to glucose, ready for the blood. (This break-down of starch is aided by heat, as in cooking.)

During this process of breaking down starch to a single sugar it passes through two other states, dextrin and maltose.

FRUCTOSE (Group 2)

Another single-molecule sugar is fructose found in fruit and juices and honey.

GALACTOSE (Group 3)

This single sugar is a constituent of lactose which occurs in milk.

The foregoing three groups of sugar are natural to the body and are proper food for it.

However, it is important that nothing hinder the digestive processes because delay gives time for fermentation of these sugars before they reach the blood. (163)

THE MOST COMMON SUGAR

The sugar most commonly used is not included in any of the foregoing groups, and is not natural to the body, and is a very unfavorable food. It is "sucrose," a double-molecule wherein two single molecules similar to the diagram already given, are linked together, like one molecule of glucose and one of fructose tied together. (To separate these two molecules twice the number of water molecules as of the sucrose present are required.) These two single sugar molecules when separated are natural to the body, but when linked together they irritate any tissue they contact. They cannot be separated by the saliva in the mouth or the gastric juice in the stomach, and while they are finally separated in the small intestine and enter the blood as simple natural sugar, their separation is made after considerable delay, and with difficulty; and until they are separated they are strong irritants to the cells of the mucous membranes of the mouth, stomach, duodenum and small intestine. This irritation often causes serious trouble.

We do not like to say,—but it is necessary in order to be faithful to the welfare of the readers of this book,—that the sugar described in the above paragraph is the common sugar which is made from sugar cane, beets, and the sap of the maple tree.

CANE SUGAR AN IRRITANT

In an experiment with cane sugar in the stomach, a solution of which 5.7 per cent was sugar produced reddening of the mucous membrane; with a 10 per cent solution the membrane became dark red, and a 20 per cent solution produced pain and distress. (164)

Cane sugar acts upon the tissues like a chemical substance, such as an acid or caustic. A bit of raw flesh placed in a strong solution of sugar soon becomes shrunken in appearance because of the abstraction of water which the sugar absorbs. Candy injures the mucous membrane of the stomach, and candy eaters often suffer from gastritis." (165)

Cane, beet, maple sugar and sorghum all are irritants and contribute to gastric catarrh, acidity, various forms of indigestion, ulcer of the stomach, hyperacidity, congestion, etc. (166)

Sherman states that sugar in quantity or concentrated form is an irritant to the stomach. (167)

SUGAR IS THE WORST FOOD

"The daily consumption of sugar in the United States, most of it refined sugar, averages per capita approximately five and one-half ounces. The addition to the diet of this material, representing more than six hundred calories, or one-fourth of all the calories of the diet, and carrying no vitamins and no minerals, is a major nutritional error. Nutritionists agree that of all food, sugar unquestionably is the worst." (168)

SWEET FOODS SUBSTITUTE BETTER FOODS

There is still another phase of this question of sugar. Not only is cane sugar an irritant to the digestive tract, but it often becomes a substitute for better foods by satisfying the appetite before the better foods are taken and so results in impaired nutrition.

THE LESSON

The sugars derived from sugar cane, beets, and the maple tree are all unfavorable foods. The trouble is not caused by the refining of the sugars but by the nature of the sugar.

The writer has not found any satisfactory explanation of why this particular double molecule of sugar is irritating while others are not,—only the fact that it is thus.

The molecules of the unrefined sugars are the same as in the refined. They also contain impurities which are said to be irritating. It is true that the refining process removes useful minerals, but this is not the cause of the irritant effect of the sugar.

A minor exception should be made to the above statement concerning the unrefined sugar molecules, in that when unrefined sugar is allowed to stand, inversion takes place to some extent and hence some invert sugar is contained in the common brown sugars found in the market.

There is one bright spot in the cane sugar question. When it is united with water and acids and boiled, it is separated into single molecules the same as is done by digestion. Therefore when it is used in canning fruits, it is, in the canning process under the influence of water, heat, and acid, inverted to single molecules and so, used in that way is an acceptable food. The same is true in case fruit is canned without sugar and the sugar is added and the fruit heated when it is opened.

A summary of the points to be remembered is as follows:

(1) The natural sugars and starches as they occur in natural foods are the most healthful sweets.

(2) Of the concentrated sweets, honey and corn syrup are to be given preference.

(3) The lower we can reduce the use of cane sugar, brown sugar from which it is derived, and sorghum in our foods (except when it is cooked into fruit) the better it will be for us. The best way is to make fewer of those foods which require cane sugar, another way is to substitute honey and corn syrup in its place in recipes where they will be acceptable. This will require a bit of experimental cooking and perhaps some adjustments in our appetites, but we will be abundantly rewarded.

Sugar Substitutes

Some people who crave sweets and realize their harmfulness, or perhaps have disabled the pancreas and so cannot use them, and have not learned to re-educate their appetites, turn to sugar substitutes as a way out of their dilemma. Such a course is not safe, as the following citations will show.

There are a number of products on the market which are used in the place of sugars, but they are harmful to the digestive tract and should not be used. Among these are saccharin, dulcin, and glucin. These sweeteners are not allowed to be used in food products. (135)

"Saccharin belongs to the great family of coal tar products, many of which are active heart poisons, hence it is not surprising that careful observation has shown it to be a highly injurious drug." (136)

"Under its influence the heart's action is lessened in vigor and its continued use may give rise to serious injury." (137)

The re-education of our taste desires is easier than many people think. It begins by securing a knowledge of that which is good for the health of the body. It is then followed by a balanced ration of good foods which in time becomes so satisfying that the appetite is satisfied without the former usual amounts of sweet foods. From that point forward the interest in concentrated sweets declines until, with many people, they cease to be sources of special temptation; the desire for them has been superseded by desires for better foods. That the reader may achieve this high ideal is the purpose of this chapter.

HONEY

Most nutritionists regard honey as a more favorable sweet than the refined sugars. Believing that those who read this book will be interested in the following article we include it here after discussing sugar. Sometimes the price of honey is high. There is one way to cut the price,—move to the country and keep your own bees.

"The almost universal craving for sweets, especially in children, best proves that there is a true need for them in the human system. The two invert sugars that honey contains (75 per cent in most grades) have many advantages as food substances. Ordinary sugar, also starch, must undergo digestion, a process that changes them into simple sugars the same as, or similar to, those found in honey. The sugars of honey, therefore, may be considered as predigested; hence the use of honey takes a load of work off the stomach and pancreas.

"Dr. G. N. W. Thomas of Edinburgh, Scotland, says: 'In heart weakness I have found honey to have a marked effect in reviving the heart action and keeping patients alive. I had further evidence of this in a recent case of pneumonia. The patient consumed two pounds of honey during the illness; there was an early crisis, with no subsequent rise of temperature and an exceptionally good pulse. I suggest that honey should be given for general physical repair, and above all, for heart failure.'

"Dr. B. F. Beck of New York City declares that during his nearly half century of medical practice he has met many surprisingly energetic folk of advanced age with remarkably healthy complexions. In taking their histories, the report of a liberal daily dose of honey was often a part of the story.

"Many nervous states can be attributed to excessive sugar consumption. Our swift modern life requires rapid metabolism to create and to replace the much-needed physical and mental energy. Simple sugar can supply this need much better than can the ordinary refined products, which are not only hard to digest, but tend to cause such ills as gastric ulcer, renal diseases, and diabetes. Dr.

Beck states that 'sugar is just as habit-forming as narcotics, and its use, misuse, and abuse, a modern nutritional disaster. Viewing the many channels through which we find refined sugar getting into the alimentary canal, such as candy, ice cream, soft drinks, syrups, pastry, jams and jellies, besides the sugar bowl, it is not hard to believe." (169)

Juice Therapy

Juice therapy can be a great blessing in certain cases if properly used. Some cleansing procedures are somewhat severe and lower the energy. For those who need a cleansing program, the following is suggested, taken from the *Madison Health Messenger*, Madison College, Tenn., Vol. 4, No. 1. (43)

VITALITY CLEANSING REGIMEN

Spring housecleaning for our physical bodies is just as advisable as for the homes in which we live. Some people do this by fasting and turning to the out-of-doors for a few days, while others who are unable to take this time from their work do it by following a cleansing diet procedure. Various cleansing diets have been found effective aids in the treatment of rheumatism, arthritis, sinusitis, catarrh, hay fever, eczema, constipation, colitis, ulcers of the digestive tract, colds.

The splendid results obtained from this Vitality Cleansing Diet, which enables one to continue working, prompts us to publish it for those who are interested in a vitality cleansing regimen.

1. One 8-ounce glass of unsweetened, undiluted grape juice at night before retiring. If any discomfort results, dilute the grape juice, using half water and half grape juice. If this is not satisfactory, heat the diluted grape juice and drink it hot. For those who cannot tolerate unsweetened grape juice, add a little honey. Prune juice may be used to substitute grape juice, and if laxative effects are not obtained from the use of either grape juice or prune juice, use an 8-ounce glass of sauerkraut juice.

2. Upon arising in the morning, drink 4 ounces soy milk mixed with 4 ounces of carrot juice—total 8 ounces.

3. In two hours drink one 8-ounce glass of orange juice.

4. In two hours repeat the soy milk and carrot juice.

5. In two hours take one 8-ounce glass of tomato juice.

6. In two hours repeat the soy milk and carrot juice.

7. In two hours take one 8-ounce glass apple juice.

8. In two hours repeat the soy milk and carrot juice.

9. Before retiring, repeat the grape juice, prune juice, or sauer-kraut juice, whichever has been effective as a laxative. This laxative drink at night may be continued as long as its effects are normal.

10. In the course of the day, one teaspoonful of honey may be added to each of the four soy milk and carrot juice feedings.

It is important that liquid food be taken at least every two hours. If the energy is not kept up to requirements, the amount of soy milk and carrot juice and honey may be increased. The other liquids should remain the same.

This may be followed for several days or longer, as desired, after which vegetable soups, made of finely ground vegetables, and cream soups made of soy milk, should be the first food taken. Solid foods, such as whole wheat bread, raw carrots, spinach, etc., should be added gradually.

As solid foods are added, special attention should be given to the quantity of fresh fruits and vegetables used each day. Most people do not eat enough fresh fruits and vegetables. If the vegetable salads are eaten first, the chances are that more raw foods and less cooked foods will be eaten.

11. During the cleansing period all animal foods are eliminated. Soy beans, soy bean products, wheat gluten, nuts, and the proteins of other vegetables and grains serve to provide the body with adequate protein for optimum nutrition.

12. Eliminate the use of all forms of tobacco.

13. Eliminate the use of all alcoholic beverages, the so-called pop drinks, tea, coffee, etc.

It will be observed that liquid food is taken every two hours, beginning with soy milk and carrot juice, alternating with fruit juices. The soy milk provides the vegetable protein, and the juices provide the necessary minerals and vitamins. The kinds of juices may be varied as best suited to the individual; however, some orange juice, lemon juice, grapefruit juice, or tomato juice should be taken for the necessary amount of Vitamin C. Do not mix any other juices except carrot juice with the soy milk, as other juices may curdle the milk. It is permissible to drink other juices with the soy milk, but in this case the soy milk should be taken first, after which other juices may be taken.

THE SOYBEAN
The Wonder Food of the World

The soybean is rapidly coming to the front as a human food in the United States as well as other countries. There are good reasons for this. It has been the chief source of protein for Oriental peoples for millenniums. It is called the "meat without bones."

A Protein Food

The soybean is an abundant source of protein,—the richest of all foods except dried egg white.

Another authority gives the range from 34.1% to 46.9%. (138)

One ounce of soybeans contains 28.4 grams of protein.

Beans vs. Beef

Beef is 14.5 per cent protein while the soybean is 42.8 per cent protein. Some authorities rate them even higher.

Supplements Meat, Milk, and Eggs

Statements like the following are finding their way into medical literature more and more:

"Soybeans are one of the most valuable and tasty additions to modern menus. They are rich in protein, vitamins and minerals and are readily adaptable to large scale use as a supplement food to meat, milk, and eggs.

"There is an infinite variety in the ways soybeans may be utilized for food and in cooking. They may be served as a vegetable or in the form of flour, soy oil margarine, soy sauce, or soybean vegetable milk. Soy flour is being added to baby foods, dehydrated soups, ice cream, cakes and cookies in order to increase the nutritive values of these foods." (139)

Its Protein Is Adequate

"The protein of the Soybean was found to be adequate for promoting normal growth and to be 'physiologically good.' " (140)

"As Good As Meat, Eggs, and Milk"

The proteins of the soybeans "are as good as the proteins of milk, meat and egg. . . . Some nutritional experts go so far as to say that the soybean protein is akin to human protein and superior to any other known protein . . . an unequalled source of protein substances for human needs." (141)

In an article describing the soybean a recent writer said,—"It is thus no longer necessary to keep a cow to enjoy a quart of milk a day or to have cheese or meat." (142)

Infant Feeding

"Soybean protein is an excellent substitute for animal protein, and, therefore, is valuable to those who are allergic or hypersensitive to animal proteins.

"Since the proteins are about 85% digestible, soybean products have also given very good results in infant feeding. Macey F. Deming, who has made an extensive study of soybeans, says that when properly prepared in suitable combination, they make one of the best foods for infants.

"According to Dr. T. Brooke, Fort Health Officer at Singapore, soybeans contain the essentials for a perfect diet and in better proportions than found in any other commonly used foods." (143)

Milk Shake To Steak

News items like the following are frequent:

Magazine "Time" in its issue of Sept. 27, 1943, science department, carried an article entitled "Down With Meat." It referred to government warnings that there is a shortage of meat protein, and to the efforts of food scientists to find supplementary and substitute foods.

It reported that Harvard workers announce that we can get along nicely with not more than one ounce of real meat daily, i.e. only a tenth of one's daily protein need come from meat, eggs, and milk.

It also stated that Yale workers assert that soybeans rival meat in protein; that from soybeans one may secure a great variety of foods from milk shakes to steaks.

Thus there is a sharp trend toward supplementing meat, eggs, and milk with the soybean.

Such announcements reveal a rapid change in the thinking of scientific nutritionists who are now demonstrating the soundness of the highest standards taught in this book, i.e. that it is not necessary to use meat, eggs, or milk if we have a variety of the natural foods, including the soybean, and learn how to balance them.

Wheat and Soybean Combined

When the soybean is combined with wheat in proportions of 20 to 80 the efficiency of the wheat protein is increased from two to three times. (144) (170)

This indicates that we should find as many ways as possible of working it into foods where wheat flour is used. This is an ideal way of "enriching" wheat flour.

Economy

The most economical way to secure protein is in the soybean where it costs not more than one-fourth as much as in beefsteak, when purchased in the form of beans or flour.

Rich in Oil

The soybean is from 14% to 24% oil of a very high quality.

"Another of the unique nutritive qualities of green vegetable soybeans is the richness and digestibility of the oil. It is interesting to note that the oil is more highly digestible than most food fats and oils. Thus in spite of the high oil content present in the soybean, the tissues and organs readily oxidize this oil instead of storing it as excess weight. For this reason the soybean is considered as a nonfattening food and therefore recommended as a food that is valuable in reducing body weight.

"Some nutritional experts claim that the quality of the soybean oil is akin to the fat of animal origin and even superior to butter fat.

"Because of these unique qualities, the soybean oil, for human consumption, occupies a place of distinction when compared to other fats and oils." (145)

Lecithin

The soybean is rich in this important nerve food, one pound of soybean flour containing as much as from 4 to 6 eggs. (146)

Base-forming; Saves Protein

It has been established that when there is a big excess of bases over acids in the food and in the body the protein in the food is used more efficiently, and that a real minimum for protein requirement can be found only when such an excess of base elements is present.

This excess of base elements over acid in the soybean is given by different authors from 31.24 c.c. of N solution (per 100 grams) to 42.00. (See A. A. Horvath on "The Nutritional Value of Soybeans" in "The American Journal of Digestive Diseases" May 1938). Others give a lower figure; nevertheless, it is granted by all that the alkalinity of the soybean is high.

"The conclusion to be drawn from these findings is that the alkalinity of the soybean ash is a highly important factor for causing a saving in protein, and this is probably the main part of the explanation why experimental data showed that a human organism is able to store three times as much nitrogen from soybean food as from meat." (147)

Base-forming; Anti-fatigue

This high alkalinity of the soybean has given it the reputation of being a very potent anti-fatigue food, possibly the very best. Experimental data is given by Horvath. (148)

Vitamins

The chief contribution of soybeans to our vitamin needs is in B-1 and B-2. The sprouts are, of course, rich in vitamin C.

Iron; A Blood Builder

The soybean is very effective in regenerating the hemoglobin of the blood and therefore stands at the head of the list of foods to protect against anemia.

"It has been established that the iron in soybeans is 'available' to over 60 per cent, being equal to beef and pork liver, superior to beef muscle, and twice superior to spinach." (149)

Minerals

"Calcium is one of the most difficult things to get in any adequate quantity in any low cost diet. . . . Soybean flour is one of the cheapest sources of calcium." (150)

This food is rich in all of the other essential minerals as well as those already mentioned.

Easily, Quickly Digested

"Soya flour does not act as a strong stimulant for gastric acidity, but is rather acid reducing, does not overburden the stomach, and does not affect the normal course of gastric motility. The digestion of soya protein goes remarkably rapid, and the soya meal leaves the stomach mostly in 2½ to 3 hours, and in some cases even in 80 minutes." (151)

Digestibility of Protein High

Not only is its protein easy to digest but it is well digested so that it is nearly all used,—from 80 to 97 per cent; meaning that this percentage of the protein is made available for use in the body. The protein of soybean milk and of cow's milk have been found to be 84.9% and 86.6% respectively. (152)

Raised With Less Effort and Soil Depletion

The soybean can be grown "with less expenditure of human and motor power, as well as with soil depletion" than other foods. "Considering its high and fine nutritional value, an acre planted in soybeans gives the largest and greatest yield of any single source of food known." (153)

Varieties

There are more than 2000 distinct types of soybeans which have maturities ranging from 75 days to 200 days.

The larger part of them are used for commercial purposes and for animal feed.

Certain varieties have been used for human food. Those which require the least cooking are said to be: Easycook, Rokusum, Hokkaido, Chuesi, Kanro, and Jogun. Those next easiest to cook are Mammoth Yellow, Dixie, and Hahto.

Some people do not care for the flavor of soybeans. Some varieties have stronger undesirable flavors than others. The variety which this author enjoys the most is the Hahto. Nearly every one likes this variety. Try them. They are also known as soy limas. If they are hard to find, write to us.

Soybean Milk for Babies

Proper nourishment for babies and children is one of the most important phases of nutrition. Not only does their present well-being depend upon it, but their foundation for the future is now being laid, and they are now preparing either for long or shortened lives.

Therefore we must know for sure if the soybean milk is a satisfactory food for babies and children. To provide a basis of confidence in this matter we present the statements of authorities, research workers, experimenters, hospitals, doctors, and mothers who relate their experiences with the milk.

In the Orient

"If the dried beans . . . are soaked for a few hours, then finely crushed and boiled for about 30 minutes in the proportion of 3 parts of water to 1 of mash, a milky emulsion is obtained which is very similar in appearance and properties to animal milk. This liquid, separated out by means of a very fine sieve or cloth strainer, is the soybean or vegetable milk so extensively used in China. . . . In the absence of animal milk, soybean milk is used extensively in the fresh state and as the basis of various kinds of vegetable cheeses in Oriental countries." (154)

Soy Milk vs. Cow's Milk

"A great deal has been written and said indicating that the proteins of soybeans and soybean products are of exceptionally high order in human nutrition. . . . Kung and Fang have conducted nitrogen metabolism trials with preschool children comparing the proteins of soybeans to the proteins of cow's milk. The result of these experiments showed no marked difference for the children studied in the protein utilization of mixed diets when supplemented with soybean milk or cow's milk." (155)

Infants

"Soybean milk has been found useful in the feeding of infants who cannot tolerate cow's milk because of individual hypersensitivity." (156)

Hospital Work

"We use soybean milk as a substitute for cow's milk in feeding milk sensitive infants. . . . It is helpful in conditions of eczema. . . . It would be a satisfactory substitute for cow's milk for a normal child." (157)

Hospital

"It is good food. I use it only for children who cannot handle milk—such as severe infantile eczema." (158)

Hospital

"In cases in which infants are sensitive to cow's milk, soybean milk has been used with success." (159)

A Child Specialist Medical Doctor

A most enthusiastic user of soybean milk for babies is Dr. Samuel J. Levin, of the Children's Hospital in Detroit, Michigan. The Journal of Pedriatics, July, 1940 published an extended article from him describing his work. In a private letter he says:

"I use soybean milk exactly as I would whole milk. In other words, if a baby is getting a dilution of whole cow's milk, say twenty ounces of cow's milk, plus ten ounces of water, we would substitute soybean milk for the cow's milk in the same amount. If the child is getting undiluted cow's milk, I would use undiluted soybean milk. I have used soybean milk to pour on cereals instead of milk, when the child is on a milk free diet. . . . We are using it quite extensively at the Allergy Clinic at the Children's Hospital."

Samuel J. Levin, M.D.
Letter to Madison Foods
Aug. 14, 1939

An Enthusiastic Grandmother

"Dear Sirs:

On the advice of relatives in Kalamazoo who have used your soybean milk for their asthmatic baby for a year with wonderful results, we got some a week ago and started using it with our asthmatic grandson who is four months old. He is a fine husky big baby but had all the symptoms of a bad asthmatic condition,—

very hard labored breathing, eczema, nine boils on his head within a month's time, severe wheezing a great deal of the time, especially after taking his feeding; also had bad colic caused by severe gas pains, especially at night. Within twenty-four hours after starting the soybean milk there was a very definite change in him, and now, after using it for one week and two days he is a different baby. All the wheezing and labored breathing are gone entirely, the eczema is all gone, and no new boils, and no more gas. He is utterly relaxed and quiet and happy, which is the first time in his life. He has turned from a crying, restless, uncomfortable baby to the best baby I ever saw, and I have had six of my own. He still has plenty of 'pep' which shows he is well nourished. We all are so grateful for this wonderful food, and you can rest assured we will pass the good news along to the parents of other asthmatic babies." (Letter on file)

For Well Babies

If soybean milk makes sick babies well, would it be a good food for babies who are now well? Would it not help to protect them from future illness?

The writer believes in soybean milk for young and old.

Later in this book the reader will find instruction concerning calcium when the change is made from cow's milk to soybean milk. Careful attention should be given to this matter.

The Formula for Babies

Whatever formula has been provided based upon cow's milk will apply to soybean milk of a similar consistency.

An 8-oz. glass of the brand of soybean milk most familiar to the writer contains about 148 calories.

It should be supplemented with fruit juices and vegetable juices, the same as cow's milk.

It is slightly laxative whereas cow's milk inclines somewhat to constipation.

Soybean milk is very rich in iron where dairy milk is very low in that mineral.

Soybean milk is alkaline to about the same degree as human mother's milk. Its calcium content is right without dilution.

Analysis of Kreme O' Soy, A Standard Brand of Soybean Milk

	Kreme O'Soy Milk	Human Milk	Cow's Milk
Protein	3.5%	1.4%	3.5%
Fat	3.9%	3.7%	3.9%
Carbohydrates	4.9%	7.2%	4.9%
Ash	.7%	.2%	.7%
Calcium	.34%	.34%	1.22%
Phosphorus	.469%	.15%	.93%
Iron	4.4 mg/k	1.8 mg/k	2.4 mg/k
Copper	8.7 mg/k	.6 mg/k	.2 mg/k

Makes Costly Foods Cheap

"The most expensive food constituents are minerals, vitamins, proteins, and fats. Soy bean flour is rich in all these constituents, and yet relatively cheap. The moderate cost of soy bean flour makes it possible for people of small incomes to obtain the maximum of these essential constituents required by the body which in the form of other foods might be beyond their reach." (44)

Every family should study ways of making soy bean products a regular part of the menu. There are many ways of doing this; a few are suggested here.

How to Use Soy Beans

(1) *In Baking*

Soybean flour may be used in combination with wheat flour up to 30% of the mixture. Breads large and small may be made with 20 to 30% soybean flour. Such a mixture is truly an "enriched" flour.

(2) *In General Cooking*

Anywhere that flour is used, soybean flour may be included as a part of the mixture.

(3) *As Beans*

The dry beans may be cooked as other beans are cooked, except they require more cooking and need special flavoring. A cook book of the right sort will be helpful here. There is a great difference in the flavor of the different varieties. In the writer's home the Hahto variety is considered to be the best; it really tastes **good.**

(4) *As Beans Ready-Cooked*

Pre-cooked and flavored canned soybeans are appearing in the market in increasing variety, particularly may these be found in specialty health food stores.

(5) *As Vegetable Meat*

Very delicious "meat substitutes" are being made from soybeans and sold in the leading food stores of most of the large cities and many of the smaller ones. These come in cans like canned meats and are ready to serve. A cookbook will tell you many ways to prepare and serve them. When you buy them you get no bones or gristle to throw away, and no animal toxins or disease but get pure food. Many people say their flavors are superior to those of meats; others say "Just as good as meat!" which with them means a high compliment.

(6) *As Milk*

Very tasty and highly nutritious soybean milk is now sold in tin cans like canned cow's milk. It is also sold in powder form, made by dehydrating liquid soybean milk.

These various forms of vegetable milk are sold in Health Food stores and are finding their way more and more into regular trade food channels. They are not labeled "Milk," but use names such as Soyalac, Soya Malt, Kreme O'Soy, Soyagen, etc.

Several recipes are here given for making soybean milk for the benefit of those, who, for any reason cannot purchase it. Home recipes cannot produce as fine flavored milk as is done by experts and machinery, but it is quite acceptable.

Soybean milk may be used in almost any place where cow's milk is used, in cooking as well as a drink and on cereals. A new type of cooking is thus developed which grows more delightful as one proceeds with it. A special cook book for this kind of cooking is helpful. The writer is earnestly looking forward to the time when soybean milk will be made and sold in a volume which will make it possible to purchase it in every large city at the same price as dairy milk or even less.

SOYBEAN MILK

Recipe No. 1—Use Flour—The simplest of all
12 cups boiling water
  3 cups soy flour   }beaten with egg beater
3½ cups cold water   }and stirred into boiling water
  1 Tablespoon salt
  3 Tablespoons dark Karo
Put into double boiler and cook for 1 hour.
Strain when cold.

This milk will cost much less than cow's milk.

Recipe No. 2—Use Flour—Kloss Formula

2 Tablespoons soy flour (heaping)
2 Cups cold water
2 Tablespoons soy oil
1 Tablespoon malt or cellulose sugar

Place the flour into a frying pan, add the cold water and stir until a smooth paste is made. Cook over a slow heat until it thickens, stirring constantly to prevent sticking onto the pan and burning. To this cooked mixture add the soy oil and beat until it disappears. Salt to taste, add the sweetening and enough water to make the consistency of milk.

Recipe No. 3—Use Beans and Liquifier

Soak two cups soybeans over night. Wash and pick over after soaking. Liquify beans as follows:

Put a cup of water and a cup of the beans in the liquifier, turn on motor until fine, then add another cup and a half of water, let run until well pulverized.

Strain through a cloth sack. Place to cook in a double boiler. In order to handle the amount of milk this will make, it is best to use a large pan with something in the bottom such as a few nails, then a smaller pan to hold the milk.

Let cook gently for about twenty minutes (after boiling starts in the outer pan). Take a cup of the cooled milk, put in the liquifier, slowly add ¼ cup oil (soy preferred) beat only enough to emulsify the oil, then put in the milk, adding 1 tablespoon Karo or honey, 1 teaspoon salt. If raw taste is gone remove from fire and cool at once. If not, cook a little longer. After adding the last ingredients if additional cooking is necessary you must stir frequently. It may curdle if it is not stirred.

Recipe No. 4—Use Beans and Grinder.

Wash the dry soybeans and soak overnight. In hot weather keep them cool with ice while soaking. Remove the skins and grind them into a coarse meal. It is well to let a little water trickle through while the beans are being ground. Put the ground beans in a cheese cloth bag, place in a bowl of lukewarm water, using three quarts of water to each pound of dry beans. Work thoroughly with the hands five to ten minutes. Wring the bag of pulp until dry. Boil the milk on a low fire for thirty minutes and stir to prevent scorching; or a double boiler may be used and avoid danger of scorching. Add dextrose and salt to taste. Keep in a cool place, like milk is kept, until used.

The pulp left after making milk from the beans may be used in a variety of ways as a base for vegetable roasts and other meat substitute entrees. This pulp has a high food value. When making milk from flour as in recipes No. 1 and No. 2, more of the content of the bean goes into the milk and less by-product is strained out than when using recipes No. 3 and No. 4.

(7) *As Cream*

Home-made cream can be made by using the milk recipe and greatly reducing the amount of water, and adding extra oil.

(8) *As Cheese*

A very satisfactory soybean cheese is now available in the health food stores. It has a texture something like cottage cheese, and may be used in many ways similar to cottage cheese. Here again a special cookbook is helpful.

(9) *As Oil*

The oil from the soybean is of excellent quality; it is an excellent cooking oil and can be used wherever cooking oil is used. It has a flavor which some people do not like.

(10) *As Home-made Soy Butter*

4 tablespoons of soy flour
4 tablespoons of water

Mix well, and cook four minutes or less

Add one cup soybean oil and beat with a rotary beater till the oil disappears

If color is wanted add a little of some kind of butter color

Add a little salt to suit taste.

This so-called butter is very satisfactory as a spread for bread, but cannot be used in every way that butter is used. It is a very wholesome food, can easily be made at home and is very inexpensive.

(11) *As Home-made Soy Mayonnaise*
To above Soy Butter
Add 1 to 3 drops of garlic juice, to suit taste
One-half teaspoonful celery seed
One-fourth teaspoonful celery salt
Paprika to give a little color
Juice of one or two lemons, depending on how acid it is wanted.

If less color is wanted, leave out the color when making the butter at the beginning.

This mayonnaise will be found to be a very satisfactory, practical, and economical food.

(12) *As Soy Acidophilus Milk*
The following formula for making this health drink at home is taken from the Madison Health Messenger, published by Madison Foods, Madison College, Tennessee.

Pour contents of 29 oz. can of soy milk into a 1 or 2 quart glass jar, and heat to body temperature (98.6 degrees—lukewarm) by placing the jar into a large vessel containing warm but not hot water. Stir constantly. Then add 2 teaspoonfuls liquid acidophilus culture and put in a warm place about body temperature (98.6 degrees), placing cap on jar but not air tight. The milk will be thick and ready in about 10 hours. Then stir, add salt desired to taste, and place in refrigerator. Out of this milk save 6 tablespoonfuls and use this in the next batch of milk instead of the culture, and it will require only 6 hours to prepare the milk. Three or four batches of milk may be made this way as long as it is kept well refrigerated after it is made. As soon as the flavor of the milk is too sharp, start over, using the pure culture.

In the preparation of soy acidophilus milk, it is important that the area in which it is prepared be clean and free from air currents that may carry dust laden with contaminating germs. Everything used should be as sterile as possible. The top of the can of soy milk should be placed in boiling hot water and then held over a hot plate till the water is dried off. Puncture two small holes in the top of the can with an ice pick or can opener that has been immersed in boiling hot water. When the milk is poured into the jar, the can should not touch the jar nor should the can be held over the opening of the jar any more than is necessary to pour the milk into it. The lid of the jar should be boiled. The surfaces worked on should be scrubbed with strong soap solution, and absolutely clean cloths and towels should be used to dry hands, etc. No cloths or towels should be used that have been used for anything previously. Spoons and implements used for stirring, etc., should be boiled first. Foreign bacteria are present almost everywhere, and due care must be exercised to prevent the transfer to the milk. With reasonable care in following the directions given, the soy acidophilus milk can be prepared successfully from the very first attempt.

The acidophilus bacillus is the healthy bacteria in the intestinal tract that destroys the putrefactive bacteria. The acidophilus bacillus in the normal intestinal tract will take care of the putrefactive bacteria without any aid; however, in most cases the intestinal tract is not normal and therefore needs some assistance, which can be given in this way.

The bacteria which are sought in acidophilus milk grow more vigorously in soybean milk than in cow's milk so that they are 50 per cent larger, exceed the number by 50 to 100 per cent, are more robust, and live longer, which means they do the user that much more good.

Acidophilus bacillus culture may be obtained from large drug stores.

NOTICE—Soy acidophilus milk is often called soy buttermilk.

(13) *As Greens; Sprouts*

The sprouts of soybeans make a very popular and nutritious food throughout the Orient, and should become popular here. They rank very high in vitamin C.

They add to the variety of greens, and they make it possible to have greens when one may not obtain them in other ways, regardless of season or conditions.

They are good as a salad, or cooked slightly with a little soy sauce added.

We give below the Chinese method of sprouting the beans:

Prepare a receptacle over which to stretch several thicknesses of cheese cloth, which will catch water which drips through the cheese cloth. Spread the beans on the cloth. Cover them with other layers of cheese cloth. Sprinkle with water several times each day. Do not let them get dry. Keep at ordinary room temperature. When the sprouts are small they may be eaten beans and all. As the sprouts grow longer, eat only the sprouts. They will start sprouting quicker if first soaked over night.

The University of Illinois College of Agriculture suggests this:

"Soybean (sprouts) can be grown indoors, and with the equipment usually found in the home kitchen. They require from ten to twenty minutes cooking and can be served in a number of ways to add variety and interest to winter menus.

The first requisite for sprouting soybeans is to select a variety that will germinate readily. Soak the soybeans over night, then put them into a flowerpot, a sink strainer or colander, or any utensil that has holes in it for drainage and that can be covered. Be sure the container is sufficient in size, for the beans swell to at least six times their original bulk as they sprout. Cover the container and leave them in a warm, dark place. Light seems to make them develop an undesirable color.

At least four or five times each day during the sprouting period, flood or sprinkle the beans with lukewarm water. In four to six days the sprouts should be from two to three inches long and ready to use.

"Soybean sprouts can be used in salads, steamed and seasoned, panned with a small amount of onion or other seasoning, as chives or parsley, or combined with other vegetables."

(14) *As Soy Sauce*

This is a delicious flavoring which is very helpful in soups, stews, gravies, certain vegetable dishes like cooked greens, vegetable baked beans, lima beans, string beans, salads, and many other things.

It is especially helpful when people are making the change from flesh-eating to vegetarianism.

(15) *As Coffee*

Coffee substitutes made largely from the soy bean are now available. Some people cannot tell the difference between them and coffee; others say they are better. They contain no caffeine. They, of course, contain very little food value and perhaps their chief use is to make it easy to discontinue the use of coffee and tea.

(16) *As Substitute for Egg-white*

There is a soybean protein preparation that will whip like egg-whites. It will not make a meringue. It is used commercially in making cream nougats and similar products. It is not yet available to the general public.

The Ideal Vegetarian Regimen

There is an increasing number of people who wish either to entirely discard the use of all animal products as foods, or who wish to work toward that end. They look with increasing suspicion upon not only the flesh of dead animals, but upon eggs, butter, cheese, cream, and milk.

Their leading reasons for wanting to eliminate all flesh and animal products are that flesh, even of healthy animals, is filled with toxic wastes on the way to the excretory organs, kidneys, lungs, and pores,—and that disease is rapidly increasing among animals, making not only their flesh unsafe, but also increasing the dangers of using the products of the animal kingdom.

Concerning the non-use of meat, fish, and fowl, the chapter "Eating for Strength" of this book gives an abundance of evidence that, as a rule, better health and greater endurance can be obtained without them in those localities where grains, vegetables, legumes, fruits, and nuts are available. By discarding flesh no problem of nutrition is raised other than that of learning how to organize a balanced ration from the other foods,—the direct products of the earth. How this may be easily done has been abundantly shown in the previous chapters of this book.

But the ideal which is taking shape in the minds of many people goes farther than the non-use of flesh.

One writer said in 1902 that "disease in animals is increasing in proportion to the increase of wickedness among men," which is in harmony with Holy Writ; and that because of it "the time would come when there will be no safety in using eggs, milk, cream, or butter, and that the people should be taught how to prepare food without those things." (45)

The same writer in the same year expressed the thought that the knowledge of natural foods and their preparation without any animal products will be, to those who make use of them now in these days of multiplying diseases, what the manna was to Israel in the wilderness of which the Scriptures say He "rained down manna upon them to eat, and had given them the corn of heaven. Man did eat angel's food. . . . And there was not one feeble person among their tribes." Ps. 78:24, 25, Ps. 105:37. (46) It seems that the manna was a factor in the good health program in those days of extremity, and that natural foods are to perform the same sort of a ministry today for those who are open to the fullness of light concerning healthful living and have set their hearts on passing triumphantly through the closing days of earth's history.

This manner of living is not urged upon anyone, but the information given here merely points the way to those who wish to follow it, and makes suggestions to those who are interested in this way of living, and gives the scientific solution of the nutritional problems which arise in making the changes to a strict vegetarian regimen.

Each one of the foods in question will now be briefly discussed. They are recognized as having valuable food qualities, and their advantages will be placed against their disadvantages so the reader can make his decision intelligently.

EGGS

Advantages	Disadvantages
1. High quality of protein	1. Acid-forming
2. Vitamins A, B1, riboflavin, nicotinic acid, and D	2. Adds to an excess of protein
3. Iron and phosphorus	3. Quick to putrefy in the digestive tract
4. Fat	4. Aids growth of germs
	5. Potential carrier of animal disease
	6. Source of allergy

Inasmuch as the desirable factors of eggs all came originally from the natural food products of vegetation, it is possible to secure them from their original sources. If one will study and follow the teachings of this book on the selection of foods and a balanced ration, the disuse of eggs will be no nutritional problem. The factors to be especially safeguarded are the vitamins. Study the list of foods providing the same vitamins. A change in cooking methods is necessary.

BUTTER

Advantages	Disadvantages
1. Fat	1. High content of cholesterol
2. Vitamins A,* B1, riboflavin, nico-tinic acid, D, and E.	2. Difficult to digest, hinders digestion of other foods
	3. Stimulating
*90 per cent of the margarine sold in the U. S. has the vitamin A potency of good butter.	4. High bacteria count
	5. Potential carrier of animal diseases to man. Tuberculosis germs have been found in butter six months old.
	6. Source of allergy

Its elements were first derived from vegetation and may now be secured there by those who have access to the natural foods listed early in this book. Sufficient fat is easily secured from other sources; so may the vitamins if careful attention is given to the matter.

CHEESE
(American Cheddar)

Advantages	Disadvantages
1. Excellent protein	1. Product of putrefaction
2. Fat	2. High bacteria content
3. Minerals, calcium and phosphorus	3. Aids growth of germs
4. Vitamin A, riboflavin	4. Potential carrier of animal disease to man
	5. Difficult to digest
	6. Contributes to constipation
	7. Source of allergy

CHEESE
(Cottage Cheese, Sweet Cream Cheeses)

Advantages	Disadvantages
1. Excellent protein	1. Aids growth of germs
2. Fat	2. High bacteria count
3. Minerals, calcium and phosphorus	3. Potential carrier of animal disease to man
4. Lactic acid	4. Source of allergy
5. Vitamin A	

Once more we must say that inasmuch as the valuable elements contained in the cheeses came originally from vegetation it is apparent that they still may be secured there if we will take the pains to do so, and if we have access to the variety of natural foods. A little study is required, but the necessary information will be found in the pages of this book.

MILK—CREAM

In the opinion of scientific nutritionists the most difficult food to be spared from the list of animal products is milk. Each year that passes it is made by some teachers, an increasingly important item in human nutrition. And yet, the foregoing pages have given plenty of scientific evidence that the milk of cows is not a necessity to humankind, and that better health may be enjoyed from another way of living.

The following discussion is not an effort to insist that the use of milk be discontinued by those who wish to use it, but it is intended to give the latest information concerning the advantages and disadvantages in its use, and to provide scientifically adequate balanced rations without milk for those, who, for any reason, may wish to exclude it from the diet, so that no nutritional deficiency will result. The objective is better health, not weakness and disease.

MILK—CREAM

Advantages	Disadvantages
1. Excellent protein	1. High bacteria count
2. Fat	2. Aids growth of germs
3. Vitamins A, B1, riboflavin, nicotinic acid	3. Potential carrier of animal disease
4. Minerals, calcium and phosphorus	4. Contributes to constipation
	5. Source of allergy

It is granted that these food factors are of great importance, which is the reason this book carefully teaches how the same elements may be secured without the disadvantages named above.

Milk and Constipation

There is a difference of opinion here, but there are so many workers of such wide clinical experience who hold that, especially with adults, it often causes fermentation, constipation and biliousness, that this tendency of milk can hardly be ignored.

Milk and Allergy

That milk is a common source of allergy will be denied by none. There are large numbers of children who have an aversion to milk. Authorities in London reported that with such children it caused nausea, vomiting, diarrhea, headache, catarrh; others report abdominal pains, asthma, and eczema. Kellogg reported—"Another point to which attention should be called in the interest of both infants and invalids is the fact that certain persons become sensitized to milk as well as to other forms of protein; and in a person who is sensitized, even the smallest amount of milk may give rise to dangerous or even fatal symptoms. Many infants die annually from this cause." (53)

See the chapter on "The Animal Kingdom" for more information about milk.

Concerning eczema, see the page in this book devoted to that subject.

Calcium in Milk the Last Stand

In the opinions of some scientific nutritionists it is easier to spare eggs, butter, cream, and cheese from the diet than to spare the milk, and that the greatest danger in removing milk from the diet is from a deficiency of calcium, especially with children and with expectant and nursing mothers. Therefore this is the most serious problem in connection with this group of foods.

We shall now undertake to show how an adqeuate supply of calcium can be secured, by young or old, without milk.

Calcium Study No. 1

The minimum daily calcium requirement is said to be .45 grams for an adult and .90 grams for children, expectant and nursing mothers; and it is claimed that it is necessary for an adult to take a pint of milk daily and the others a quart to make sure of these respective amounts of calcium. Therefore we will take the cow's milk as the basis from which to work. Here are the figures on the calcium content of three kinds of milk.

Cow's Milk	Human Milk	Soy Bean Milk
		Approximates human milk, but is not standardized.
.120	.034	

Cow's milk contains three and a half times as much calcium as human milk. Which one is right for a human baby? He who believes in God as the Creator will accept human milk as the standard, not the cow's milk.

There are reasons for this difference in calcium content in the two kinds of milk—the calf grows to full size in two years while the baby takes twenty years, and the calf grows into a much larger animal than does the baby; for these reasons the calcium requirement is larger.

Prominent workers have contended that milk is too rich in calcium for the good of the child. Dr. J. H. Kellogg held that view for years. A typical statement of his follows:

"Dr. Rosamund contends that a quart of milk gives a child more calcium than it needs. A pint and a half would be enough, even if there were no calcium in other foods. Other articles of diet, like eggs, celery, oatmeal, beans, cabbage, and carrots, contain considerable amounts of this mineral." (54)

Dr. Kellogg recommends that in feeding cow's milk to infants it should be modified. "Cow's milk contains a large amount of protein, and lime to support the rapid growth of the calf which attains puberty at the end of two years, about one-seventh of the time required for the human infants to reach the same stage of development . . . Various formulas have been recommended for the modification of cow's milk in artificial feeding . . . A good formula is equal parts of full milk and boiled water with an ounce of malt sugar for each pint of water added to the milk." (55)

The above facts, and the growing practice in children's hospitals to use soybean milk in place of cow's milk, place this matter in a very different light from that of former years.

Calcium Study No. 2

In a preceding chapter figures were given from U. S. Government chemists to show that two-thirds of the calcium in wheat is removed when it is made into white flour, which is the main ingredient in nearly all of the baked goods of today. A similar loss is met in many of the refined breakfast cereals in common use.

Those who advise a pint and a quart of milk daily, consent to the people eating largely of these refined flours and cereals, and this book teaches young and old to use entire grain products. Manifestly, those who "rob" certain natural foods of calcium must "spike" others with it from unnatural sources to make up the loss; but those who use whole foods will not need to do so.

Calcium Study No. 3

It is taught by many that the next richest source of calcium, after milk, is the leafy vegetables. The teaching of this book is to give more prominence to those foods, which further lessens the necessity to secure it from cow's milk.

Calcium Study No. 4

The University of Wisconsin made an exhaustive study of the loss of each kind of mineral from all kinds of vegetables by various methods of cooking. The most common method is that of boiling in water, which entailed losses varying, according to the mineral, the amount of water, and the length of cooking time, all the way from 10 per cent to 75 per cent. If vegetables are cooked in that manner, naturally it will be necessary to supply the deficiency of minerals from some other source. Those who have fixed the standard for calcium consent to the vegetables being boiled in water, and this book does not. Those who cook properly will not need as much extra calcium as those who do not.

Calcium Study No. 5

It is now known that an alkaline diet causes the calcium to be retained in the body and absorbed into the blood whereas an acid-forming ration causes the calcium to leave the body through the feces. (56)

The chief acid-forming foods are meats, eggs, and grains. Usually those who hold that it is necessary to use milk to get enough calcium advocate the use of more meats, eggs, and grains than are recommended in this book, and therefore those who follow this book will not need as much extra calcium as will those who do not.

Calcium Study No. 6

Cocoanut oil in the food increases the efficiency of calcium in the body so that a given amount will accomplish more work—the body makes better use of it. (57)

Who knows but that it will yet be discovered that when the diet is composed entirely of natural foods, the various parts help each other to become a perfect whole?

This fact concerning cocoanut oil is of interest in view of the fact that certain margarines have a high content of cocoanut fat.

Calcium Study No. 7

Recent experiments have shown that the use of orange juice increases the retention and deposit of calcium in the bones from 8 to 10 per cent, and that this work has opened a new phase of the subject of growth. The amount of orange juice fed to rats in these experiments would equal two glasses a day for a boy weighing 100 pounds. (58)

An extensive experiment was made in 341 school children among whom the addition of orange juice to the diet decreased tooth decay 57 per cent and increased the growth rate 75 per cent. (59)

Calcium Study No. 8

It is reported that the inclusion of 20 per cent fresh cranberries or apples increased the retention of calcium in white rats. (60)

Calcium Study No. 9

"One fifth to one fourth of the calcium of milk is utilized and retained by children." (61) This point alone brings us back to the calcium content of human milk.

Calcium Study No. 10

Sodium bicarbonate (baking soda) tends to restrict the absorption of calcium from the intestine. This book does not grant the use of soda in any food whatsoever and therefore this loss is not entailed. (62)

Calcium Study No. 11

"Soy flour is one of the cheapest sources of calcium known. One hundred grams of calcium in soy flour costs one fifteenth as much as it costs in wheat flour and one third as much as it costs in milk." (63) Why not use more of it?

Calcium Study No. 12

The hundreds of millions of Oriental peoples who until recent times made no use of milk and yet had a well-balanced diet, constitute ample evidence that milk is not necessary in human nutrition if one has access to natural foods and will give some special attention to the subject.

Calcium Study No. 13

"It is possible to construct a complete dietary without the use of even milk or eggs." (64)

"It is possible, if the food is selected with a thorough knowledge of the defects of individual foods, and of their supplementary values—their power to make good each other's deficiencies—to secure a human dietary which would be fairly satisfactory without either milk or eggs, but there is a certain hazard to health in attempting to do so without expert knowledge." (65)

Apparently the "hazard" to health in entering into this way of living is lack of information, or inability to secure the natural foods. Have we not here removed the hazard for those who really want to live the cleaner way?

However, the reader is warned that where milk and eggs have formed a part of the regular dietary, it is unsafe to discard them unless their food values are replaced from other sources. To do so is to incur the danger of malnutrition with its ensuing consequences. The authority upon which the present writer depends most when offering the public this "Ideal Vegetarian Regimen" wrote in 1902,—"Let the diet reform be progressive. Let the people be taught how to prepare food without the use of milk or butter. Tell them that the time will soon come when there will be no safety in using eggs, milk, cream, or butter, because disease in animals is increasing in proportion to the increase of wickedness among men." (171)

This statement, and related ones, have caused some of our food manufacturers to devote much study and skill to the preparation of soybean milk and other protein foods to replace animal products. The same statement has spurred the present writer on to put into printed form in this book sufficient instruction to make it possible, for those who will study it carefully and follow it, to secure a better and more healthful ration than they were having before. This cannot be done in a haphazard manner. It is necessary to know food values as taught throughout this book and then to learn to arrange meals from nature's foods. It is very easy to do, but it must be done with care. Probably it will be well to use soybean milk as freely as dairy milk has been used in the past.

In view of the foregoing thirteen side-lights on calcium it seems evident that those who are allergic to milk, or who, for any reason, do not wish to use it, can have a balanced ration without it, if they will.

To make such a step easily possible and practical, a table is given on an earlier page of this book as a guide in selecting foods to make sure of an adequate supply of calcium.

It is urged that free use be made of soy beans and their products, and that, with children, soy bean milk be used in place of the dairy milk. With children the use of vegetable juices, raw and cooked, will aid in making sure of the calcium and other minerals.

PRIMARY AND SECONDARY FOODS

Primary, Original Foods	Secondary Foods
Grains	Flesh
Vegetables	Eggs
Legumes	Milk
Fruits	Cream
Nuts	Butter
	Cheese

The secondary foods are made by animals from the primary foods, and in doing so the animals get the first benefit of these foods, and therefore when man eats the secondary foods he gets only the second benefit of the primary foods—or what is left.

The primary foods protect man from disease, while the secondary foods subject him to disease in three ways: (1) by bringing him the diseases of animals, and (2) by being carriers of still other diseases, and (3) by providing the most favorable foods for the growth of germs.

The primary foods are the best foods for the man and the poorest for the germs, whereas the secondary foods are the poorest for the man and the best for the germs, so that he who learns how to live on the primary foods is building up himself and holding down the germs at the same time.

When the ration consists exclusively of the primary foods, well balanced, such a ration provides a degree of immunity to disease which it is not possible to secure otherwise.

Shall We Feed Human Beings or Animals?

A Basic Food Economy

Two Philosophies of Nutrition

All food comes from the soil, whether consumed by human beings or fed to animals. The food values in animal flesh, eggs, milk, butter and cheese, were eaten in vegetation by the animals, so that in eating flesh and animal products vegetation is being eaten second hand. In this case the animals get the first benefit and the humans get the second. The animals add nothing to what they ate, but only take from it.

By giving it first to the animals and then eating the animals and their products to get what they ate, nearly all of the food value the animals ate is lost before it reaches human beings.

That round-about method of getting human nutrition from the soil is a gross waste of food and of the use of the land.

The correctness of the foregoing paragraphs has been demonstrated for many hundreds of years by millions of people in China, Japan, and India where such a wasteful procedure cannot be tolerated. Their better way is now being loudly proclaimed by modern investigators and scientists. Here are a few of them.

Take China for instance. Here is still in process the best large-scale experiment in vegetarianism of which the people of our generation have any knowledge. Their ration excludes milk and its products, eggs, and meat,—all foods from animal sources,—to such an extent that less than 5 per cent of their protein is from animal sources, while in the United States 55 per cent of our protein comes from animals.

The Chinese nation of several hundred million people has survived for forty centuries without milk or a dairy industry. One does not have to look far for the reason.

The amount of ground required to raise feed for cows that people may eat the cow's flesh along with her milk, butter, and cheese, if devoted to raising food which the people themselves can eat without the "cow converter," will feed three times as many people. The Chinese never could waste food like that nor allow land to be used so unprofitably.

Humans First

100 acres in	Will supply energy for one year.
Potatoes	269 persons
Wheat	91 "
Barley	161 "
Oats	99 "
Potatoes fed to hogs	47 "
Grass fed to beef	5 "

(172)

One acre of corn will feed one person 635 days. The same corn fed to hogs will provide food in the form of pork for only 125 days.

(173)

Waste of 85%

"We in the United States have had a diet composed of 40% (in calories) of meats and live stock products only because we could afford that luxury. We like to eat these products better than the things from which they are produced. But converting one into the other is wasteful. Meat production represents a caloric waste of probably 85%; if we feed 100 calories to animals, we get perhaps 15 calories back in the meat produced." (174)

The same report states that,

If only our corn crop for one year were all fed to the people it would meet the total calorie needs of the whole nation for one year. The corn calories fed to live stock is four times the calorie content of all meat and live stock products consumed by our entire human population. The same principle applies to other cereals and forage crops.

The Report summarizes as follows:

"This indicates how many calories are lost in converting food into meats and live stock products. . . . Converting one into the other is wasteful. Meat production represents the caloric waste of probably 85%. If we feed 100 calories to animals we get back perhaps 15% in calories from the meat produced." (175)

"Live stock feed takes calories equivalent to nearly three times our annual food needs." (176)

"Most of our corn is used as live stock feed. The caloric content of the part so used is nearly four times the caloric content of all meat and live stock products in our entire national consumption." (177)

A Change Is Necessary

"We have about reached the place now where we cannot expand our meat production any more, because we are not going to have enough of the basic element,—feed,—to support more increase. And we are going to have to start with some of these grains (as substitutes) eating them ourselves rather than feeding them to animals and then eating the animals. That is a change in the diet of this country. . . . We are getting people to do it gradually, and we are doing all we can in that direction. . . . The great demand is for proteins and fats,—meat, dairy products and some oil crops. We are going to use our peanuts and soy beans increasingly, it seems to me, for human food. There may be some chance of our doing there what other nations have had to do, and that is live on vegetable fats and proteins more than we have been doing." (178)

The Direction of the Change

"If we were to go the limit and reduce live stock so far that no human food products would be converted into meats and live stock products, we could, with continued favorable crop weather, feed about one-fourth of these one and a quarter billions Europeans on a continuing basis. Such an extreme shift is unlikely. But that is the direction of change in our agriculture production and in our diets that will have to occur, if we are to supply much food to other countries. How far we will go depends on the extent of the encouragement or discouragement given to live stock production. So far, live stock production has been encouraged." (179)

Note that the report from which we have taken several of these statements is titled "Food in War and in Peace" which report was made as a result of conditions produced by a world war. But let it be remembered that wars have not yet ceased, and that there is a point of both individual and national economy involved in these two philosophies of nutrition.

Other parts of this book reveal the great benefits to health to be secured by living on the natural, cheaper food,—grains, legumes, vegetables, fruits, and nuts,—which were the diet of the human race for the first 1656 years of its existence when they reached ages running into five to nine centuries.

A New Type of Farm and Garden

The minds of some of those who are planning for the future in harmony with the principles already set forth, turn to a new type of farm and garden in which "animal husbandry" does not hold the first place.

With the animals out of the reckoning, the gardener will face a serious problem to fertilize the soil. He must use either commercial fertilizers or turn to the development of vegetable humus. The well informed gardener will strongly favor humus which restores to the soil the elements taken from it by plant growth while the chemical fertilizer does not, and will study the developing science of modern gardening. One of the basic principles of replacing the losses of the soil, resulting from its production of food, is the simple fact that plant life is nourished principally by the air, sunshine and water, while only five parts in a thousand are drawn from the soil itself. Therefore, when decayed vegetation is put into the soil, or a crop turned under to decay and make humus, more is thereby put back into the soil than was taken from it by the growth of plants. That is the value of animal fertilizer,—decaying vegetation. Doing this results in building up the soil so that it can again produce plant life containing the elements needed in the human body. Plants can grow even though deficient in some elements, but they will not sufficiently nourish the body. For instance, a pinch of manganese added to the soil about tomatoes, it is said, will increase the vitamin C content of the tomatoes three fold. The present author is not trying to give gardening instruction, but merely to indicate the importance of basic principles and to interest the reader in looking farther into the subject.

MODERN GARDENING

The nutritional value of the foods, for man and animals, raised in gardens and on farms, varies according to the composition of the soil, and will reflect its deficiencies.

As an example: in some sections of the country the soil is so lacking in calcium that calcium must be fed to the cattle or they die. Other soils are lacking other minerals.

It is now claimed that where cattle are infected with Bang's disease the addition of manganese, copper, and cobalt to the soil will prevent further infection and will overcome the infection in cattle already sick. Crushed rock is added to the soil in some instances to make up its mineral deficiency.

It seems clear that if such soil deficiencies can be determined and corrected, and if the vegetable humus required for plant growth is provided, this procedure would go a long way toward restoring the nutritional value of foods grown for mankind and for animals.

The question of soil fertility and how the soil should be nourished is coming rapidly to the fore and experimental work is being done in various places. Literature is being written on it. Writers do not all agree, but help can be gleaned from most of them.

For instance, in 1938 the U. S. Department of Agriculture published a book of 1200 pages entitled "SOILS AND MEN" which contains an abundance of useful information. However, it should be understood that its first objective is to help growers of crops to secure the highest possible financial returns. This plan does not always insure the highest nutritional value of such produce. It may be standard in size, and profitable, and yet be seriously deficient in vitamins and certain valuable minerals. The book mentioned gives much advice on soil management, erosion, cover crops, and many other points. But to increase the nutritional value of foods grown, one should study the literature on "Organic Gardening" to learn the procedures by which to build up the humus in the soil and the right ways to fertilize it.

Then study the science of restoring the deficient minerals and trace elements. These two lines of soil building when combined with soil management may some day be called "Modern Gardening." Some of the plans suggested may be practical only in home gardens for family use. Other plans will be suited to large gardens and farms.

The book "SOILS AND MEN," of course, lays first emphasis on animal manure well composted. This includes droppings from sheep and fowls. (page 516) Old straw or hay composted three to four months is valuable. (page 516) Peat moss is recommended for improving the physical condition of the soil but it is not very valuable as a plant nutrient. (page 517) "Leaves alone, when dry, are about twice as rich per pound in plant food as barnyard manure." (page 516) Therefore no leaves should be burned or allowed to be wasted in any way.

Wood ashes, corn-cob ashes and ashes other than coal are good soil nutrients. (pages 518-519) Coal ashes provide no nutritive elements but in heavy soil they lighten it and improve its drainage. (page 516). Wood sawdust is a good fertilizer after it has lain in the pile till it takes on a dark color. It can be spread on the top to a depth of one or two inches any time of the year and worked into the soil the next time it is cultivated. (180)

Hulls of various seeds such as cottonseed, peanuts, or chaff, weeds, stubble or any discarded vegetation, all make good compost material. (181)

For a small home garden it is easy to make compost of all sorts of waste such as garbage, leaves, grass cuttings, weeds and everything that will decay and make vegetation grow. Often neighbors do not have gardens or do not know the value of these wastes and will give them away, particularly the falling autumn leaves. Nothing makes better fertilizer than leaves.

Cover crops are plowed under while green; they add humus to the soil and some of them add nitrogen. They can be plowed under in the fall or left during the winter to protect the ground and turned under in the spring. This is a subject by itself and is too much for this book. Get bulletins from Washington or your state department of agriculture.

The gardener should know the right depth to plow the ground to cause the soil to absorb moisture rather than shed it. The surface of the soil must have proper care to prevent erosion and the consequent loss of the precious minerals provided. These features must be worked out according to the nature and depth of the soil and underlying conditions in each locality. Here again government bulletins will help you.

The publishers of the book you are reading are continually collecting literature on these various phases of gardening and will gladly assist readers to know where to get source material.

Immunity: What Is It? How Obtained?

Dr. Alexis Carrel for years with the Rockefeller Institute, in his book "Man the Unknown," says there are two kinds of health and immunity—one natural and the other artificial; that to date the trend of medical science has been toward the artificial; that medicine has been following the easiest road of building artificial health through the use of pharmaceutical products, chemicals, drugs, antitoxic sera, hospital technique, etc.

He says we ought to learn the secret of natural immunity to disease; that the future advance of medicine will not come through better hospitals, or more and better pharmaceutical products, but through having sound nervous systems, immunity to infections, and through the prevention of degenerative diseases. For instance, instead of giving a man a substitute for the secretion of some gland, we ought to find out how to make his own glands secrete their proper juices. (66)

Perhaps another way of saying it is that we need to build up health rather than to cure disease.

In following out his thought he states that in the Rockefeller Institute mousery the incidence of pneumonia was 52 per cent on a standard diet, but that by improving the diets they could reduce the incidence of pneumonia to zero. (67)

"Good Health" of February, 1937 reported a paper read by Sir Robert McCarrison, M.D., to the British Medical Association, which summed up meant,—"Faulty food, faulty nutrition, faulty function, faulty structure, faulty health, disease.

"Concerning tuberculosis and nutrition, the example was cited of the Papwroth Village Settlement. The children born there are the offspring of parents with tuberculosis, yet in twenty years not one of them has contracted any clinical form of the disease. The families have all dwelt together. This achievement has been brought about by adequate nutrition, which maintains the child's resistance to infection, and by the absence of mass dose infection."

Dr. McCarrison's work in India has conclusively shown that animals will have health or disease, according to their food and other conditions.

Why then, do we not study and work more diligently to produce natural health?

Many authorities have said that disease cannot attack perfectly healthy tissue. Here is a sample citation:

"Living cells resist the attacks of micro-organisms. A raw apple or potato remains intact for months, while a cooked apple or potato is in a very few days covered with mold and in an active state of fermentation and destructive change. Living cells resist germs." (68)

He also reports that germs placed on cooked cabbage increased in number enormously, while those on raw cabbage diminished in number. (69)

One Hundred and Sixty-five Parasites

There are more than fifty varieties of animal parasites that attack the interior of the human body. There are more than fifteen varieties of insect parasites that attack the exterior of the human body, and there are more than a hundred varieties of vegetable parasites that attack either the exterior or interior of the human system. (70)

What a host of foes! Manifestly one of our great problems is to learn how to hold the natural immunity of the body so high that these enemies from without cannot enter the blood stream either through the skin or the mucous membrane, and in case they do enter, to have the means for destroying them strong enough to do battle successfully. This section is devoted to a few suggestions concerning that problem.

The first precaution, of course, is that we shall use good judgment and not deliberately, unnecessarily put into the body foods or other things laden with living germs. But after having done our best, there will be many battles to fight within. It is well therefore for us to know something of the body's defenses and how they are maintained. Among them are these:

First: The skin outside of the body and the mucous membrane inside will not allow germs to enter the body itself if the cells of the skin and membrane are normal. This defensive power is impaired by a deficiency of vitamins.

Second: The saliva contains substances which inhibit the growth of germs.

Third: The hydrochloric acid in the gastric juice is a strong disinfectant.

Fourth: Bacteria usually thrive in acid media while alkaline media inhibits their growth. An alkaline condition of tissue and blood aids in fighting bacteria. See chapter on acids and bases for more data on this point.

Fifth: The blood contains substances which hinder the growth of germs.

Sixth: The blood contains white corpuscles which devour germs.

Seventh: Certain minerals assist in combating germs, as when calcium walls off the tuberculosis germ in the lungs.

When these defenses are normal they are adequate, but they are dependent for their vitality upon, (a) sunshine, (b) air, (c) water, (d) a perfect ration, (e) exercise, (f) rest, and (g) a serene mind—the very things about which many people are careless. For instance—

(a) We are not particular about the outdoor life in the sun.

(b) We are careless about fresh air and good ventilation.

(c) Few people take a sufficient amount of water.

(d) Hardly a person gets a balanced ration, as you have already learned in this book. Just to emphasize one item: "The discovery of vitamins may some day be regarded as rivaling in importance the discovery of micro-organisms as causative factors in disease."— Dr. R. R. Williams. Who knows the extent of protection from germs we might find in vitamins if we made a real business of getting the full supply of them in natural foods as the Creator intended? Professor H. C. Sherman has said that "to get full protection against infections requires four times as much vitamin A as to prevent typical eye disease." (71)

This means that with the amount of vitamins and the degree of health with which most people are content, we are not prepared to fight germs, but need four times as much. And yet we refine our grains, bake, boil, fry, and stew everything, put in soda and baking powder, and do everything possible to cut down our supply of vitamins, except drink milk and take cod liver oil, and then wonder why we are not immune. We know we are missing our vitamins in many ways, but someone has told us that we can make up the losses in other ways, and we believe it and act accordingly. We cannot make up that loss! We need all of the vitamins which God put in all of our foods to get enough to protect us against infections.

(e) Talk about exercise! Too many people today will not even walk a block; they must ride in automobiles and streetcars. Exercise has almost disappeared from their mode of life. . . . "More people rust out than wear out."

(f) It is not possible to properly rest unless one has first exercised. But many people today do not even try to make proper use of the night which God provided for quiet repose. Night has been made as bright as day, and half of it, more or less, is used for gaiety and pleasure, and to do numberless things which further lessen the vitality of brain, nerves, and body, so that the next day is "the morning after" instead of the body having been replenished with new vigor for the day's tasks. And then what? They resort to a variety of concoctions in never-ending quantities to pep up the lagging energies, some of which are said to rest you in five minutes. These restore nothing to the tired body but further whip up its remaining forces to action. Tomorrow these will be required in larger doses than today, and so the merry-go-round of the vicious cycle, which will end in disaster, has become the daily experience of millions of people.

(g) Serene mind! We live in a world full of troubles and worries for which there is no human remedy; solace comes only from above whence millions of people will not accept it though it be freely proffered.

Few people can be found today who even want a serene mind —they want to be thrilled all of the time; they are not happy unless they are continually keyed up to the highest pitch—on the "go," and going fast.

Then because we have failed to build up natural health we get some "shots" to give us "immunity" to this and to that. What shame that we treat ourselves and the will of our Maker thus!

But that is only half of the story. This we have just told relates mostly to common failures to build up the body defenses. There is also a long list of popular indulgences which tear them down. They have already been named in this book but must be reviewed here. They are:

Indigestion and constipation, both everywhere present, fill the body with toxins which lower the vitality of all cells.

Not content with the above, people deliberately put poison into their bodies in the form of tobacco, alcohol, tea, coffee, cola drinks, spices, pain-killing remedies, many drugs commonly used, and other things too numerous to mention.

Then, too, most people use foods which are literally loaded with living germs, like trichinae in pork, and other meats filled with germs as described in the chapters on "Eating for Strength," and "The Animal Kingdom a Reservoir of Disease."

Other less potent sources of germs in foods are eggs, cheese, butter, cream, and milk. Eternal vigilance is required on the part of authorities to keep these dairy products clean enough so they are considered eatable. And some workers who are searching out new ways of combating the growth of germs within the body reason like this: If we have to fight so hard to keep down the growth of germs in these dairy foods while they are still outside of the body, the same fight must go on after they are eaten, only now it is within and so becomes the body's fight against these hordes of bacteria. On this reasoning it is contended that a higher state of immunity can be reached without these foods than with them, provided one learns how to secure a balanced ration without them. On this point the reader is referred to the section on "The Ideal Vegetarian Regimen."

It is true that there is a marked difference in the heritage we individually have received in the physical constitution and tendencies from our forbears, but even so, the degree of immunity and health we each have depends very largely upon our personal adherence to the laws which govern life.

It is the height of absurdity for the people to follow their present practices and then expect to possess immunity to disease, or to hope that "shots" or serums will restore the protection and vitality they have literally thrown away.

The principles in this section cannot be gainsaid, and yet they are so widely ignored that the very existence of the human race is at stake.

Why does not someone get at these fundamental things and inaugurate a reformatory movement which will carry a knowledge of the first principles of the preservation of human health and life to every man, woman and child in America?

The Common Cold

Public Malady Number One

First. It is agreed that germs are a factor. Arctic explorers have no colds until they return to civilization.

Second. A germ being involved, it is a matter of infection and resistance. Manifestly, if the immunity is 100 per cent perfect, infection can not "take."

Third. Inasmuch as we all live and associate with other folk we cannot get away entirely from infection unless we go to the Arctics. Therefore our main defense must lie in our own personal resistance. What, then, are the factors in raising and lowering the resistance?

Resistance is RAISED by	Resistance is LOWERED by
Vitamins	27 varieties of indigestion
Minerals	Constipation
Alkalies	Deficiency of items in first column
A balanced ration	Chilling*
Good digestion	Fatigue
Proper elimination—a clean state throughout the inner man	Worry
Rest	Tobacco
Sleep	Alcohol
Fresh air	Too much clothing
Sunshine	Overheated rooms
A serene mind	Poor ventilation

See the preceding chapter on immunity.

The highest degree of immunity to infection is secured by using the strict vegetarian ration as directed in the Automatic Menu Planner, without the use of milk, cream, cottage cheese, butter, or eggs.

---

*For every degree Centigrade of loss of body temperature the activity of the protoplasm of the cells decreases ten per cent, which lowers the immunity. (72) A draft of cold air on the calf of the leg reduced the temperature in the muscles 11 degrees F. "Health," May, 1941, page 12.

Vaccines and inoculations to prevent colds are of questionable value. "Approximately 20,000 employees of a telephone company were given injections to prevent colds and their susceptibility remained unchanged." (73)

There are also other physical handicaps which may contribute to taking cold, but in the main, one's condition is the direct result of his habits and practices.

If one is so unfortunate as to take cold, the first thing to do when the first symptom is noted is to clean the entire digestive tract, go to bed, drink water and fruit juices copiously until the cold begins to yield, and when hungry again, eat fruits and vegetables for a day or two, and then come back to the regular alkaline ration.

There are some medications for nose and throat which may be helpful. Hydrotherapy is the best sort of treatment, and it can be administered at home by those who know how to do it. Every home library should contain a book giving this instruction.

Allergy

Leading Forms of Allergy

Under this heading are included many conditions today. It is defined as "altered reactivity" meaning an altered or abnormal reaction of some part of the body to substances entering it through the air passages or through the mouth to the stomach.

The leading classifications are: Hives, eczema, migraine, hayfever, and asthma.

These are conditions which often baffle the best of medical workers. When writing about them they do not always agree. Manifestly this book can only deal with a few general principles which are basic to these altered reactions. I am first of all anxious to help the readers of this book discover the things they are doing to cause any of these reactions. Sometimes it is a simple matter, and at other times it is almost impossible to know where to lay the blame. An incident may be to the point. I once saw a person suffering acutely with hives at bed time with weals three and four inches across, all over the body. His supper had been largely of watermelon. He took a liberal enema and in less than an hour the weals and discomfort were gone and he went to sleep. That was a simple matter. Again, I saw a man who was continually suffer-

ing indescribable agonies from migraine headaches. He was talk-
ing of suicide as the only possible relief. Some one told him of the
principles set forth in this book. He was willing to try all of them
except to stop using cigarettes. Finally, upon persuasion he prom-
ised to try the entire plan. For a number of weeks he had no
headache. Then his craving for cigarettes got the better of him
and his agonies at once returned. That, too, was simple to understand, but he thought it was too hard to do. I knew a man suffering with asthma who said he became well by following the principles in this book, which excluded the use of tobacco. Again, I
saw a case of asthma in a teen-age girl who always got immediate
relief by merely going for a ride,—a change of environment and
thinking. I have seen so many things occur of this nature that I
cannot refrain from placing a few principles before the readers of
this book. Some of the sufferers should be helped even if not all
of them are made well.

The Approach

There are two ways to approach the subject of allergy. One
way is to search for the offending food and eliminate it, or if it be
something in the air, flee from it. The other way is quite different. Let us reason about it.

(1) All will agree that it is an individual's over-sensitiveness—
that is, one person is sensitive to certain foods while people all
around him are not. That person, then is different from the others—he is abnormal. If he could change himself by doing something to restore his body to normal, allergy would cease. This is
the aspect of the subject that interests us most at this time.

(12) The part of the anatomy that is sensitive to anything is
the nerves—that, everyone knows. It is said the sensitized people
usually have "an unbalanced condition of the nervous system."
(74) Manifestly, one thing to do, at least, is to undertake to restore normalcy to the nervous system. That may be a big order,
but it is worth the effort. Among the steps to take are the following:

Nerve builders are—a balanced, highly alkaline ration, with
extra minerals and vitamins, fresh air, sunshine, exercise, rest, and
a serene state of mind.

Nerve destroyers are—coffee, tea, cola drinks, tobacco, alcohol,
foods deficient in minerals and vitamins (these have been ex-

plained in the early part of this book), indigestion, constipation, and worry.

Both the sick and the well will always do right in stopping every bad habit and adopting a normal balanced program. Many of our ills disappear when we do so. Allergic people will be surprised at the results. But there is still more to do.

(3) All will agree that the substance to which the nerves most often are sensitive is a protein. In that case it must be plain that the allergic person does not take care of the proteins as normal people do; in other words, it is not the fault of the protein, but the fault of the person. If he will make the changes in his eating and other habits as suggested in this chapter so that his "altered reactivity" comes back to normal, it should be possible for him to handle the proteins in a strict vegetarian diet. There may be exceptions, but the writer doubts it. At least it is worth trying.

Proteins are handled by two processes—(a) digestion, and (b) absorption. We will consider digestion first.

(a) Digestion is carried on by four digestive juices, mouth, stomach, pancreas, and liver. These juices all have to be made of substances which their respective glands elaborate from the blood, and each juice has a high mineral content. Manifestly, if the allergic person is robbing his body of minerals by living on demineralized food, as explained in the early chapters, how can he expect to have normal digestive juices? In that case he has a right to expect to get undigested proteins into his blood,—and there is nothing much more poisonous in the blood than proteins in that condition. On the point of inefficient digestive juices, one famous clinician has said that allergy is often relieved by giving extra pancreatic juice. (75) Perhaps the patient cannot make his own pancreatic juice because his food does not contain the necessary elements,—a balanced ration. Or perhaps he is guilty of some of the twenty-seven varieties of indigestion already treated in this book.

(b) Absorption takes place in the small intestine. The blood absorbs what it can get from the small intestine—it must take what is there, even if it be undigested or decayed proteins. Manifestly we must overcome not only indigestion, but constipation if we would properly handle our proteins. This is proven by the fact that allergic people often get relief by taking an enema. The con-

dition of the blood will be influenced by the condition in the small
intestine, and its condition depends upon good digestion and good
elimination as well as good food.

Therefore under this head of "absorption" the reader is now
asked to study the entire chapter on constipation where the causes
and correction are discussed in detail. All causes of putrefaction
must be eliminated. If the proteins are to be prepared for the
blood they must be well digested; there must be no putrefaction,
and there must be prompt elimination.

The larger part of what has gone into this chapter has been
found in the writings of medical workers. Some of their statements are now given. The first of them is the subject of eczema.

Eczema

"Eczema and most other forms of skin diseases are greatly influenced by diet. Various skin maladies are commonly associated
with chronic intestinal toxemia and are apparently due to lowered
vital resistance resulting from the absorption into the blood of
large quantities of putrefaction products developed in the intestine.
. . . These eruptions may occur in persons who are sensitized to
some particular food stuff. The food substances most often incriminated are oysters or other shellfish, pork, mutton, veal, strawberries, buckwheat, eggs, sometimes milk and even tomatoes. In
all cases of eczema and other forms of skin eruptions, a strict antitoxic diet should be adopted. Meats of all sorts should be eliminated and a search made for the particular substances to which
the body may be sensitized. . . . Gershun (Vratch) calls attention
to the fact that skin diseases in infants are frequently due to poisons in the mother's food. Psoriasis and eczema have been shown
to be due to this cause, the disease disappearing when the mother
discards meat. . . . Special attention should be given to the bowels,
which should be made to move three times daily. . . . Certain infants are sensitized to cow's milk."

Dr. Kellogg cites many years of successful experience in following these methods by Dr. L. D. Bulkley of the New York Skin and
Cancer Hospital. (77)

Cod liver oil and butter have been known to be offenders. (78)

Marvelous success is being attained of late in treating infantile
eczema with soybean milk; in fact, it is rapidly becoming a standard regime in many children's hospitals. The most of these cases

are allergic to cow's milk. One pediatrician, Samuel J. Levin, M.D., reports seventy-one cases out of eighty-six, making rapid recovery by using soybean emulsion (soybean milk) as the principal part of the treatment. (79)

From all of the information available it seems that when all the causes of indigestion are avoided, constipation corrected, and a highly alkaline, strictly vegetarian diet is followed, bad habits stopped, as taught in this book, there should be no eczema. At least it is worth trying. If one knows that he is sensitive to certain foods, they may be avoided. There seems to be no doubt that the elimination, not only of all flesh foods, but of all animal products, will be helpful.

Migraine

Medical authorities agree that this is difficult to relieve; that certain people have a tendency toward it, and that the tendency may be hereditary. In that case the sufferer is handicapped, and may have to be more strict in his way of living than the normal person who can tolerate some indiscretions and not suffer immediately for it.

The reader who is afflicted with migraine headaches is asked to make sure that any eye-strain is relieved, and then carefully study the way of living propounded in this book from the beginning, and to follow it. Make sure of a balanced, alkaline ration, of good digestion and good elimination. Indulge absolutely in no bad habit. Of special importance are tobacco, tea, coffee, alcohol, and cola drinks.

He will do well to study the portions of this book devoted to nerves, asthma, hay-fever, and allergy. Everything must be done that can be done to restore nerve vitality to normal and relieve the body of toxins. The person who is willing to make every correction will be repaid.

Hay Fever and Asthma

(Read the section on "Allergy" before reading this section)

"Asthma is based upon a decided nervous predisposition in all cases. The exciting cause may be a cold, hay-fever, the inhaling of dust, or the odors from animals such as the horse or the cat. Fright or other sudden emotions may bring on an attack." (80)

"In the writer's experience fully nine-tenths of all cases of asthma may be attributed to intestinal toxemia, or auto-intoxication. . . . Changing the intestinal flora, and normal colon activity will secure prompt and permanent relief in a great majority of cases of chronic asthma of adults. The bowls must move three times a day and the colon must be kept thoroughly free from decomposing residues that the stools will be free from putrid or ammoniacal odors. . . . Meat must of course be discarded. Eggs, if eaten at all must be eaten sparingly. . . . A warm enema should be taken at night to make sure that the colon is completely evacuated. . . . In many cases the asthmatic is found to be sensitized to certain foods. . . . These foods should be avoided and by carefully graduated training, the sensitivity should be overcome." (81)

Hay-fever. "Those who are highly nervous are most susceptible."

"This disease may end in an attack of bronchial asthma, and the two are often associated, as both are based upon a nervous predisposition and an unusual susceptibility to small amounts of albumins." (82)

"Asthma generally is curable. There are at least three kinds of asthma. One kind is due to intestinal toxemia. Poisons absorbed from the colon, excreted through the lungs, irritate the air passages and cause them to contract and produce a spasm.

"Another form less common is due to bronchial catarrh.

"Still another form is due to a diseased condition of the heart so that the organ is not able to carry away the blood from the lungs, and they become congested." (83)

Asthma can be caused by the incomplete digestion of proteins. (84)

Some people get relief from asthma by changing from a high protein to a low protein ration. (85)

The above statements strike at the root of these twin ailments, and therefore to deal merely with the exciting causes does not get at the root of the matter. When the system is cleared of toxins and the nerve energy is restored to normal the exciting causes do not exist. They do not trouble normal people.

CORRECTIVE PROCEDURES

First—Negative Items

Every practice which has been indulged that develops toxins or lowers nerve vitality must be discontinued absolutely and entirely. Among these are the following: the use of alcohol, tobacco, tea, coffee, cocoa, coca-cola, spices, rich desserts, meat, fish, fowl; beware of an excess of sugar, and eggs to be eaten only moderately, if at all. The use of cow's milk is seriously questioned. Soybean milk is safer. Use salt sparingly.

It is necessary to obtain good digestion and have no sour stomach. See chapter on Indigestion.

It is necessary to bring the bowel elimination up to two or three eliminations each twenty-four hours.

Worry must not be indulged. It is one of the most destructive forces entering into the human experience.

Everything that disturbs the nerves should be avoided as far as possible.

Second—Positive Items

Nerve energy is supplied by certain elements as definitely as houses are built out of certain materials.

(a) Get an abundance of all of the minerals in the food, particularly phosphorus and calcium. This means that all of the cereals and grains eaten should be whole grains. It also means that vegetables should be cooked waterless so there will be no loss of minerals. Tables of foods highest in minerals are found in this book.

One physician of high repute advises all of his allergy cases in his particular region to take calcium tables regularly because the foods there are deficient in calcium.

(b) All of the vitamins are necessary but particularly thiamin. For detailed information about the sources of vitamins, see the chapter entitled, "The Mysteries of Life."

(c) At least 75 per cent of the foods as spread out on the table should be alkaline and 90 per cent would be better. For instruction concerning these items see the chapter on "How Acids and Alkalies Affect the Health."

(d) The person must have fresh air day and night. As much out-door life as may be obtained will be helpful.

(e) Sunshine is helpful.

(f) Quietness and relaxation are very beneficial.

(g) Menus for all meals should contain the variety and arrangement set forth in the Automatic Menu Planner. The variety suggested here should be used in the dinner. In the dinner the most important groups are numbers two and five. The Menu Planner is the base for the planning of all meals but it should be modified to harmonize with the sections on vitamins, sour stomach and constipation. In other words, foods rich in phosphorus and other minerals must be stressed. Foods rich in vitamins, especially thiamin, must be stressed. If constipation exists, the laxative foods must be emphasized.

If the above program is followed, hay-fever and asthma will usually be relieved and often disappear.

Summary

Before we close this chapter which we hope will be helpful to a large number of sufferers we want to review it in a different manner which will simplify both the subject and the procedures to follow. For this purpose we will separate all of the foregoing material into seven divisions and deal with each one by itself.

(1) *Focal Infection*

Good sense indicates that the body should be examined by a thoroughgoing doctor for any possible focal infection. This should be done for the protection of the whole body regardless of allergy.

(2) Orris root, cosmetics, dyed goods, wool, silk, feathers, animal dusts, house dust, and the pollen of plants constitute one section of the possible causes. Each one of these can be considered separately and such steps taken as seem best for the time being. It may be that allergy to these items will not always continue. It is not natural for us to be sensitive to these things, and therefore when the condition of the body is brought up to normal these allergies should disappear like falling leaves. The writer used to suffer with hay-fever in a certain town. After learning more about how to live he returned to the same town for three years without any signs of hay-fever.

(3) Tea, coffee, spices, chocolate, alcohol, and tobacco make another list. All of these are injurious and should be discontinued now and forever for many reasons, only one of which is allergy. See other chapters dealing with these articles more fully.

(4) Pork, all sea foods, chicken and all other flesh foods are a group of very likely offenders. These are but second hand foods which only give the eater a small part of the original value of such foods as they ate, (some of which we cannot mention in a clean book like this) and we have already abundantly shown that human beings are much benefited by omitting all of them and living directly on the clean foods of nature. When living the better way flesh foods as a cause of allergy are automatically eliminated so we do not need to give further thought to them here.

(5) Next we come to a group consisting of eggs, milk, cream, butter and cheese. Will the reader please now study the chapter on "The Ideal Vegetarian Regimen" where these foods are especially considered, and to the portions of this book expounding a balanced ration without these foods. In case the reader decides to practice this cleaner way of living, these foods are eliminated from the field of allergy from this time forward. If these foods are to be retained we feel that we have done our part concerning allergy by mentioning them. It may be they can be retained if all of the other instruction is followed.

(6) The following list of foods has been held back until now for a very good reason. They are wheat, buckwheat, potatoes, celery, cabbage, onions, legumes, nuts, peanuts, strawberries, tomatoes, citrus fruits, raw fruits, and seasonal fruits. These all are good, wholesome, natural foods,—first class. We do not want to incriminate one of them unless we have to do so. We also know that most food allergies arise from the items mentioned in sections three, four, and five, unless it be from wheat or buckwheat in section six. The foods in section six should not cause an allergy, although if any one of them is proven guilty it can be discontinued until the body condition has been brought up to normal. This brings us to the next section.

(7) Remember the watermelon which caused the severe case of hives. The watermelon was all right but the man ate too much of it, causing a digestive upset. Therefore in section seven we must consider indigestion and constipation as often being basic causes of allergy even while eating foods from group number six. Will the reader at this point please consider again the chapters on digestion and constipation and then give the body every opportunity to take good care of good foods eaten so they will reach the blood in proper condition to be used to build up the cells and their functions and not produce any unfavorable reaction.

If these seven sections are carefully followed the writer believes that most allergies which are not hereditary will be overcome, and those which are inherited will become less severe. The Automatic Menu Planner will help in planning balanced meals.

Why So Much Allergy?

A recent study of the prevalence of allergy indicates that three-fourths of the people are allergic to a greater or less extent. Why should they not be when nearly every person is doing so many things to disturb the life processes within the body and throw them out of balance and cause "altered reactivity" which is allergy? The Book says, "The curse causeless shall not come."

Underweight—How To Gain

After age thirty-five if one is in good health, underweight is not considered to be an unfavorable condition.

To Gain Weight

(a) Eat three good meals a day according to the Automatic Menu Planner, with extra large servings of fats—cream, butter or its substitutes, olives, vegetable oils, nuts, soy beans, other beans; extra servings of sweet fruits—bananas, dates, raisins, and other fruits, fresh, cooked, or dried; liberal servings of potatoes; whole grain breads and cereals as liberally as can be done and keep within the limit of 25 per cent acid-forming foods; drink milk freely or soy bean milk.

It should be understood that fats can add weight to the body ounce for ounce; that starch and sugar can add three or four times their weight because they hold water with them, and salt retains 100 times its own weight of water. The best sort of weight to add is muscle tissue. (86)

(b) A half hour before meals, particularly breakfast, a glass of orange juice or some other fruit juice.

(c) Use raw fruits liberally.

(d) Get the standard amount of water daily but as directed in the Menu Planner.

(e) Conservative desserts may be used but avoid rich ones.

(f) Do not eat candy even though it does add weight; the sugar is an irritant.

(g) Do not eat between meals other than the fruit juices as already mentioned.

(h) Get an abundance of sleep in fresh pure air.

(i) A daily rest period is helpful.

(j) In case of a child, go to a competent physician and make sure that no insidious disease is beginning to work.

(k) Be sure of some exercise each day, but be conservative about it, and avoid over-fatigue.

(l) Avoid all the causes of indigestion given in this book.

(m) Live above constipation.

(n) Maintain a serene, care-free mental poise. Remember that a very active mind tends to speed up all of the body chemical processes. Don't "drive"; learn to relax. No forecast can be made as to how successful you will be, but this is the program.

Overweight and Reducing Suggestions

"People who are past forty-five years of age and weigh 20 per cent more than the average person have a death rate greater by one-half than the average for their age. If they have a persistent 40 per cent overweight, the rate is almost double that of the average."

"Excess weight may be a forerunner of high blood pressure, heart disease, diabetes, kidney trouble, hardening of the arteries, or apoplexy." (87)

McCollum has said that those who are slightly underweight will usually live longer than the so-called normal weight person or the overweight. (88)

In no case use weight-reducing remedies; they are dangerous.

Many people deplete the blood of necessary life-giving elements when trying to reduce. They go on a starvation diet and are continually hungry. Some become victims of tuberculosis and others become anemic. All this is unnecessary.

A person who is overweight has laid by his food in fat and should reduce his total daily caloric intake to a point that is less than he requires to produce heat and energy, and so FORCE the body to draw upon its surplus. One can find this point only by checking his calories daily and his weight frequently. Some people can lose weight on 1500 calories daily, while others have to come down to 1200. This can be done and still keep the blood well supplied with nourishment for every organ and with protective agencies against disease. If one secures a good supply of minerals, maintains the proper alkaline balance, gets all of his vitamins, and his 10 per cent of protein, the quality of his blood will be maintained and he will feel energetic and well even though he is reducing, and will not open his system to the danger of anemia or tuberculosis. This means that he should live largely on fruits and vegetables. One may eat freely enough of these to satisfy his appetite.

The Procedure

The order in which one should eliminate certain elements from his ration is as follows:

(1) Stop all artificial sweets and cut sweet foods to a low minimum, or eliminate them altogether.

(2) Reduce all fats to a very low point or stop their use entirely, according to the urgency of the case. This applies to butter, cream, salad oils, mayonnaise dressing, fats of all kinds, olives and olive oil, nuts. If one is constipated and needs the ripe olives he can keep them by reducing other items more severely.

The reason for reducing fats before starches is this: Fat is disposed of by oxidation, and starches (carbohydrates) are used in the process of burning the fat; therefore a given amount of carbohydrate is used in disposing of a given amount of fat. For this same reason the reduction of fats in the foods should be greater than the reduction of starches. (89)

(3) Stop or reduce the starches of the acid-forming class, namely the cereals and breadstuffs.

(4) As a last resort reduce the alkaline carbohydrates—potatoes, bananas, etc.

The above is a safe, sane method of reducing.

The following rules have been compiled from the best authorities:

1. Upon arising, exercise at least five minutes and gradually increase the time each day. Do bending and twisting exercises.

2. Follow the exercise with a cold bath.

3. Eat regularly two or three meals a day and do not go hungry.

4. Use salt sparingly. A low salt intake facilitates a loss of weight.

5. Eat slowly and chew food well.

6. Do not drink with the meals, but drink freely between meals, not closer than one-half hour before or two hours after.

7. Never eat between meals.

8. Take exercise every day. Walking is a good exercise.

9. Get eight or nine hours of sleep every night. Sleep will help to maintain the vitality and vigor and aid you in sticking to the regime.

10. Make sure of getting the iron-yielding foods and so keep the blood in good condition.

Fasting Hazards

There are certain dangers involved in fasting which are not commonly understood. Because of these, fasting is not the right method to follow to reduce the weight.

Starvation reduces the muscles, heart, glands, and other essential structures.

Calcium, phosphorus and iron are continually eliminated so that in a fast of five weeks one-half of the body's supply would be lost. The same is true of the vitamins.

While fasting the body lives on its fat as long as any is left, and the oxidation of fat without carbohydrate produces acidosis.

One should engage in a prolonged fast only under the care of a physician versed in this procedure.

It is seldom necessary to go beyond a juice therapy fast.

Best of all is to live every day so that the body will always be free from toxins so that no fast is needed.

Diabetes

These pargraphs are not written to disturb the procedure now being followed by the diabetic reader, but to give a few suggestions to go along with his program to make it more effective.

The chief cause is said to be overfeeding; that it is never seen in people over fifty whose weight is normal; that it almost disappeared in Germany during the first World War; that diabetics nearly always have a history of chronic constipation; that such constipation causes the pancreas to become infected which renders its cells inefficient. (90)

One authority says to cut down the amount of food, clean out the intestines and give the liver a chance and the diabetes will take care of itself.

Kellogg holds that a purely vegetable diet is best; that vegetable proteins are well tolerated but that meat sends up the sugar in the urine at once; that if one stays off meat and eggs he may use some bread and even sugar. (91)

Surely it is safe for the heavy eater to reduce the amount of food eaten, and to correct constipation.

Manifestly the Alkaline Diet, without sugar, low in acid-forming starches, is the right program for the diabetic. Soybean foods are useful.

All bad habits should of course be corrected.

Kidney Stones

Kidney stones have been produced in guinea pigs by feeding a diet deficient in vitamin A. Other factors involved were understood to be unbalance of minerals, infections, and excessive alkalinity of the urine. (92)

The Cleveland (Ohio) Clinic reports (Dr. C. C. Higgins) a series of over forty cases of kidney stones having been dissolved by dietary measures. It required from fifty to a hundred days. Their procedure is an excess of vitamin A, and a higher than usual acid-ash diet. (93)

Other workers, including H. C. Sherman, Hindhede, strongly advise a high alkaline ration to make the urine alkaline. (94)

McCarrison lists stone in the kidney among the conditions he produced in animals by abnormal feeding.

When all of the information is combined it seems clear that when one lives on a normal ration, kidney stones will not form.

Gallstones

Gallstones are known to be caused by bacteria which may arise from chronic constipation. (95)

They are formed of cholesterol, consequently those who have had trouble should not use foods high in cholesterol, like eggs, butter, fats, and meats. (96)

Anemia

(How to Build Up the Blood)

Anemia is usually divided into two groups. The first is known as ordinary or secondary anemia, and is a temporary, easily corrected condition, in which the hemoglobin has suffered more than the red corpuscles, and when the person supplies the needed iron the blood condition is quickly corrected. (98)

Pernicious anemia is much more serious. In this type the red blood corpuscles have suffered more than the hemoglobin; they are degenerated, and are not being reproduced fast enough to replace the normal losses. There may be changes in the spinal cord shown by numbness of the hands and feet and weakness in the legs. To correct this, the processes by which the red cells are manufactured must be accelerated. The study of recent years has added much to the knowledge of these processes so that the prospect of recovery is regarded with more encouragement than formerly. McCarrison says it is "almost invariably curable."

A number of factors seem to be involved. The following outline of the subject has been made from the work of Dr. J. H. Kellogg, Dr. Robert McCarrison, Dr. William Dameshke of New York, and others. To make a complex matter simple, each factor will be discussed by itself.

First

Manifestly red corpuscles cannot be made without protein and iron. The danger of iron deficiency is much greater than that of protein. The average American diet is deficient in iron but contains an excess of protein.

The anemic person needs three or four times as much iron as the normal person. See index for a table of food sources with means of measuring the amounts eaten daily.

Second

Usually there is a serious deficency of hydrochloric acid in the gastric juice, from which two bad results arise.

(a) The hydrochloric acid is the agent that splits the protein in the stomach so that the small intestine may prepare it for absorption into the blood. It also does something which liberates the iron in the food so that it may pass into the blood from the intestine. When these do not occur, the consequences must become serious.

(b) The hydrochloric acid is a strong antiseptic. When it is weak, germs are allowed to pass into the intestine where they increase the intestinal putrefaction and hinder the completion of digestion and the absorption of nutrient into the blood, a further result of which must be that an extra load of toxins will go into the bloodstream and pass to the liver to be de-toxicated, which will hinder the liver in work, to be discussed presently.

This problem of deficiency of hydrochloric acid has several features. A list of habits which could cause these glands to fail is given in the chapter on "Twenty-seven Varieties of Indigestion" in the section on "Low Acid." Every bad habit mentioned there should be corrected. Then, a balanced ration low in fat should be secured to make sure the blood gets the necessary elements out of which the glands may elaborate the hydrochloric acid. To help the weak acid to digest the balanced ration, it may be necessary for a time to supplement the acid. The physician may prescribe free hydrochloric acid, but it should be taken only under the direction of a physician. Some authorities give two ounces of lemon juice with each meal instead of the free acid, until the glands improve in their function. In the absence of lemon juice, pineapple juice or grape juice will act somewhat the same as the lemon juice.

Third

Next we must consider the condition in the intestine. It is said that severe intestinal putrefaction nearly always accompanies anemia, and that the blood improves when the intestinal condition is corrected. This, therefore, is very important. The reader should now consult the chapter on "Constipation" and follow it until the needed result is obtained. Now we are getting good absorption into the blood. The toxins which were injuring the spinal cord are no longer going from the colon.

Fourth

Red blood corpuscles are manufactured in the red bone marrow, but this can be done only in the presence of a hormone manufactured by the liver. If the liver is not getting hordes of bacteria and loads of toxins from the intestine it will have a better opportunity to do its legitimate work and produce this hormone.

Proof that these are the factors involved is offered in the following:

Feeding ground pig's stomach is said to help the stomach and so help the anemia.

Feeding liver to the patient helps the liver and so helps the anemia.

Feeding normal gastric juice helps the anemia.

Feeding hydrochloric acid or lemon juice helps the stomach and the anemia.

However, some of these procedures may help one organ and not be good for the whole man. For instance, feeding of liver is highly injurious to the kidneys. Rats fed on a high liver diet developed Bright's disease—some of them in ten days—none of them survived a year, although they grew fast and looked sleek. (99)

Manifestly eating liver is not the best procedure, although it was in vogue for a number of years. There is now an extract of liver which secures the hormone and leaves out the tissue and toxins. Even this may not be necessary if every correction is made in the manner of living and the best diet is taken.

Eating meat cannot be the best procedure because its iron is poor in quality and because meat leads to putrefaction in the intestine, a condition which must be overcome.

A vegetarian regimen is the most successful one. The foods high in iron should be given prominence in the daily menu. The iron in certain foods is especially helpful. This is true of the soy bean. The iron in whole wheat has been found to be as efficient as liver in feeding rats, and was better than the iron in egg yolks.

Favorable reports have been made on bananas and grape juice. The legumes are very helpful, as are the leafy greens.

The diet should be richer in protein than the average. See chapter on "Eating for Strength" for tables by which to determine the amounts of protein eaten.

See Thiamin in "The Mysteries of Life" early in this book.

Blood Destroyers

Not only must every effort be made to build up the blood, but every practice which destroys it must be abandoned. Among these destroyers should be mentioned tea, coffee, cola drinks, alcohol, and tobacco. Eliminate everything not found in the Automatic Menu Planner.

A word should be said here about alum baking powders and aluminum cooking utensils. See the section on "Light on the Aluminum Question."

Aluminum is what the chemist calls a very "active" metal and has the power to displace all metals which are less active. Iron is one of the less active metals. Therefore the chemist says aluminum can displace iron in the liver and red blood corpuscles, as has been demonstrated by animal experiments. That it does the same in humans and is a common cause of anemia is believed by many doctors. A few of their statements are in this book and many more are on file.

Arthritis

This term is applied to a group of afflictions differing somewhat from each other. One type is said to be caused by infection, the source of which is found in tonsils, teeth, appendix, colon, gallbladder, sinuses, etc.

Much can be done in the early stages, but the more advanced the conditions the more difficult it becomes to secure restoration to health.

If there be infection, that, of course, should have attention. There is no doubt that a faulty diet lowers the resistance to infections, as is discussed in the section on "Immunity"; this may even be the most important factor.

This book is most concerned with the manner of living which prevents this group of unfortunate afflictions. In the program of prevention, diet must hold first place.

A typical medical comment, which sheds much light on the subject, follows:

"Arthritis offers a difficult and important problem to the physician. It is of frequent occurrence and is often painful and disabling. Many approaches have been made toward the secret of its cure. One such contribution is described by Dr. Lovell Langstroth, of San Francisco (California and Western Medicine), who made a study of one hundred cases. Seventy-seven of these were of the degenerative type, eight of the infectious and the rest intermediate. A diet rich in protective foods, particularly vegetables and fruits, was given to seventy-two patients with degenerative arthritis, five were not improved, thirty-nine were much improved, and fifteen were completely relieved.

"It was found that improvement was greatest in the cases where bread had formerly been eaten in the largest quantities. Dr. Langstroth does not blame this cereal specifically for having brought on arthritis, but believes that its free use lessens the intake of protective foods and is thus indirectly injurious. Where the patient was middle age, inactive, and overweight, he was placed for a time on a diet consisting wholly of fruits and vegetables. After a few days other foods were added. There was usually a loss of from eight to ten pounds, with increasing freedom from pain, stiffness and disability. The patients felt generally better, and had a clearer skin. Actinotherapy, heat, diathermy, massage and postural exercises were employed to suit individual needs.

"In infections or proliferative type, a protective diet is prescribed likewise, but sun bathing is almost indispensable. The patient should live where this is possible for eight months in the year. He should be as active as his condition permits. Later, massage is indicated. It is suggested that the disease may not invariably be due to focal infection, as is generally believed, but may be a deficiency tissue disease related to vitamin D." (100)

It is quite clear that a diet chiefly of vegetables and fruits is the right plan. This is the "Alkaline Diet" discussed in this book. If people had always lived on the alkaline diet they would not have arthritis of the diet deficiency sort, and the alkaline diet would be one factor to protect them against the type caused by infection.

If one holds his acid-forming food down to 25 per cent of the total food that will automatically keep the amount of bread down to a low point.

One should make sure of all of his vitamins and the full supply of minerals. Some people are helped by taking dicalcium phosphate tablets daily.

Use nothing not given in the list of "Natural Foods."

Discontinue every bad habit like tobacco, alcohol, tea, coffee, cola drinks, etc.

Correct indigestion and constipation.

Colitis

Colitis has been shown to be a deficiency disease, the diet being lacking in vitamins and minerals. It often is an aftermath of years of constipation and the use of cathartics.

The one-time "bland" diet is not the correction because it is still deficient in the vital elements.

The ration must contain the minerals and vitamins.

Study the chapter on "Constipation." That program may have to be modified by taking out some of the irritating fibers, but the general plan is the same.

Very likely there is infection, which can be conquered only by the minerals and vitamins in the "Alkaline Diet," and by correcting the intestinal condition. Dr. Kellogg says that the coarse foods are needed even though they do cause some pain. (101)

It is important that all foods which quickly putrefy be avoided. These are meats of all kinds, eggs, and cheese.

Sometimes cultured buttermilk helps the intestinal condition. Soy bean milk will be the best milk for most cases.

Bananas are rich in vitamins and minerals and are non-irritating. Ripe olives are in the same class, and both are good for constipation.

Employ as nearly a normal ration as the colon will tolerate.

Staying Young While Growing Older

Age Fifty

The study of geriatrics—how to extend good health into the upper brackets of life—is receiving the attention of certain workers in the health field.

Only seven per cent of Americans live past age 65. About three-fourths of the people die before the age of fifty. Many more years should be added, when cares might be lessened and people could enjoy the things they have done; their interests in life might ripen, and they give to others the benefits of their experience and so add much to the sum total of human happiness.

The experiences which come to us from ages 40 to 100 cannot be separated from those which have gone before, because they are the direct result of them.

Three Periods of Life

There are three periods of life which must have careful attention if we are to have good health the first forty years and then the second forty or more.

The First Period

(1) The first period is prenatal. Many children are born handicapped with mental or physical inferiority, or both; some have unstable nervous systems; others have weak eyes, or are "predisposed" to this or that condition. There are reasons for these things. One or both parents may have indulged in practices which made the production of normal children less likely. If we name a few we must mention the use of tobacco, alcohol, and other narcotics; also licentiousness. Deficiencies of minerals and vitamins are liable to give a trend to their offspring from which they can hardly, if ever, recover. As an example, calcium is necessary to a sound nervous system with both parents and children, and it is now understood that the most common and greatest deficiency in the American diet is calcium. And yet, men and women in every walk of life daily unwittingly rob themselves of calcium in numerous and unnecessary ways, as set forth in other portions of this book.

The consequence of these practices upon the offspring is almost wholly ignored. Most parents seem only to care for the pleasure of present indulgence regardless of the future effects upon either themselves or their progeny. This is hereditary. This is a crime against the race—race degeneracy.

A writer, regarded by the author of this book as an unquestioned authority, has stated the matter in the following plain language:

"Fathers as well as mothers are involved in this responsibility, Both parents transmit their own characteristics, mental and physical, their dispositions and appetites, to their children. As the result of parental intemperance, children often lack physical strength and mental and moral power. Liquor-drinkers and tobacco-users may, and do, transmit their insatiable craving, their inflamed blood and irritable nerves, to their children. The licentious often bequeath their unholy desires, and even loathsome diseases, as a legacy to their offspring. And as the children have less power to resist temptation than had the parents, the tendency is for each generation to fall lower and lower. To a great degree, parents are responsible, not only for the violent passions and perverted appetites of their children, but for the infirmities of the thousands born deaf, blind, diseased, or idiotic." (182)

This matter is so fundamental and of such far reaching importance that the present writer has thought best to reproduce another statement from Ellen G. White, which presents the subject in a wider setting and vastly increases its seriousness and significance.

"Man came from the hand of God perfect in every faculty of mind and body; in perfect soundness, therefore in perfect health. It took more than two thousand years of indulgence of appetite and lustful passions to create such a state of things in the human organism as would lessen vital force. Through successive generations the tendency was more swiftly downward. Indulgence of appetite and passion combined, led to excess and violence; debauchery and abominations of every kind weakened the energies, and brought upon the race diseases of every type, until the vigor and glory of the first generations passed away, and in the third generation from Adam, man began to show signs of decay. Successive generations after the flood degenerated more rapidly."

"All this weight of woe and accumulated suffering can be traced to the indulgence of appetite and passion. Luxurious living and the use of wine corrupt the blood, inflame the passions, and produce disease of every kind. But the evil does not end here. Parents leave maladies as a legacy to their children. As a rule, every intemperate man who rears children transmits his inclinations and evil tendencies to his offspring; he gives them disease from his own inflamed and corrupted blood. Licentiousness, disease, and imbecility are transmitted as an inheritance of woe from father to son and from generation to generation, and this brings anguish and suffering into the world, and is no less than a repetition of the fall of man." (183)

A New Kind of Parents Needed

The foregoing takes us back to the beginnings or origins of the conditions which confront us with increasing severity, after sixty years of age, and show us what must be done if the desired health is to continue after sixty. The first necessity is a generation of parents who will understand and observe the laws of life, and teach their children to do the same. Naturally we do not expect ever to see the time when all of the parents in the world will follow this way of living, but we do hope that this book will aid a few people in doing so.

Surely it is now plain that we have found the right starting point for our study of geriatrics, and we will proceed with our subject.

The Second Period

The second period with which we must deal is from birth to age forty. If we can get some parents to live as taught in this book and rear their children to do the same, the situation for them will be entirely transformed, and age forty will not with them be as it now is with many—"the dangerous age." Today it is dangerous to live after forty, not because of the dangers we meet after forty, but because of the dangerous way we have lived during those first forty years, so that we are unfitted to continue the journey of life as we should do.

The average father does not wish to be bothered with learning how to live to be well. If he gets sick he will go to the doctor. Neither does he wish to curtail his indulgences, nor will he give the needed attention to training his children. He may tell John not to smoke, but he smokes, and John will more than likely do as his father did rather than as he said.

Another common attitude with both parents and youth is this: Many indulgences do not cause any immediate suffering; if they do, the suffering is not seen to be related to habits. For instance, smoking is the usual cause of Buerger's Disease which is a condition of the feet, or hands, or both, and unless the smoker has been told about it he will never suspicion that smoking is the cause, and so the smoker continues his habit until the surgeon takes off some of the toes, or one or both feet. Then the end is not far away. This is one of the "end products" of smoking, but it took many years of smoking to produce it, during which the smoker was unaware of what it was doing to him. And so it is with many other things. Here is another example; Two-thirds of one kidney can function sufficiently to sustain life. The Creator gave all of us a kidney and a third to spare, like our spare automobile tires. People commonly indulge in many practices which destroy the cells of the kidney, but as they cause no pain they are not aware of the slow degeneration of that vital organ; there is no way for them to know until the kidneys begin to fail to do their work, and then they are near the end of life. Thus it is with many other organs. "Man cannot know to what extent the factors of safety of these silent partners have been reduced."

If these facts of life are not known by parents and taught to the youth by parents, schools, and churches, there is no way for them to know about them, and at about age forty many of them will begin their years of suffering for which there often is no remedy.

But if the right example is set by adults, and the proper instruction given by parents, educators and spiritual instructors, so that the youth grow up living in daily harmony with life's laws, they may come to age forty with all organs unimpaired. They may then enjoy a goodly number of years of great usefulness and much satisfaction. To this they have now added twenty years of experience, and they are now ready for the greatest of undertakings. If they can have good health now for another forty years what wonderful things they can do and how happy they can be!

The Third Period

This brings us to the third period of life where the study of geriatrics is being applied today with the hope that some of those who are more or less disabled may be helped to meet at least a portion of life's responsibilities. And here let it be said that often it is possible to accomplish a great deal. The manner of living can be changed so as to lift the load off the worn kidneys; there are ways by which the heart load may be lessened. In case of overweight, the heart will be greatly helped by bringing the weight down to normal. Tired nerves must be rested. A wornout stomach may, well it is hard to say; if it is given the right kind of food and only at proper times instead of eating everything and at irregular hours, it may recover part of its ability to function; it is worth trying. There are usually things which can be done to lower the blood pressure and ease the load on the hardened arteries and the heart. The use of tobacco, alcohol, tea, and coffee can be discontinued; a vegetarian regimen can be adopted. The daily schedule can call for more rest and less work. Changes can be made in the entire pattern of living.

The dietetic errors of former years can be corrected so the foods eaten will be rich in calcium, iron, and vitamins. Bread is an example of the point. To make white flour from wheat, two-thirds of the calcium, four-fifths of the iron, and five-sixths of the phosphorus which nature put there for our benefit have been removed and sold, in the bran, shorts, and middlings. Finely ground whole grain wheat flour retains all of these valuable elements. One authority, in writing about this food for those past middle life says—"No nutrition student interested in the welfare of the aged will advocate any other bread than that made with flour of the greatest possible natural nutritive value." (184)

The same author urges that "there is need for constant education of those in the latter half of life to induce them to broaden their food likes rather than to increase the number they dislike."

One geriatrician says that a deficiency of calcium is one of the causes of aging, and that an abundance of calcium "extends the prime of life in later years. It is one of the secrets of youth prolongation." (185)

Not only may a calcium supplement be needed, but some may need extra iron and vitamins. The geriatrician can first correct the daily living and then direct in the use of remedies or supplements as may be needed.

These principles apply, of course, to both men and women but with more force to men than to women because they ignore life's laws more often than women do and as a consequence death comes to them a few years sooner than to women.

"While there is life there is hope." Study all parts of the book you are now reading. Make every change indicated. Avoid extreme fatigue as a subtle enemy. Acknowledge your violations of life's laws, physical and spiritual, to your Maker and ask for His blessing to rest upon you as you now do His will; then trust and hope for a great deal. The writer of this book was supposed to have died by the doctor's orders over fifty years ago, but is now writing this book with glee, enjoying both mental and physical work during these upper brackets of life, happy in the service of God and humanity.

As we close this chapter the reader is asked to remember that the foundations of life are laid in the prenatal period; that the next most important step is to keep life's laws from birth until age forty arrives. Then, if you continue for the remainder of life after the same pattern, barring accident, you have no need to fear the years, but will enjoy every one to the full as long as they keep coming, perhaps to age one hundred.

Light on the Aluminum Question*

There are many rumors and stories current concerning ill effects arising in the body from the use of aluminum where it comes in contact with food and drink. Often it is apparent that these stories are based upon supposition or hearsay, and therefore are not reliable. I have traced some of these reports against the use of aluminum to the source and found that they were not true.

A great deal of scientific work has been done with aluminum to protect its reputation against these attacks.

I have read widely on both sides of the subject from authors in various countries. The wide disagreement over the matter is at least confusing. The great difficulty is that science seems to be arrayed on both sides of the question, which makes it impossible for the average person to arrive at the truth of the matter.

For a number of years I relied upon the scientific work done in defense of aluminum and paid little heed to the rising chorus of warnings against the popular metal. The time came when these repeated challenges to investigate the other side of the question could not be ignored. I concluded that where there is much smoke there must be some fire.

Knowing that truth never contradicts truth, it was apparent

---

* The material on the following pages is a portion of a more extended treatise on this subject bearing the same title as this section, prepared by the same author.

that something was wrong in the contentions made for and against aluminum. Science cannot rightfully be marshaled on both sides of a question and made to contradict itself.

A wide and extended study of the subject reveals two uses made of scientific knowledge of aluminum. One use is made by scientists who are working to protect the reputation of the metal, who may be paid for doing so. Often these writings are published and circulated at the expense of those interested in aluminum. Manifestly such writings must be regarded with some suspicion because of their origin; they may be biased and "tainted."

A different use is made of science by another sort of workers, namely those who are working to protect the health of the people. It is possible that these workers do not have as much money available to conduct their researches and to publish and circulate such vast amounts of literature as do those in the first class. There is such a thing as error having the advantage over truth for a time. I have found such to be the case, more or less, in other fields of investigation. As an example: In making a digest of the writings of fourteen hundred authors from fourteen different countries, on the subject of tobacco, I often found that science is used in an attempt to prove that the moderate use of tobacco is not harmful. Again, a great deal of scientific work has been done to prove (?) that refined white flour is a health food. The same is done with coffee, tea, and even alcohol.

When writing scientific articles it is as easy and human for an author to be biased as when dealing with non-scientific themes. Many times I have seen authors meet views which were unwelcome to them by saying, "There is no scientific evidence," or, "The evidence submitted was not satisfactory," or "It has never been satisfactorily proven." In that way one can readily brush aside any findings or opinions which he wishes to discredit or undermine.

Therefore, when science is used to prove two opposite views it becomes necessary to look behind the scenes and discover who is using the science—whether its users are working in the interest of the people or in the interest of some organized industry. If this can be discerned it will greatly help the investigator to know how to properly weigh the conflicting testimony.

It is regrettable to find that much of the current scientific literature concerning alumnium comes directly or indirectly from those who are interested to have aluminum used. It is likewise regrettable to often find that those who should be working for the health of the people accept at face value the reports of the research work done by the vested interests, and repeat and reprint such reports as their own final conclusion and put their influence behind them. When this occurs, the public becomes almost helpless.

Inasmuch as there is plenty of literature extant in defense of aluminum and not so much to be found in defense of the people, the following material is offered for consideration. "Safety first" is always recognized as the best rule, and there is no other motive back of the publication of this material than a desire to protect the health of the people who will be influenced by that which is here presented.

Some of the testimony to follow pertains to the use of alum in baking powders. Being salts of aluminum, it belongs in this discussion. Other testimony will be concerning the use of aluminum cooking utensils. All phases of the subject will be covered.

SUMMARY FROM ABROAD

That which seems to be a fair-minded summary of both sides of the subject, published in London, will make an appropriate beginning of this study. It is a work entitled

"THE CLINICAL ASPECT OF CHRONIC POISONING
BY ALUMINUM AND ITS ALLOYS"

by Leo Spira, M.D., with a Foreword by Prof. Dr. Hans Horst Meyer, University of Vienna. Parts of this summary follow:

"FOREWORD"

"In the following paper Dr. Leo Spira communicates the results of his observations over a period of ten years. He has, in my opinion, made a very careful medical study of a disease picture which exhibits considerable variety and yet, on the whole, presents a uniform complex of chronic signs and symptoms. The author has pursued to eventual cure and, as it appears, has correctly comprehended the puzzling and prolonged course of this disease, both in his own case and that of numerous patients. By systematically examining all the possible causes Dr. Spira has recognized, as a hitherto hardly considered source of this chronic poisoning, the use of aluminum utensils in the kitchen. He has actually proved this by the success of the treatment which he based on his findings in cases in which every other method of treatment had failed, and in which patients who had already been cured suffered a relapse when the prescribed special regime was temporarily interrupted.

"The publication of these experiences, particularly as a bibliography of the very comprehensive literature on the subject is appended, appears to me to be very valuable, not only for the medical profession and the general public but also for the industry. The latter will be stimulated to discover a resistant alloy that, like some iron compounds, will not be attacked by the ordinary oxidizing and dissolving agents.

Vienna, Sept., 1932   PROF. DR. HANS H. MEYER."

"Three main groups are distinctly discernible, namely: gastrointestinal, cutaneous and general.

"In the first group the outstanding feature is constipation. It appears that this complaint is present in almost every patient, and even amongst those who do not suffer from it habitually it is present from time to time. Few are found who are not obliged to use an aperient, however small the quantity. Constipation is invariably accompanied by flatulence and colicky pain of such severity as in some cases to suggest the possibility of gastric or duodenal ulcer, cholelithiasis, nephrolithiasis, colitis or even 'acute abdomen,' and resistance of the abdominal wall associated with tympanites appears to be extremely common. Some patients complain of dryness in the mouth and throat. The appetite is considerably impaired or entirely lost and there is retching during or after meals, with, in some cases, a distressing hiccough. Attacks of nausea set in and, in more advanced states, also vomiting of every kind of food soon after it has been taken. X-ray examination reveals in these cases only colonic stasis.

"The obvious change presented on examination concerns the condition of the mouth. The tongue loses the natural aspect of a flesh-colored, moist, smooth surface, with the papillaevallatae and foliatae only slight elevated. There appears a thick white or dirty grey fur, with the papillae vividly red and enlarged. The patients at first attribute this condition of the tongue to a slight attack of indigestion, caused previously by some article of food. The changed appearance, however, persists, and different methods of treatment, dietetic as well as mechanical, fail to remove the fur. The only method which temporarily restores the normal aspect appears to be scraping the surface with a soft toothbrush dipped in bicarbonate of soda. This action seems to be chemically neutralizing rather than mechanical.

"Later on, in much advanced cases, the tongue becomes indented by the teeth, raw and excoriated. Deep fissures appear on the surface and constitute the condition of superficial glossitis.

"In acute exacerbations the whole mucous membrane of the mouth is involved and presents the complete picture of stomatitis. Herpetic ulcers develop and the gums appear red and swollen, with pus collecting under them, and thus a condition of severe gingivitis closely similar to, if not identical with, alveolar pyorrhoea is established.

"In the meantime, the initial gastro-intestinal symptoms progress steadily towards a chronic condition, in spite of most careful dieting.

"Certain skin conditions also appear to be present with greater frequency in this country than they were on the Continent up to ten years ago. Acute and chronic urticarias, and the various eczemata usually attributed to idiosyncrasy for certain foodstuffs occurred but rarely in my continental experience. In this country, on the other hand, in the acute cases the signs and symptoms are often of such unusual severity, as immediately to suggest their being due to a highly potent irritant which, in its action, is closely similar to arsenic and belongs probably to the same group of poisons although arsenic itself has not been found. Cases of pruritus generalized all over the body, of unknown origin, appear also to be extremely common. Sometimes it is more pronounced in the hands and feet, and especially in the interdigital spaces. In more advanced cases, a skin disease develops, which, when affecting the fingers and hands, is diagnosed as cheiropompholyx and dysidrosis and generally attributed to a vasomotor neurosis, the lesions being in anatomic relation with the sweat-structures. Between the toes, and more especially in the third and fourth interdigital spaces, a condition makes its appearance which is very similar to, and in fact is often diagnosed, as "dhobi-itch" or "foot-tetter," if a fungus is found. Excoriations and rhagadae between the toes develop, and a normal skin in the interdigital spaces showing no peeling is hardly ever seen. Very often, however, no fungus can be detected by any method and then the condition is diagnosed as being due to gout or to so-called "soft corns." In some cases the skin of the whole or parts of the body is affected by a rash which, when attacking children, is identical with "infantile eczema," and often attributed to allergy. In other cases recurrent attacks of herpes situated on any part of the body, or the occurrence of persistent furunculosis, are a striking feature. Scattered over the skin of the chest and abdomen, multiple pin-head or larger sized telangiectatic naevi are often observed. Loss of hair, keratosis of the palms and soles, and so-called "chillblains" on the fingers and toes are met with quite frequently. The fingernails become soft and brittle, lose their lustre and appear opaque and thickened, while longitudinal striation in varied degree is usually present. When associated with onychia and paronchia, their appearance is very similar to onychomycosis, but a fungus cannot always be detected.

"Turning to the third group in the symptom-complex, frequent attacks of neuralgia and twitching of the legs must be mentioned. They occur mostly at night during sleep, and are sometimes so painful as to alarm the patient. Pain in the fingers and toes, paraesthesiae of the whole hands and more especially along the ulnar nerve distribution of the fingers, associated with the sensation of numbness and deadness, in some cases even gangrene of the toes, resemble very much Raynaud's disease and ergotism. Arthralgiae of the most severe type, diagnosed as being of rheumatic origin are a very common occurence. Giddiness and excessive perspiration are frequently observed and anemia is a regular feature. In the urine, traces of albumen and a few red blood corpuscles can be found and the regularity with which a slight reduction of Fehling's solution is detected in practically every patient, often perceptible only after the tested material has cooled down, is most remarkable. A systolic blood pressure as low as 80 mm. Hg. among middle-aged and even older patients is met with very frequently. Nervous symptoms comprise depression, and even melancholia, loss of energy and general lassitude.

"It must, of course, not be assumed that all the symptoms are in each case developed to the marked degree which has been described, or that they run concurrently in every patient. In some patients a few or all symptoms of one group, for instance, gastro-intestinal or cutaneous, predominate. Others may complain at one and the same time of symptoms described in two of the groups given above, for instance, gastro-intestinal and cutaneous.

"These latter, however, or even those suffering from all the three groups, were met with so often that a common cause suggested itself as aetiological factor. It was curious that patients who left England temporarily to live abroad improved in health rapidly, even without any medical attention, and that they suffered from recurrence of their symptoms within a very short time of their return. On the other hand, people with previously perfect health who came to live in London complained of illness after a stay of a few months, or even weeks. It was therefore to be suspected that the casual agent must be looked for in this country, and some of the cutaneous manifestations, when accompanied by symptoms of the other two groups, were chosen as a starting point of the investigations.

"It has already been mentioned that the dermatoses under discussion were attributed in many cases to a vegetable fungus, which however, could frequently not be detected. Where a fungus was found local treatment often failed to cure the condition. If these dermatoses were actually due to infection, then, it was thought, severe gastro-intestinal disturbances occurring at the same time might likewise be caused by the same or a similar fungus, introduced into the body by food or fluid contaminated by it, thus constituting a mycotic gastro-enteritis. The food would have to be such as was most indispensable in everyday life, since patients suffering from these groups of symptoms belonged to different spheres of life and lived in different parts of London. Bread and its ingredients, meat, milk and butter, vegetables, fruit, coffee, tea, sugar, salt and water had to be considered.

"The empiric method of elimination was chosen for the investigation. One article of food after another was struck off the list of diet, and it was recommended that water be taken only after being boiled. The results, however, were always negative, and it was concluded that experiments in this direction were fruitless.

"To make certain that water could not be suspected of contamination, the cisterns in my house were emptied and cleaned under my personal supervision. Contrary to expectation, only a mineral, and no organic matter visible to the naked eye, was found, and thereupon the theory of an organic poison was given up and the possibility of the presence of a mineral or metallic poison accepted. This again led to the belief that the symptoms might be traced back, not to the different articles of food, but to the utensils in which this food was prepared.

"From the fact that all the cooking utensils used in the house were made of aluminum, attention was especially directed to the possible occurrence of a poison therein. This suspicion had to be maintained for the particular reason that subsequently, in several cases, lead was found in the excreta, and in some tin as well.

"To keep aluminum utensils clean, soda or a material containing it, such as soap, special cleaning powders, etc., are used. For the sake of experiment the aluminum utensils were not removed altogether from the household, but the order given that instead of cleaning them with soda, only water and brush should be employed, with the result that not only the rebellious skin disease diagnosed as cheiropompholyx and dysidrosis and the affection very similar to "dhobi-itch," but also all the gastro-intestinal symptoms came to a standstill within a few days. The improvement was still more marked when the aluminum utensils were removed altogether. It must therefore be assumed that all the symptoms were due to a poison contained in the aluminum utensils.

"At this point emphasis is laid on the fact that nothing was known to me at the time (i.e., 1928) in regard to the discussion in the medical press of different countries about the possible toxicity of aluminum. The literature concerning this metal was gone into only after the above conclusions were arrived at, and it showed that a dispute had been proceeding for many years and had led, in some cases, to a controversy between the medical profession and powerful industrial interests.

"It is true that the described condition was not entirely cured by the elimination of aluminum utensils. Although the cutaneous manifestations disappeared altogether, the gastro-intestinal symptoms, though considerably alleviated, persisted in appearing shortly after meals. The possibility of the presence of some additional irritant had therefore to be pursued with a view to finding further sources containing injurious substances, such possible sources being tinned foods and hard aluminized or chlorinated tap water running through lead pipes, to which attention had again to be directed.

"A diet was now chosen which excluded everything prepared in tap water. Only raw fruit, or fruit and potatoes baked in their jackets, soft-boiled eggs, etc., were given, and tap water replaced by a pure and wholesome natural mineral water, which was also used for boiling food wherever possible.

"To absorb and eliminate the poison accumulated in the body, large doses of a high-grade charcoal and an aperient were given.

"This regime was applied with the strictest perseverance in all the cases included under the three headings given at the beginning of this paper, and it resulted in the most rapid disappearance of all the symptoms, including the skin manifestations. A complete cure, not obtainable by any other of the many methods of treatment applied hitherto, was maintained as long as the patients persevered with the regime prescribed to them. They were put gradually on an ordinary diet, but were not allowed to use aluminum utensils, tap water or other likely sources of metallic contamination, and remained perfectly well as long as they took small doses of charcoal and an aperient. In cases, however, in which for some reason they omitted these precautions, the symptoms again made their appearance, to disappear as rapidly as before, when the regime was again strictly followed.

Conclusions

"(1) The extremely common manifestations of the skin, such as pruritis, dermatitis, herpetiformis, cheiropompholyx, dysidrosis, infantile eczema, etc., are of gastro-intestinal origin, and accompanied by gastro-intestinal symptoms and those of disturbed metabolism.

"(2) The symptom-complex described is caused by one or several irritants contained in aluminum utensils and in chlorinated or aluminized tap water, since it disappeared when further intake of poison was stopped and the amount ingested was eliminated by charcoal and aperient.

"(3) As the skin manifestations disappear under the described treatment, without any local applications, it seems likely that the prevailing theory that they are caused by a fungus is not tenable. It is probable rather that this infection, where present, is of a secondary nature . . .

(Eight case histories have been omitted here.)

"(1) Aluminum.

"The controversy concerning the dangers arising from its use is an old one, but the first classical experiments on animals were performed in 1886 by Siem under the direction of the well-known pharmacologist Hans Horst Meyer. When injecting small doses of sodium aluminum tartrate subcutaneously at intervals of a few days, he found that the animals died after 2-4 weeks, the lethal dose being an amount of the salt which corresponded to 0.25-0.30 g. (i.e., 4-5 grains) aluminum oxide per kilogram of the animal's weight By injecting, however, a single large dose in cats, death resulted after only 5-11 days, the lethal dose being then as little as 0.15 g. (i.e., 2½ grains) per kilogram.

"The first symptom noted, as early as the third day after the commencement of the injections, was severe disturbance of the digestive tract. Anorexia, even complete refusal of food, and very severe constipation, with one single defaecation in the course of five days, were the outstanding features. With the cumulative action of the injections which were superadded at intervals, frequent behement vomiting of bile-stained mucous masses and diminished excretion of urine developed. Albuminuria was not always present. Small ulcers appeared on the buccal mucous membrane and the animals lost weight rapidly. The blood pressure and the bodily temperature became low, owing to paralysis of the center of the nerve supply to the vascular system. Towards the end of the experiment the central nervous system became profoundly disturbed and the animals developed signs of acute bulbar paralysis. General tremor, with tonic and clonic convulsions of the head and extremities, accelerated death, which was due to paralysis of the respiratory center, the heart being the ultimum moriens.

"In the case of the cat, peroral daily administration of the salt corresponding to 0.1 g. (i.e., 1½ grains) alumina per kilogram of the animal's weight for four weeks produced behement diarrhoea, but with the beginning of the second week the animal again recovered its normal state.

"The post-mortem examination showed hyperaemia and swelling of the mucous membrane of the stomach and small intestine, especially the duodenum, and small ulcers were found in the gastric mucosa. The kidneys were hyperaemic and deep red in color and showed signs of parenchymatous nephritis. In some cases the cortical substance was much infiltrated by fat and exhibited a few pin-head sized extravasations of blood. The liver was dark red in color but the outline of the lobules was quite distinct. The lobules themselves appeared opaque and slightly yellow. The heart muscle was invariably soft and flabby. Microscopically the liver showed finely granular degeneration and the vessels of the cortex and medulla of the kidneys were engorged with blood. The epithelium of the convoluted tubules showed signs of hyaline degeneration and their lumen was filled with hyaline casts.

"Siem classes the mode of action of aluminum with that of mercury and lead, since all these metals are readily absorbed from the gastro-intestinal tract.

"The ensuing controversy concerning the dangers arising from the use of aluminum compounds seems to have ceased for a time but was resumed once more in America before the War, when the question of the aluminum contained in alum baking powder came under discussion. In this way the possibility of the aluminum contained in kitchen utensils being detrimental to health came to the fore. The discussion in medical circles in several countries, among them England, France, Germany, Switzerland and the United States, was protracted, being chiefly concerned with the element aluminum alone. As a result two sets of opinion developed which were diametrically opposed to each other. On the one hand the opinion has been expressed that, as the result of scientific investigation on animal and man, aluminum has been found to be innocuous. On the other hand, it was claimed with equal emphasis that scientific investigation had proved aluminum to be definitely poisonous. Between the parties were those who declared that although it was in general harmless, aluminum was found to be detrimental in some cases. Even the correctness of the methods employed in laboratory analyses and the value of the chemical and physiological experiments and pathological findings were disputed.

"One set of investigators, amongst them Lehmann in Germany, Mackenzie, Schmidt and Hoagland, McCollum and his collaborators in America, stated that aluminum derived from a scientifically aluminized food was either not soluble and therefore not absorbed at all, or only in minute quantities which were perfectly harmless to the body, and that since there was no absorption there was no deposition of the element in the tissues. They contended that the amount of aluminum in aluminized food was very small in comparison with that taken regularly in the great variety of articles of food which contained it as a natural constituent. The sulphate of different metals was injected by Bertrand and Servescu under the skin of animals, and they asserted that aluminum was less toxic than, for instance, nickel or copper, since an injection of 100 mg. (i.e., about 1½ grains) of the aluminum salt per kilogram of the animal's weight killed the animal only after 8.34 hours. The statement was even made by Myers and Mull to the effect that the injection of aluminum salts into animals raised their growth and reproduction. According to them, no abnormalities were to be noted in the animals at the autopsy and all the organs appeared to be healthy apart from a marked increase of the aluminum content in the liver.

"Contrary to these findings, Gies, Steel and Kahn, all in America, found (each of them in independent investigations) that aluminum phosphate was dissolved by the hydrochloric acid of the gastric juice; that the aluminum chloride, thus formed, owing to its astringent and protein precipitating properties, attacked the mucous membrane of the stomach, passed from the alimentary tract into the blood circulation and, without manifesting any tendency to accumulate in the blood, was deposited to some extent in various parts of the body, whereas another part was excreted in both the bile and urine.

"The conversion of aluminum phosphate into the chloride under the influence of the hydrochloric acid of the gastric juice was demonstrated in the excellent experiments made on animals by the French investigators Schaeffer and his collaborators. They too showed that aluminum was absorbed, in comparatively large amounts, into the blood circulation and deposited in the tissues of the body. Animals fed on aluminized food gained weight more slowly than control animals. The younger they were, the more sensitive were they to aluminum. They suffered from severe diarrhoea immediately after being fed on aluminized food, and showed a definite retardation of reproduction. The anatomical changes produced by aluminum were demonstrated by necrosis of the epithelium of the gastric mucosa in the region of the fungus and pylorus and also the duodenum, comparable with erosion seen in man; further by congestion and oedema of the mucous membrane of the intestine, especially the colon descendens and the sigmoid. There was glomerule-nephritis and considerable atrophy of the ovaries. All the control animals escaped injury.

"In a very comprehensive series of experiments the American physiologists, Underhill and his collaborators, described the metabolism of aluminum. In animal experiments they found that the aluminum content in the blood tended to increase after ingestion of aluminized food. Aluminum was deposited in the various tissues and the main places of storage were the liver, kidneys, brain, spleen and muscles. The bile and spleen contained more than eight times, the brain more than five and a half times and the liver and kidneys more than four times as much aluminum per unit as the blood. On examining the tissues of dogs at different ages they ascertained that there existed a direct relationship between the age of the animal and the quantity of aluminum stored in the tissues, and that this same tendency for aluminum content to increase with advancing age existed in man.

"In the clinical aspect of aluminum poisoning produced in experimental animals, loss of appetite was noted as the first symptom. They soon appeared inactive and depressed and lay quietly in their cages, manifesting no interest in their surroundings, and, if forced to move, they were slow and clumsy. In addition, on feeding dogs for twelve weeks with aluminized food, a skin disease developed in one of the animals, which was covered with abscesses that became large bleeding sores. When given milk, a quart at a time, by stomach tube for a few days, improvement started at once; by the end of the experiment it was eating all its food, the skin had healed, and new hair was growing.

"The post-mortem examination revealed marked congestion in all the viscera, especially in the mesenteric vessels. The stomach was greatly distended, the mucosa somewhat swollen and containing a few pin-point to pin-head sized hemorrhages. In a few animals the intestinal mucosa contained a few small greyish superficial ulcers. Intestinal contents were greenish in color and contained no blood or mucous. The liver showed extensive tissue changes consisting of congestion, central necrosis and fatty infiltration. The kidneys were pale and soft, the principal site of damage being the convoluted tubule, although the glomerular tufts were also sometimes swollen.

"According to reports in the German literature of the last few years, diseases are making their appearance which have hitherto been unknown on the Continent. Gonnermann attributes the increasing number of disturbances of metabolism and also increased incidence of amenorrhoea to aluminum found, amongst the German population, in different parts of the body in recent years is due to the fact that unusual amounts of alum were of necessity given in food during the War.

"Considering the more extensive use of aluminum utensils in the households abroad, the increasing incidence of disease is not surprising, and the results obtained from a comparison between the health conditions in this country during the last ten years and those on the Continent previously are no longer valid. It is therefore interesting to learn that in Germany too, within the last two years, some diseases have been traced directly to aluminum.

"Putensen, in Bavaria, from personal observation on patients describes the signs and symptoms of aluminum poisoning in practically all details, as reported by me in 1928. He, too, lays special stress on constipation, flatulence, low blood pressure and giddiness as the main characteristics. Eczema and pruritus as well were observed by him in one patient. Moreover, he described the case of a dog whose persistent rash and sores associated with intense itching did not respond to local treatment, but disappeared eight days after the aluminum utensils from which the dog was fed were discarded.

"Von Halla records twenty-five cases of patients suffering from severe constipation and dermatoses, which did not yield to any treatment on orthodox lines, but were cured after the aluminum utensils had been removed from their households.

"Kazil, in Prague, described, as the outstanding symptom, diarrhoea followed by severe constipation, colicky pain, neuralgiae and anaemia. In post-mortem examinations performed on workers in aluminum factories he observed that the lymphatic glands had become impregnated with minute particles of aluminum, and that this had led to proliferation of the connective tissue and atrophy of the pulp. Similar changes had occurred in the spleen and the bone marrow, and the deposition of aluminum and consecutive irritative action had taken place also in the liver and the glands of generation. The digestive tract showed signs of hyperaemia and mucous catarrh, both of which were of chronic nature.

"It would appear impossible, though it has been done in certain quarters, to minimize or to consider as valueless findings which have been arrived at after most careful and painstaking researches. The chemical properties of aluminum seem, however, to be established beyond dispute. It is readily attacked by acids and soluble in alkalies.

"It is attacked slowly by cold acetic acid, but the rate of attack increases markedly with rising temperature and with progressing dilution of the acid. It is attacked with great rapidity by hydrochloric acid, hydrogen being evolved and aluminum chloride formed. Hydrofluoric acid in all concentrations acts rapidly upon aluminum and its alloys, but lactic acid only slowly. The metal is attacked even by fairly pure atmospheric air, and all the more rapidly by impure air such as that in large industrial cities.

"Aluminum is readily soluble in alkalies, alkaline waters and water to which alkalies or soap have been added. The blackening and corrosion of aluminum kitchen utensils is often traced to alkalies which have come in contact with them.

"'In 1928, I expressed the opinion, though without being able to give any proofs, that diverticulosis of the colon, which is a disease occurring in ever-increasing frequency, might have some relation to the increased use of alumnium cooking utensils. As early as 1925, however, Odier in Switzerland reported, without adducing any scientific data, that a few persons, hitherto in perfect health, had developed cancer of the digestive tract some months after the introduction of aluminum utensils into their households. He suggested the possibility of a connection between the alarmingly increasing incidence of cancer and the widespread use of aluminum for cooking purposes. This suggestion was refuted by Lehmann, Frank and Blumenthal in Germany, and Bordas in France, in each case without any scientific argument being put forward. To judge, however, from the observations described in the German literature by two independent observers, Buerstenbinder and Merk, the hypothesis of Odier seems to be gaining ground as one more theory of the causation of cancer of the digestive tract. No explanation was put forward by Odier, but it may be fruitful to investigate whether the development of cancer of the gastro-intestinal tract cannot be traced to chronic irritation by the particles of carbon which are present in practically all grades of aluminum utensils as an impurity. They are derived from the carbon lining, made of petroleum coke with an oil or tar binder, which constitutes the electrodes that come in contact with the materials used in the furnace during the process of manufacture of aluminum.'"

(Three pages of bibliography have been omitted.) (102)

It would almost seem that the foregoing summary would be sufficient to settle the matter with the average reader; but inasmuch as the use of aluminum is widespread, and it is in popular favor, and "protected" from every standpoint, it seems wise to provide enough scientific information to satisfy the most doubtful reader. Therefore we now present four statements from standard medical reference books concerning alum and aluminum.

Alum—U. S. Dispensatory

"Alum is a powerful astringent with very decided irritant qualities, and when taken internally in sufficient quantities is emetic and purgative, and may even cause gastro-intestinal inflammation. It is widely employed in various conditions in which an astringent or styptic is desired. . . . When small quantities of the soluble salts of aluminum are introduced into the circulation they produce a slow form of poisoning characterized by motor palsies and areas of local anesthesia with fatty degeneration in the kidney and liver. The nervous symptoms have been shown by Doelken to be due to anatomical changes in the nerve centers. There are also often symptoms of gastro-intestinal inflammation which is presumably the result of the effort of the glands of the intestinal tract to eliminate the poisoning." (103)

ALUM

"Physiological action. This agent is actively astringent coagulating the albumen of the tissues and of the blood and produces a local constriction of the capillaries. It is mildly escharotic (burns) and produces a hardening of the skin and tissues in general. It excites and later diminishes the salivary secretions as well as those of the mucous surfaces, it diminishes the gastric fluid and precipitates pepsin. As a result of its action on the intestinal secretions, constipation is produced. Through its irritating properties which may be in excess of its astringent properties gastroenteritis may result." (104)

Aluminum Hydroxide

"Physiological Action. This agent produces profound prostration with irritation of the mucous membranes with diminished secretions and as a result there is constipation and inactivity of the bowels. The nervous system is affected as is indicated by the extreme prostration with numbness of the parts and paralysis of the involuntary muscles." (105)

"Lancet" reported tests in 1913 as follows:

(1) Aluminum loses its luster when water is boiled in it.

(2) When cold water was let stand in aluminum for twenty-four hours, a white gelatinous substance sweated from it which proved to contain alumina and silica.

(3) A 1 per cent solution of common salt in tap water left overnight gave the same result.

(4) A 1 per cent solution of acetic acid, representing household vinegar, when boiled for several hours, showed nothing.

(5) Common salt and acetic acid were boiled several hours and then contained traces of aluminum salt. After standing cold overnight "some soft white aluminum rust appeared in several places, and the metal was pitted."

(6) When tartaric acid, which occurs in fruits and vegetables, was boiled and let stand for twenty-four hours, it "produced patches of white aluminum rust."

(7) With common salt and tartaric acid the saucepan remained clean and "apparently unaffected, but on testing the fluid, traces of aluminum salt were found."

(8) With citric acid, "there were signs of the aluminum being attacked."

(9) With a solution 1/100 per cent carbonate of soda the aluminum was affected, the saucepan was darkened and the solution responded decidedly to the tests for aluminum. "It is here noted that 'it is desirable to exclude alkaline soda salts in cooking operations in which aluminum vessels are used, and that it has been noticed that in the price lists of aluminum goods the warning was generally issued that soda should not be used.' "

(10) Beefsteak fried showed distinct traces of aluminum.

(11) Tomatoes, butter, salt and pepper, fried—showed slight indications of soluble salts of aluminum.

(12) Soup made of extract of beef, with carrots, onions, salt, pepper and vinegar, showed traces of aluminum.

Brussels sprouts showed traces of aluminum, but when carbonate of soda was added "there were signs of the metal being attacked and aluminum was found in small quantities in the liquor."

It was stated as not advisable "to leave water for long in aluminum water bottles," and that "it is desirable also not to scour cooking vessels to such an extent as to remove any thin coating which forms on the surface, for this coating subsequently becomes protective." An additional precaution advised to "keep the vessels perfectly dry when not in use, and coat them with a film of hydrocarbon oil to protect the metal from the combined action of moisture and air."

This series of twelve tests were reported in London "Lancet" in 1913 and are recorded by Cooper in "Danger of Food Contamination by Aluminum," pages 10-13.

Doctor Cooper repeated these tests. His report follows:

(1) One thousand c.c. London tap water stood twenty-four hours; 2.45 gr. of aluminum, silica, and iron per gallon of water detached from the dish.

(2) One thousand c.c. tap water boiled in dish for twenty minutes was cloudy, and on standing a while, a white voluminous precipitate was deposited. The water contained a trace of metallic aluminum. The white precipitate contained alumina and calcium. Silica was present and a trace of iron. The darkening was due to iron impurities in the aluminum which became exposed when the surface of the aluminum was removed.

(3) On heating milk, a considerable amount of material was taken up by the milk, 140 gr. per gallon, the most of which was aluminum. In this case the milk did not stand in aluminum after heating.

(4) When gooseberries were stewed 31 to 85 gr. per gallon was taken from the pan.

(5) Rhubarb when cooked gave 7.7 gr. per gallon.

(6) Three lemons were put in 500 c.c. of water. The liquid dissolved 26.6 gr. per gallon.

(7) Soup of mutton, potatoes, onion, carrot and 0.5 grm. of salt was made and let stand twenty-four hours. Three hundred gr. per gallon was taken from the metal.

In above experiments allowance was made for the quantities of aluminum occurring normally in these foods. The same foods were cooked in enamel to check against the aluminum, and only the normal amounts were found in the foods cooked in enamelware. (106)

Aluminum-Poisoning Symptoms

"Besides its irritative, inflammatory, ulcerative and paretic effects upon the gastric and intestinal mucosa, it apparently seriously deranges the nervous system. It has a strong affinity for fibrous, tendinous and ligamentous tissue, and tends to cause subacute inflammatory conditions of the gums, strongly suggesting a possible influence in pyorrhoea." (107)

Aluminum Not Normal in Human Body

"One scientist has gone so far as to say the life itself of the animal body is actually dependent on the presence of aluminum in it, but this is definitely and finally refuted by F. P. Underhill and F. I. Peterman (Yale University, *American Journal of Physiology*, Sept. 1929) already referred to, who, using tests capable of detecting the remotest trace of the metal, prove that it is not found in the foetus." (108)

Aluminum Stored in the Body

Reported in *American Journal of Physiology*, Sept., 1929. Work done by Frank P. Underhill and F. I. Peterman of Yale University.

"Using the sensitive Alizarine test they found it chiefly in the liver, brain, kidney and spleen, and that it was mainly excreted in the bile, which holds eight times the quantity of the blood. Its peculiar affinity for nervous tissue is shown by the fact that the brain holds a larger store per 100 grm. of tissue than the liver, and more than 5½ times as much per unit as the blood. Muscular tissue generally holds relatively small amounts, but when the total mass of muscular tissue in the body is considered the total aluminum stored in this may reach an important figure. Their researches amply show that aluminum, though found in animal organisms, is not essential to those organisms, that it is a foreign substance which is being continually eliminated, that such elimination puts a strain on the organism, and that when more is forced upon the system than it can deal with disastrous results follow." (109)

Cooper Reviews Objectors

"That it is harmful is amply proved, and can be constantly re-proved by anyone who cares to do so, on his sick acquaintance, by stopping using aluminum cooking utensils and watching the effects. No proof could be better than this. This is the final and absolute proof of proofs, because it evidences the effects on the human body. Yet Dr. Burns puts aside all such evidence, provided by myself and other medical men (as for example the cases which have been recorded in the British Medical Journal of late) with no better argument than that such evidence is a figment of the imagination and consequent on suggestion; weakly likening it to the imaginary benefit derived from inactive patent medicines . . . He can only exonerate aluminum by shutting the door to the only evidence that really matters."—"Danger of Food Contamination by Aluminum," Cooper, p. 36. (110)

Indefensible

"It is to be noted that in their critical explanations McCollum and his two workers do not discuss the physiological lesions observed by us and affecting the mucous membrane of the alimentary canal, nor do they discuss the effects proved on the ovary of the mouse. To affect the mucous membranes with which it is in contact it is to be noted that (salt of) aluminum does not need to be absorbed. As for the action of the element of aluminum on the ovaries shown by us, it proves clearly the absorption of the metal which does not need to be in considerable doses in the organisms in order to be physiologically active. . . .

" 'Our observations on the work of Shaeffer and his co-workers,'' writes McCollum, 'are not presented as a defense of alum baking powders.' We are glad of it. For every physiologist informed on questions of nutrition, these products are indefensible." (111)

Coffee Pot Test

The Massachusetts Institute of Technology, Cambridge, Massachusetts, ran a three-year test for the USA coffee trade interests to determine the most satisfactory material to use in making coffee pots. Concerning aluminum they reported—

(a) That it is impossible to make fine-flavored coffee in it;

(b) That the inner surface of the pots were corroded by the coffee;

(c) That ill effects, usually gastric disturbances, followed the drinking of such coffee. (112)

If one or two cups of coffee made in an aluminum pot are liable to cause gastric disturbance would not food cooked in aluminum be liable to do the same?

Aluminum and Blood Hemoglobin

"Seibert and Wells (1929) state that rabbits consuming 0.1 grm., of sodium aluminum sulphate (11 mgm. of aluminum) daily in their food eventually showed less hemoglobin in their blood than control rabbits receiving no aluminum."—"Death in the Pot," by Harold W. Keens, p. 38. (113)

Replaces Iron

"Dogs fed with aluminum phosphate absorbed considerable aluminum; some was retained in the body, in all probability replacing the iron of ferruginous proteins (ferratin of liver), and accompanying the iron in its cycle (circulation in the body), in bone marrow, corpuscles, liver, proteins. Still another portion remained in the bones. There is a storage of aluminum, at least temporary, which is not confined to any one particular tissue. The distribution is not uniform, however, and seems to be roughly parallel to that of iron. Much of the aluminum fed was speedily eliminated in the bile and in the urine. The dogs were not apparently affected." (114)

Various metals possess different degrees of potency of electrochemical activity. The chemist has set them up in the following order with the weakest at the bottom and the strongest at the top. Each one is more active than all of those below it and the potency increases as we climb the list. The more active ones have power to displace the less active ones,—those below it. Note that aluminum is fifth from the top. It can displace all of those below it, one of which is iron. This is offered as an explanation of the loss of iron from the body and the accumulation of aluminum when even small amounts of aluminum are introduced into the system

Potassium
Sodium
Calcium
Magnesium
Aluminum
Manganese
Zinc
Chromium
Iron
Nickel
Tin
Lead
Copper
Bismuth
Antimony
Mercury
Silver
Platinum
Gold

Dissolved by Alkalies

"It is well known that alkalies act as solvents of aluminum and therefore salt and soda and bicarbonate of soda should not be used for cleaning." (115)

Will not these elements in foods do the same?

Defense Arguments Change

"So the ground of defense has now shifted. It began by saying that little or no chemical action took place; then that it only occurred when salt and soda were used when cooking and cleaning; then that the amount absorbed by the human body when salt and soda were not used was too small to affect any but a few hypersensitive individuals."

"Each of these positions has become insecure. So the argument now is to show that in any case all natural foodstuffs contain aluminum before they are cooked. This looks like being the last, or nearly last ditch." (116)

A great deal of similar information is still in my files and accumulating every month. It is impossible to present all of it here. It is sincerely hoped that the foregoing is sufficient.

It is possible that certain readers may be critical of some of these statements and of their authors, but it will be very difficult for such readers to brush aside all of this testimony and human experience and still contend that the use of aluminum is harmless.

When health and life are involved, "safety first" is the proper measure.

Fabulous sums of money are being spent on research, to protect the health of the people. Every field is being searched to find clues to the causes of disease. Every germ is being watched and every food studied. Drugs and serums are provided in great plentitude. Elaborate surgical equipment is found in every hospital, and the medical colleges are training surgeons in the latest technique to remove or repair the various "parts" of the body.

Can it be that those whose profession is to warn against health hazards and to cure disease will continue to ignore the rapidly multiplying testimony of chemists, doctors, and authors who are lifting their voices in sincere, earnest warning against the use of aluminum?

A Few High Lights on the Cancer Problem

This is not a treatise on the subject, but an attempt to bring together a few items which may help those who have not had the opportunity of reading as widely on the subject as some of us have done.

Cancer is one of the gravest health problems confronting all civilized peoples. It is now the second cause of death, and in the United States takes a toll of 150,000 lives each year. One person in every five and a half over forty years of age will die of it. It has increased 25 per cent in ten years.

The main hope cannot be in curing cancer after it has formed, but rather in discovering the cause and applying preventative measures. Frantic efforts are being made to find methods of control and to learn its origin. This section is chiefly concerned with cause and prevention.

The Theory of Micro-Organism

There are two theories regarding the source of human cancer— (1) a micro-organism, (2) some, as yet, unknown influence brought to bear upon cells which causes them to "go wild." The latter is more commonly accepted by medical authorities but it is not by any means unanimous. From a somewhat wide range of reading on the subject, the following points have been gleaned.

The study of the history of the microbe theory, which has been conducted by the Murdock Foundation in New York City, reveals that for over a half century many workers in various countries have recorded having observed in malignant tumors minute bodies which have been called by different names as "sporozoa," "coccoid-like bodies," "spore-like bodies," "parasitic cell inclusions," "fuchsine bodies," "coccidia," "foreign parasite," "blastomycetes," "saccharomyces litogen," etc. One worker states that over a period of six years he examined microscopically 1,278 cancers, and that in 1,130 of them found "parasitic bodies." One worker says they are in every cancer and in the peripheral blood. (117)

Every now and then reports like the following find their way into public print:

"Cancer by Virus"

"Cancer, at least of certain types, may be caused by filterable viruses, and in that respect resemble a numerous and varied group of human ills including smallpox, influenza, and infantile paralysis. Three converging lines of evidence pointing to this idea have been set forth by Dr. James B. Murphy and Albert Claude of the Rockefeller Institute for Medical Research, by Drs. Jacob Furth and Elvin A. Kabat of Cornell University Medical College, and Dr. F. Duran-Raynals of Yale University."

"In one line of research, fluids from malignant transplantable tumors of chickens were whirled in the ultracentrifuge, passed through fine-pored filters, and otherwise treated after the manner of virus-containing fluids in known animal and plant diseases. Materials obtained from these cancer-fluid filtrates, injected into the tissues of healthy chickens, produced typical cancerous growths." (118)

Cancer an Infection

An eminent American physician and surgeon, a student of the cancer problem for many years, wrote the following in a letter to J. Ellis Barker, which was published in "Fortnightly Review," and republished in "The Motive," Chicago, February, 1925:

"Dear Sir:

"In the issue of the 'Evening Standard' of July 8th I read your reference to a review of your recent book on cancer, wherein you say that you have been 'reproached for failing to deal with the microscopical and biochemical characteristics of cancer cells.'

"Aside from the very good reasons which you offer for not having thus treated the study of the subject, perhaps you would be interested to know that Prof. D. B. Roncalli (formerly professor of surgical pathology in the ancient University of Padua and now holding the same position in the University of Naples), in his classical work published ten years ago, declared that in his opinion the cause of cancer is an infection pure and simple sui generis.

"Prof. Roncalli is one of the foremost pathologists in Italy, a distinguished surgeon also, and one whose microscopic study of cancer cells has been enormous. Please let me assure you as a qualified physician and surgeon in America and Italy, that in a study of Roncalli's researches and his 'slides' made from hundreds of cases of all varieties and types of cancer and his findings based thereon,

I find nothing out of harmony with your theory as to what might be termed some of the exciting causes of cancer, such as 'Constipation, autointoxication, absence of vitamines in sufficient quantities,' etc. May they not be some of the exciting causes to the infection pure and simple sui generis which Roncalli's extensive studies claim as the cause? And his opinion is based on long years of scientific research, all of which is set out in his classical work of three thousand pages. I was so much interested in his labors that I spent months with him in his clinic at the University of Padua in 1913-1914. It was my intention to translate his works into English, but the war intervened and I had to give up the thought."

(*Signed*) WILLIAM JAMIESON GAVIGAN

Cancer a Germ Disease

The following paragraphs are extracts from an article by G. K. Abbott, M.D.:

"The cause of cancer has been the subject of much controversy, and in recent years of considerable scientific investigation. As yet there is no unanimity of opinion among medical men as to its causation. The marked resemblance between the behavior of cancer, tuberculosis, and leprosy has led some very astute medical observers to urge strongly the idea of the germ origin of cancer. Among such men were Sir James Paget of England, also Haviland, and later Ballance and Shattuck, with Roncalli of Naples, and many other men."

"Dr. William B. Coley, professor of Clinical Cancer Research of Cornell Medical School writes:

" 'The main argument against the theory of the extrinsic origin of cancer is that no one has discovered the germ. This is no more an argument that the germ does not exist, than that the germ which causes smallpox or measles does not exist. We know that these two diseases are of germ origin, and the very fact that their cause has not been discovered, should be some excuse for our not having yet discovered the micro-organism which is the possible cause of cancer.' "

"In 1921 Dr. John W. Nuzum, of the University of Illinois published the results of experimental work by which he had demonstrated in transplantable cancer of white mice, the constant presence of a certain germ. This germ has grown on artificial media, injected into numerous white mice, producing cancer in them, and again recovered in pure culture. It will be recognized that these experiments satisfy Koch's laws, which are requirements original- ly formulated by Robert Koch, whereby it is proved that a given disease is of specific germ origin. Dr. Nuzum found the same germ in a case of human cancer, and produced cancer in animals by its injection. In March of this year, Dr. Nuzum reported fur- ther confirmation of his discovery through animal experimentation, and finally the production of cancer in one human being by re- peated injections of this same germ secured from another case of cancer in the human. In this case the experimental cancer was cured by early surgery. So convincing are these researches that they have led one of America's greatest surgeons, Dr. Albert J. Ochsner, to avow publicly his belief in the germ origin of cancer. He says:

" 'I am convinced that John Nuzum's research in connection with the study of cancer in a short time will be recognized as being on a par with the discoveries made in tuberculosis, smallpox, and leprosy.' "

" 'The invariable presence of this micrococcus in cancer in man and in lower animals, the fact that typical metastasizing cancer has been produced in lower animals and in man by inoculation with pure cultures of this micrococcus, and the fact that pure cultures of this micrococcus, and the fact that pure cultures of the same micrococcus obtained from these cancers thus produced, have again produced typical cancers in other animals under proper con- dition, convince me that Nuzum's micrococcus is in fact the ulti- mate cause of cancer.' "

"That the day is not far distant when the parasite, that is, the germ origin, of cancer will be as fully accepted by medical men as the germ nature of tuberculosis and leprosy, the writer person- ally has no doubt." (119)

An important step in the development of knowledge concerning the causation of cancer seems to have been taken at the University of Texas by Alfred Taylor, Ph.D., and reported in "Southern Medi- cine & Surgery" of July 1943. He is working on the theory that cancer is caused by a virus.

He has experimented with a cell-free agent which will reproduce the same type of tumor as that from which it was taken.

Dr. William G. Doern, Director of the Doern Clinic in Milwaukee reports that what "appears to be the cancer germ may be seen (with magnification stepped up to two thousand diameters), and the final detailed study of this micro-organism requires three thousand diameters magnification. If we step up the magnification three times, we must step up illumination fifteen times to get results."

He reports, as an example, that sixteen rats were injected with human cancer germ cultures and all of them developed tumors. He had conducted such experiments for several years and is thoroughly convinced that cancer is caused by a microscopic germ. (186)

The May 1949 issue of Life and Health carried an article by D. A. Delafield and Wayne McFarland, M.D., on cancer in which they reported Dr. John Bittner's experiments with mice at the University of Minnesota which convinced him that the disease is caused by a "filterable virus"; in other words, "a living virulent" organism of submicroscopic size.

They also report that Dr. Ryojun Kinoshita of Osaka University has done work with rats and mice from which he concludes that a virus is associated with cancer. With a powerful electron microscope he was able to make photographs of the virus, several of which were thrown on the screen when he gave an address at the National Cancer Institute, Bethesda, Maryland, in November, 1948.

They further reported on work done for eight years on chickens by Dr. Nelson F. Waters of the Department of Agriculture's Poultry Research Laboratory, at East Lansing, Michigan, from which he concludes that a form of cancer called lymphomatosis is an infectious disease which spreads from one chicken to another. This is similar to lymph cancer in human beings.

Meat and Cancer

Exhaustive statistical studies have been made in many countries of the incidence of cancer, which reveal that it is most often associated with eating flesh.

"At the Panama-Pacific Exposition held in San Francisco to celebrate the opening of the Panana Canal, Hoffman (probably the foremost Life Insurance statistician in the United States) presented a remarkable and very graphic statistical exhibit showing the mortality from cancer in every country in the world in which statistical studies had been made. This exhibit brought out very definitely and clearly the fact that cancer was by far most frequent in countries in which the consumption of meat was highest. The association of high mortality from cancer with high meat consumption was so constant that almost no exception could be found. Attention, however, has been called to the fact that although the native Eskimos of the Arctic region subsist upon an almost exclusive meat diet, it is not known that death from cancer is frequent among them. However, it must be considered that no studies have been made on the subject on which a sound opinion could be based."

"Another significant fact is worthy of consideration. Cancer is a disease of middle and advanced age. It may almost be said that the Eskimo dies of old age before he is old enough to die of cancer."

"Captain MacMillan told the writer that it is rare to find an Eskimo much over fifty years old. They go to pieces rapidly after middle age, and those who live to the age of fifty-five, are exceedingly decrepit and infirm." (120)

The above Dr. Frederick L. Hoffman, who is head of the statistical department of the Prudential Life Insurance Company, has written a book of one thousand pages dealing statistically with cancer.

A long list of physicians from various countries might be given, who bear positive testimony based on their clinical experience, agreeing with Hoffman. The following is typical:

Dr. Keates of India is quoted, "I have always believed that the diet of the Punjabi villager, consisting as it does of freshly ground whole-meal wheat flour, pulses, milk and ghi (butter) with fresh vegetables, renders him immune to a great many diseases. . . . such as dental caries, appendicitis, and carcinoma." (121)

Dr. Wm. J. Mayo said, "Is it not possible, therefore, that there is something in the habits of civilized man, in the cooking or other preparation of his food, which acts to produce the precancerous conditions? Within the last one hundred years, four times as much meat is taken as before that time. If flesh foods are not fully broken up, decomposition results, and active poisons are thrown into an organ not intended for their reception, and which has not had time to adapt itself to the new condition." (122)

"The intestinal secretion is almost invariably deficient, and constipation, even in early cases is so common that the toxins produced by the millions of micro-organisms generated through intestinal stasis and fecal putrefaction must be looked upon as one of the prime elements in the causation of cancer. Sir Arbuthnot Lane has spoken of cancer as one of the terminal results of intestinal stasis."

"Aborigines living simple lives, largely vegetarians, have been shown by any number of observers, in many lands, to be almost if not entirely free from cancer, while many have also reported the definite increase of the disease, and its mortality, in proportion to their adoption of the customs and diet of so-called modern civilization.

"The statistics from many countries show that increase in the consumption of meat, coffee and alcoholic beverages, appears to be coincident with a very great and proportionately greater augmentation of the mortality from cancer. In England the consumption of meat has doubled during the last fifty years, while the deaths from cancer have increased fourfold. The United States consumes one-half of the total amount of coffee handled in trade everywhere.

"In India," says Dr. Hoffman, "meat is eliminated to a point of minor importance while vegetable factors hold first place. This, in my judgment, is precisely the diet least likely to favor the development of malignant new growths in the light of such investigations as I have thus far been able to make, and while they are evidently inconclusive for the time being, it is quite reasonable to expect evidence to be forthcoming showing that races on a vegetable diet are less liable to malignant tumors than those who follow a predominating meat diet." (34)

Diet a Basic Cause

The following significant report was made by Dr. L. Duncan Buckley, M.D., while he was serving as senior physician in the New York Skin and Cancer Hospital: "Laboratory experience has repeatedly demonstrated the controlling effect of diet on cancer in animals. In one extensive series of experiments seventy-five per cent of seventy-five inoculated mice developed tumors while under normal diet, whereas only 19 per cent of another seventy-five inoculated mice developed tumors while under a diet with vegetable proteins; moreover, the tumors in the latter were hardly larger in thirty days than those in the former in ten days."

"In many reviews I have been quoted regarding meat-eating's being the cause of cancer; this is only partially true, as may be judged from what has preceded. The true cause is a metabolic disturbance arising from diverse agencies, prominent among which are errors of diet, especially along the line of meat, coffee, and alcohol, together with faulty living and imperfect action of some of the organs of the body." (124)

"The late Dr. William Parker, famous New York surgeon, declared, 'In regard to the effect of abstemiousness on cancer, I can speak with great positiveness that a vegetable or at least a very bland diet, does check the progress of the disease, and in some cases now under treatment, has been attended by an alleviation of symptoms and in a few instances even by a recession of growth.' " (125)

"Ehrlich has shown that mice living on a rice diet cannot be inoculated with cancer, while those on a meat diet can readily be inoculated, the tumors developing quickly and continuing to grow until the animal dies." (126)

"The writer saw in the laboratory of Ehrlich, who made an extensive study of diet upon cancer, rats in whom well-developed cancerous growths had very largely disappeared under special feeding." (127)

Food the Chief Factor

"I believe that the state of affairs found in this fish hatchery points very strongly to the infectious nature of this form of cancer and that the contagion is water-borne. It is possible that feeding liver into the waters of the fish hatchery has some relation to the outbreak in this case. I know of a second fish hatchery where the disease was endemic for a number of years and where the feeding of liver has been changed to the feeding of chopped sea fish and in the last three years the disease has disappeared. . . . Feeding is probably more important than any other factor. The removal of feeding or change to natural food tends toward the recovery of affected fishes, and prevents or delays the initial process." (128)

A report by Dr. J. L. Halberg of the Pearson Foundation indicates that cancer has been cured by entirely withholding all animal proteins.

A news item from Cornell University Medical School announces the cancer in mice disappeared while they were on a very restricted diet.

The discovery that cancer is caused by a living virulent organism is a step of first magnitude toward the solution of the cancer problem, but that does not reveal the steps to take to overcome the cancer in the human subject. There are those who believe that the needed help will come largely from nutrition and physical therapy. Some very interesting work which is not yet ready to be publicized is being done in several places with diet. This approach to the subject seems to be coming to the fore.

Thus two lines of evidence are accumulating. First, that the cause of cancer is an organism; second, that, to some extent at least, it can be controlled by diet.

Constipation and Cancer

"Cancer never affects a healthy organ. In every case in which I have had an opportunity of verifying it, I have found that the cancer patient was suffering from chronic intestinal stasis and that the infection by cancer was an indirect consequence of that condition. Cancer is the final stage in the sequence of chronic intestinal stasis. It is the last chapter in the story of defective draining of the large bowel, as it is in the rest of the intestinal tract." (129)

"If you wish to produce cancer with a fair degree of certainty, supply a constipated subject with plenty of meat, and endeavor to deal with his constipation by means of irritating purgative drugs." (130)

"Dr. Robert Bell of London never saw a case of cancer in which there had not been prolonged constipation." (131)

"Several eminent pathologists have called attention to the relation of mastitis, or chronic inflammation of the mammary gland, to cancer. The lumps often observed in the breasts of women, when examined under the microscope, often present appearances almost indistinguishable from cancer; and there is much evidence that in many cases these abnormalities may develop into cancer."

"Mastitis is believed by eminent English surgeons to be due in some cases to infection from the colon. When constipation and resulting colitis exist, there is a constant stream of germs passing into the blood which may disperse the infection over the entire body, and so infect the milk glands."

"English observers have recently noted that mastitis in cattle often assumes the human type and so may become a cause of infection in human beings."

"The possibility that mastitis may result from neglect of the colon, may lead to cancer, adds another reason for exercising the greatest vigilance in the supervision of milk supplies." (132)

Tobacco and Cancer

The volume of literature going to show that cancers of the lip, tongue, esophagus, stomach, and lungs, result from the use of tobacco is too great to attempt to reproduce here. Let it simply be understood that we have a mass of such documents on file.

Aluminum and Cancer

In the section entitled "Light on the Aluminum Question," will be found a number of opinions indicating a very firm belief that aluminum is irritating enough and strong enough a poison so that cancer can more readily develop at the areas of such irritation. The accumulative effect of daily eating food prepared in aluminum utensils may well be considered. Although some people scoff at the idea, it may yet be found to be a very important factor. Only a few of the opinions on file have been included in this book.

Six different factors have been mentioned in the foregoing paragraphs; still others might be added as irritants; those mentioned are—

1. Micro-organism	4. Constipation
2. Meat	5. Tobacco
3. Diet	6. Aluminum

Will the reader please ponder the thought that these may all be true and there be no contradiction? Think a moment.

(1) If a micro-organism is the enemy at work in the cells, the question of immunity comes to the fore at once and assumes a place of first importance. Working on that basis for a moment, see what we find.

(2) Meat tends to fill the system with toxins as discussed in the chapter on "Eating for Strength," which toxins weaken the vitality of the cells.

Also, the extractives of meat are an ideal medium for the growth of bacteria.

(3) Constipation fills the system with toxins which lower the vitality of cells.

(4) Tobacco contains several deadly poisons; a single drop of one of them—nicotine—put into the blood stream all at once will destroy the life of every cell in the body in a few minutes. Who can say that the daily saturation of the body with minute quantities of the poisons in tobacco is not an important factor in lowering the body immunity to all bacteria, the cancer germ included?

(5) Aluminum is classed as a poison by standard reference medical works. Even the manufacturers of aluminum utensils admit that from their use small quantities of it enter the system. Their claim is that the amounts are so small that they do no harm. Their claims may not be true. Many medical workers today are stoutly contending that they are not true. There is a strong probability that aluminum can be lined up with these other irritants as a "door-opener" to cancer.

(6) A normal ration will have in it the vitamins and minerals and a high alkaline balance, all of which are the mighty factors in the maintenance of immunity and of vitality and life in the cells. The alkalies are strong deterrants to the growth of bacteria. In the laboratories of the Murdock Foundation the workers have for a dozen years been transplanting something from cancer tissue, placing it in the incubator and later planting it in animals which in due time develop cancer. Then from these new cancers they have taken something and repeated the process with the same results. Note that the media in which these cultures grow in the incubator is slightly acid, and that if they are planted in an alkaline solution, they stop growing and die.

Note another important item in the diet. The Murdock Foundation report of January, 1940, affirms that a high blood sugar content favors the growth of the cancer organism. (133)

Dr. Dudley Jackson of San Antonio, Texas, has shown that high blood sugar is present with the higher types of malignancy.

It is well known that sugar is an excellent food for germs outside of the body, and there is no reason to believe it is not also a good food for germs inside of the body.

Furthermore, sugar is a definite cell irritant, and as such lessens the resisting power of the cells.

Therefore sugar damages the man and helps the germ at the same time.

In the light of these contributions the enormous consumption of sugar takes on a new dangerous aspect not before presented to the public, and should receive consideration in this study.

We present still another point in the realm of foods:

"The study of the effect of varying dosages of vitamin A from various sources on the growth of tumors of mice under controlled conditions showed that the tumor implants were not affected by those amounts of vitamin A in the usual diet, supplemented by as much as 500 units of vitamin A. On the other hand, when maximal dosages (1,000 or more vitamin A units) of the provitamin, carotene, were administered, varying degrees of inhibition of tumor growth were observed. . . .

"The administration of the maximal dosages of vitamin A appeared to be without harmful effect upon the animals. This suggests that the inhibited growth of tumor is the result of a specific action of the vitamin A upon the cancer cell." (134)

The usual site of cancer growth is in some epithelial tissue. Vitamin A's major function is to maintain the vitality of epithelial cells. Therefore it is reasonable to expect that large doses of vitamin A would increase the resistance or immunity of these cells to the cancer germ.

Re-study Immunity

Let the reader at this point turn and read the section on "Immunity" and then the one on "The Ideal Vegetarian Regimen" and ponder their meaning.

People Encourage Germs

People everywhere are doing everything possible to encourage cancer germs to do their worst, and are shamefully neglecting the means of defense which are waiting to be used, and which would cost them less than their bad habits.

The great tragedy of it all is that sometimes those who ought to know these things and be telling them to every person on earth are themselves practicing the same destructive habits, and then spending million of the people's money blindly looking in the wrong direction for the cause of the plague of cancer.

Who will dare to stand up and say that if men would cease every injurious practice and employ every health-building force which God has so generously placed in nature all around us, the cancer germ could keep on growing in human bodies? Is it not worth trying?

The saddest part of the picture pertains to the church placed in a sinful and dying world as a Heavenly light to lead men and women back to loyalty to their Creator's laws, the transgression of which has brought all the woe, misery, sickness, suffering, and death the world has ever seen.

To know and observe the laws of the physical life lies at the very foundation of loyalty, and yet almost every church is ignorant here, and doing nothing to learn these principles and teach them to the people; and their members and leaders are transgressors along with the non-professors of religion. They go solemnly on with their rounds of church services supposedly giving the people the genuine gospel when the vital principle is missing, and leaders and people know it not.

The church should be the place where parents, teachers, doctors, lawyers, legislators, and all others would find a guiding influence which would lead them into the light of truth, and into a right relationship to their Maker—loyalty to His laws pertaining to the physical, mental, and spiritual phases of human existence, all three of which are required to make one Christian.

The church should advocate and represent this higher order of living, and should reveal a complete interpretation, not a partial one, of what it means for man to be loyal to his Maker. If the church as the source of divine guidance in the world is negligent in this work, it fails of fulfilling its divine commission, and dark indeed will the future be. Let there be a true church, giving the gospel in all its fullness and saving power. This is the greatest need of the world today.

BIBLIOGRAPHY FOR PART II

(1) "Ministry of Healing," pages 125, 126, 128.
(2) Lamotte, page 58.
(3) "Ministry of Healing," page 272.
(4) Vol. 1, page 701.
(5) Vol. 1, page 701.
(6) Vol. 2, pages 67, 68.
(7) "Ministry of Healing," pages 272, 273.
(8) "Ministry of Healing," page 273.

(9) Vol. 1, pages 702, 703.
(10) "Counsels on Health," page 58.
(11) Vol. 2, page 530.
(12) "Ministry of Healing," page 274.
(13) "Ministry of Healing," pages 274, 275.
(14) "Ministry of Healing," pages 237, 238.
(15) "Ministry of Healing," page 238.
(16) "Counsels to Teachers," page 307.
(17) Vol. 2, pages 525, 526.
(18) "Ministry of Healing," page 240.
(19) "Ministry of Healing," page 238.
(20) Vol. 1, page 555.
(21) "Counsels to Teachers," pages 295, 296.
(22) Vol. 3, page 138.
(23) "Ministry of Healing," page 238.
(24) Vol. 3. page 153.
(25) Vol. 3, pages 489, 490.
(26) "Ministry of Healing," pages 238, 239.
(27) Vol. 2, page 529.
(28) Vol. 3, pages 77, 78.
(29) "Ministry of Healing," page 240.
(30) "Education," page 210.
(31) R. Manning Clarke, M.D., in "Signs of the Times," February 12, 1924.
(32) "How to Live," by Fisher and Fisk, pages 118, 119.
(33) How to Live, pages 120-122.
(34) Vol. 7, page 85.
(35) "Ministry of Healing," page 275.
(36) "Ministry of Healing," page 275.
(37) "Counsels on Health," pages 58, 59.
(38) "Ministry of Healing," page 275.
(39) "Counsels on Health," pages 61, 62.
(40) "Ministry of Healing," page 276.
(41) "Counsels on Health," page 62.
(42) "Ministry of Healing," page 276.
(43) "Madison Health Messenger," Madison College, Tenn., Vol. 4, No. 1.
(44) Food Research Division of the U. S. Dept. of Agriculture. Report by L. H. Bailey, R. G. Capen, and J. A. LeClerc, in "Cereal Chemistry," Vol. 12, page 441, 1935.
(45) "Counsels on Diet and Foods," page 349.
(46) "Counsels on Diet and Foods," page 269.
(47) "Newer Knowledge of Nutrition," by E. V. McCollum, page 157.
(48) "Good Health," August, 1935.
(49) "Food, Nutrition, and Clinical Dietetics," by Risley and Walton, page 53.
(50) "Food, Nutrition, and Clinical Dietetics," by Risley and Walton, pages 52, 53.
(51) "Good Health," May, 1937.
(52) "American Journal of Public Health," Vol. 27, No. 12.
(53) "New Dietetics," page 451.
(54) "Good Health," June, 1935.
(55) "New Dietetics," page 451.
(56) "Journal of American Medical Association," August 13, 1938. Article by Alfred T. Shohl, M.D.
(57) "Newer Knowledge of Nutrition," by E. V. McCollum, page 410.
(58) "The Journal of Biological Chemistry," September, 1939.
(59) "World's Dental Story," California Fruit Growers' Exchange, Los Angeles.
(60) "Journal of the American Dietetic Association," June-July, 1939.
(61) "Journal of the American Dietetic Association," August--September, 1939, page 588.
(62) "Fearfully and Wonderfully Made," Eulenburg-Wiener, page 188.
(63) "Soy Flour," "Food Research Division Contribution," No. 303, U. S. Dept. of Agriculture by J. A. LeClerc and L. H. Bailey.

(64) "Medical Papers," page 122, article by F. W. Gardner, M.D.

(65) E. V. McCollum, Ph.D., Prof. of Biochemistry of Johns Hopkins, article in "Life and Health," March, 1937, page 29, reprinted by permission of "Life and Health."

(66) "Man, the Unknown," Dr. Alexis Carrell, pages 283-314.

(67) "Man the Unknown," Dr. Alexis Carrell, page 207.

(68) "The Crippled Colon," J. H. Kellogg, M.D., page 255.

(69) "The Crippled Colon," J. H. Kellogg, M.D., page 255.

(70) "Parasites That Wreck Your Health," by L. Herbert Lanier, M.D., Chief of Staff, Meagher Memorial Hospital, Texarkana, Arkansas.

(71) "High Blood Pressure," G. K. Abbott, M.D., page 159, quoting Prof. H. C. Sherman.

(72) "The Phenomena of Life," by George Crile, M.D., page 190.

(73) "Michigan Public Health," Michigan State Board of Health Bulletin for March, 1940.

(74) "Good Health," November, 1937, pages 338, 339.

(75) "Good Health," February, 1937, page 47.

(76) "New Dietetics," by J. H. Kellogg, M.D., pages 914, 915.

(77) "New Dietetics," by J. H. Kellogg, M.D., pages 913, 914.

(78) "Good Health," October, 1937, page 308.

(79) "Journal of Pediatrics," July, 1940.

(80) "Home Physician," 1923 edition, page 490.

(81) "New Dietetics," by J. H. Kellogg, M.D., page 896.

(82) "Home Physician," 1923 edition, page 483.

(83) "Question Box," J. H. Kellogg, M.D., page 791.

(84) "The Normal Diet," by W. D. Sansum, page 62.

(85) "New Dietetics," J. H. Kellogg, M.D., page 422.

(86) J. H. Kellogg, M.D., "Good Health," September, 1938, page 280; "Question Box," page 245.

(87) Metropolitan Life Insurance Company, Publicity.

(88) "Foods, Nutrition and Health," McCollum and Becker, page 97.

(89) "The Normal Diet," by W. D. Sansum, M.D., page 49.

(90) J. H. Kellogg, M.D., in "The Crippled Colon," page 158; "Good Health," June, 1934; "Good Health," August, 1935.

(91) "The Crippled Colon," pages 159, 160; "Good Health," June, 1934, pages 9-11.

(92) "Journal of the American Dietetic Association," June-July, 1939.

(93) "Medical Annals of the District of Columbia," March, 1935, and "Journal of the American Medical Association," April 13, 1935.

(94) "Chemistry of Food and Nutrition," by H. C. Sherman, pages 273-280.

(95) "The Infected Colon," by J. H. Kellogg, M.D., page 198; "Question Box," by J. H. Kellogg, M.D., page 424.

(96) "New Dietetics," by J. H. Kellogg, M.D., page 435.

(98) "Health Question Box," by J. H. Kellogg, M.D., page 895.

(99) "High Blood Pressure," by G. K. Abbott, M.D., pages 72, 73.

(100) "Good Health," July, 1935, page 214.

(101) "The Crippled Colon," page 187.

(102) "The Clinical Aspect of Chronic Poisoning by Aluminum and Its Alloys," by Leo Spira, M.D. Published by John Bale, Sons and Danielsson, Ltd., 83-91 Great Titchfield Street, W. 1, London. 1933.

(103) "U. S. Dispensatory," 21st edition, 1928, page 109. Used in all drugstores, hospitals, physicians' offices, and recognized in Courts at law as an authority on the use and doses of medical substances.

(104) "Materia Medica Therapeutics and Pharmacology," by Alexander Blackwood, A.B., F.A.C.P., Professor of Clinical Medicine and Therapeutics in Hahnemann Medical College, Chicago, page 111.

(105) "Materia Medica Therapeutics and Pharmacology," by Alexander Blackwood, A.B., F.A.C.P., Professor of Clinical Medicine and Therapeutics in Hahnemann Medical College, Chicago, page 112.

(106) R. M. LeHunte Cooper, M.D., in "Danger of Food Contamination by Aluminum," pages 13, 14. Tests made by Doctor Eastes of the Pathological and Public Health Laboratories, Harley Street, London.

(107) "Danger of Food Contamination by Aluminum," Cooper, page 2.

(108) "Danger of Food Contamination by Aluminum," Cooper, page 2.

(109) Published in "The Danger of Food Contamination by Aluminum" (3rd edition), page 21, by R. M. LeHunte Cooper, M.D., B.S., M.R.C.S., L.R.C.P., Medical Officer of Health, Harrismith, O. R. Colony. John Bale, Sons and Danielsson, Ltd., 83-91, Great Titchfield Street, London, W. 1.

(110) "Danger of Food Contamination by Aluminum," Cooper, page 36.

(111) Translated from the French. Taken from article written by G. Shaeffer and co-workers in answer to article by McCollum, Rask and Becker, entitled "With Regard to the Physiological Actions of Baking Powders Containing Alum," and is published in "Bulletin: Societe Scientifique d'Hygiene Alimentaire," Vol. XVII, No. 2, 1929, pages 86, 87. Masson et Cie, Editeurs, Libraires de l'Academie de Medecine, 120, Boulevard Saint-Germain, Paris.

(112) Reported by Edgar J. Saxon in "Health and Life," Dec., 1938, page 460. Was published by Samuel C. Prescott and the Joint Coffee Trade Publicity Committee, 64 Water Street, New York City, in 1924.

(113) "Death in the Pot," by Harold W. Keens, page 38.

(114) A. K. Balls, Doctorial Dissertation, Columbia University, 1917. Reprinted in Mellon Institute of Industrial Research Bulletin No. 3, 1933, Pittsburgh, Pennsylvania. Above is cited by Gies.

(115) British Aluminum Hollow Ware Manufacturers' Assn., Bulletin No. 11, "Death in the Pot," Harold W. Keens, page 40.

(116) Edgar J. Saxon, editor "Health and Life," December, 1938, London, page 463.

(117) "Studies in Malignancy," by Grover and Engle, pages 8, 9; "Cancer," by J. Ellis Barker, pages 32, 33.

(118) Health News in "Health," March, 1940, page 10.

(119) "Review and Herald," Washington, D. C., July 16, 1925.

(120) "Good Health," May, 1937, page 154; and "Good Health," December, 1936, page 369.

(121) "Good Health," September, 1937, pages 271, 272.

(122) Quoted in "Life and Health," June, 1935, page 26.

(123) "Good Health," June, 1934, page 21.

(124) "Oriental Watchman and Herald of Health," May, 1938, page 26.

(125) "Good Health," March, 1938, page 86.

(126) "Good Health," March, 1938, page 86.

(127) "New Dietetics," by J. H. Kellogg, M.D., page 915.

(128) Harvey R. Gaylor and Milliard C. Marsh in "Bulletin of the Bureau of Fisheries," Volume XXXII.

(129) Sir William Arbuthnot Lane in "The Medical Record," reprinted in "Good Health," February, 1938, page 46.

(130) Sir William Arbuthnot Lane in "Modern Living," May, 1935.

(131) "Good Health," March, 1938, page 86.

(132) "Good Health," October, 1934, page 21.

(133) "The Treatment of Cancer in Man," page 14.

(134) Clifford Kuh, "A Study of Vitamin A in Relation to Experimental Cancer," in "The Yale Journal of Biological Medicine," Vol. 5, No. 2, December, 1932.

(135) Risley & Walton, "Foods, Nutrition and Clinical Dietetics," page 93.

(136) J. H. Kellogg, M.D., "New Dietetics," page 157.

(137) J. H. Kellogg, M.D., "New Dietetics," page 801.

(138) "Composition and Nutritive Properties of Soybeans." Soybean Nutritional Research Council, page 12.

(139) "Georgia's Health," State department of health monthly bulletin, October, 1943.

(140) A. A. Horvath, "The American Journal of Digestive Diseases," Vol. V, No. 3.

(141) Thomas A. Rogers, Head of the Dept. of Chemistry, Central State Teachers' College, Stevens Point, Wisconsin.

(142) Walter M. Kollmorgen, Research Director, Tennessee State Planning Commission, "The Tennessee Planner," September-October, 1943.

(143) "The Composition and Nutritive Properties of Soybeans," page 60.

(144) A. A. Horvath, "The American Journal of Digestive Diseases," Vol. V, No. 3.

(145) Thomas A. Rogers, Head Chemist, Central State Teachers' College, Stevens Point, Wisconsin, Pamphlet.

(146) A. A. Horvath, "The American Journal of Digestive Diseases," Vol. V. No. 3.

(147) A. A. Horvath, "American Journal of Digestive Disease," Vol. V, No. 3.

(148) A. A. Horvath, "American Journal of Digestive Diseases," Vol. V, No. 3.

(149) A. A. Horvath, "American Journal of Digestive Diseases," Vol. V, No. 3.

(150) L. H. Bailey, R. G. Capen and J. A. LeClerc in "Cereal Chemistry," September, 1935, page 462.

(151) A. A. Horvath, "American Journal of Digestive Diseases," Vol. V, No. 3.

(152) A. A. Horvath, "American Journal of Diegstive Diseases," Vol. V, No. 3.

(153) Thomas A. Rogers, Head Chemist Central State Teachers' College, Stevens Point, Wisconsin, Pamphlet.

(154) W. J. Morse, U. S. Dept. of Agriculture, "Farmers' Bulletin," No. 1617.

(155) "The Composition and Nutritive Properties of Soybeans," Soybean Nutritional Research Council, page 17.

(156) D. Breese Jones, Protein and Nutrition Research Division, U. S. Dept. of Agriculture, Bulletin MC-28, April, 1938.

(157) Irene Waters, Pediatric Dietitian, Vanderbilt Clinic, Presbyterian Hospital, New York. In private letter.

(158) Dr. Fred B. Smith, Union Memorial Hospital, Baltimore, Md. In Private letter.

(159) W. H. Sebrell, Surgeon in Charge, Nutrition Studies U. S. Public Health Service, Washington, D. C. Private letter.

(160) "Foods, Nutrition and Health," McCollum and Becker, pages 4, 5.

(161) "Wisdom of the Body," Walter B. Cannon, M.D., pages 98-103.

(162) "Food Nutrition and Health," McCollum and Bceker, page 16.

(163) "Chemistry of Food and Nutrition," page 11.

(164) "Cancer," J. Ellis Barker, (London), published by E. P. Dutton and Co., New York, page 333.

(165) "Good Health," January, 1938, pages 14, 15.

(166) "Health Question Box," by J. H. Kellogg, page 339.

(167) "Chemistry of Food and Nutrition," 1932, page 16.

(168) "Life and Health," August, 1942, from "Annals of Internal Medicine."

(169) Earl C. Reed in "Health," July, 1940, page 13.

(170) "Composition and Nutritive Properties of Soybeans." page 18.

(171) Ellen G. White, T. 7:135.

(172) R. D. Jennings, "Agriculture Economist Division of Farm Management and Costs," United States Dept. of Agriculture, in personal letter.

(173) Prof. F. A. Harper in "Have We Food Enough for All."

(174) Prof. F. A. Harper, Dept. Agricultural Economics, Cornell University, in "Food in War and in Peace." Report of N. Y. State Joint Legislative Committee on Nutrition," 1944, page 24.

(175) "Food In War and in Peace," in report of New York State Joint Legislative Committee on Nutrition, 1944.

(176) Ibid.

(177) Ibid.

(178) Claude R. Wickard, Secretary of Agriculture.

(179) "Food in War and in Peace," Report of the New York State Joint Legislative Committee on Nutrition.

(180) "The Southern Gardener," by Dr. Floyd Brailliar, page 30.

(181) Ibid., page 29.

(182) Ellen G. White, in "Patriarchs and Prophets," page 561.

(183) Ellen G. White, T. Vol. 4: 29, 30.

(184) Dr. Clive M. McCoy of Cornell University, Corning, N. Y.

(185) C. Ward Crampton, M.D.

(186) William G. Doern, M.S., M.D., Research Dept. The Doern Clinic, Milwaukee, Wisconsin.

INDEX

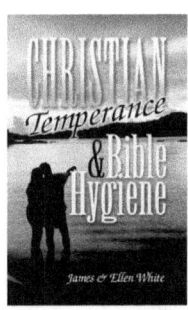

Christian Temperance and Bible Hygiene

James and E. G. White were among the first to present the subjects of hygiene and temperance in consistency with the Bible and Christian beliefs.

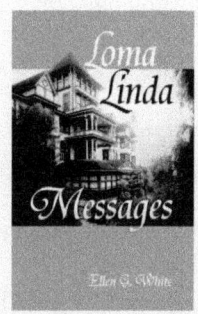

Loma Linda Messages

This 1935 collection of E. G. White's admonitions arouses God's people to follow the Divine blueprint of the medical work.

Other Titles from TEACH Services, Inc.

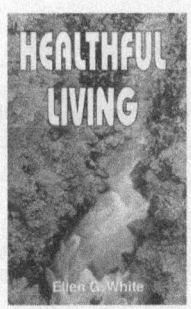

Healthful Living

Written by E. G. White, this is the most concise and condensed information upon the subjects of health and health reform.

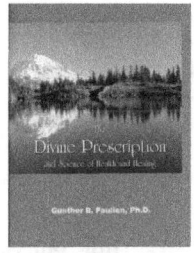

The Divine Prescription

Gunther B. Paulien, PhD presents the matter of health and healing from the standpoint of the Bible and the *Spirit of Prophecy*.